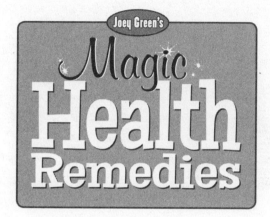

Joey Green's

Magic
Health
Remedies

Other Books by Joey Green

Hellbent on Insanity

The Gilligan's Island Handbook

The Get Smart Handbook

The Partridge Family Album

Polish Your Furniture with Panty Hose

Hi Bob!

Selling Out

Paint Your House with Powdered Milk

Wash Your Hair with Whipped Cream

The Bubble Wrap Book

Joey Green's Encyclopedia of Offbeat Uses for
    Brand-Name Products

The Zen of Oz

The Warning Label Book

Monica Speaks

The Official Slinky Book

You Know You've Reached Middle Age If . . .

The Mad Scientist Handbook

Clean Your Clothes with Cheez Whiz

The Road to Success Is Paved with Failure

Clean It! Fix It! Eat It!

Joey Green's Magic Brands

The Mad Scientist Handbook 2

Senior Moments

Jesus and Moses: The Parallel Sayings

Joey Green's Amazing Kitchen Cures

Jesus and Muhammad: The Parallel Sayings

Joey Green's Gardening Magic

How They Met

Joey Green's Incredible Country Store

Potato Radio, Dizzy Dice

Joey Green's Supermarket Spa

Contrary to Popular Belief

Marx & Lennon: The Parallel Sayings

Joey Green's Rainy Day Magic

The Jolly President

Champagne and Caviar Again?

Joey Green's Mealtime Magic

The Bathroom Professor: Philosophy on the Go

Famous Failures

Lunacy: The Best of the Cornell Lunatic

Joey Green's Fit-It Magic

Too Old for MySpace, Too Young for Medicare

You Know You Need a Vacation If . . .

Sarah Palin's Secret Diary

Joey Green's Cleaning Magic

Joey Green's Amazing Pet Cures

Dumb History

Joey Green's Kitchen Magic

The Ultimate Mad Scientist Handbook

Weird & Wonderful Christmas

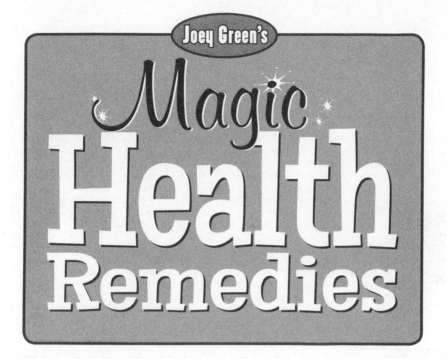

Joey Green's Magic Health Remedies

1,363 Quick-and-Easy Cures
Using Everyday Brand-Name Products

by **Joey Green**

author of *Joey Green's Kitchen Magic*

Direct and trade editions are both being published in 2013.
Rodale books may be purchased for business or promotional use or for special sales.
For information, please write to:
Special Markets Department, Rodale Inc., 733 Third Avenue, New York, NY 10017
Printed in the United States of America
Rodale Inc. makes every effort to use acid-free ♾, recycled paper ♲.
Book design by Chris Rhoads
Illustrations by Glen Mullaly

Library of Congress Cataloging-in-Publication Data is on file with the publisher.

ISBN 978–1–60961–948–0 direct hardcover
ISBN 978–1–60961–949–7 trade paperback

Distributed to the trade by Macmillan

2 4 6 8 10 9 7 5 3 1 direct hardcover
2 4 6 8 10 9 7 5 3 1 trade paperback

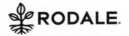

We inspire and enable people to improve their lives and the world around them.
rodalebooks.com

For Jeff and Amy

Contents

But First, a Word from Our Sponsor   ix

But First, a Word from Our Sponsor

"The art of medicine consists of amusing the patient while nature cures the disease."

—VOLTAIRE

In the Middle Ages, high-priced university-trained doctors firmly believed they could cure disease by bloodletting the patient—cutting a vein or placing leeches on the skin—to remove the "corrupt humours" supposedly causing the ailment. If a patient failed to recover from the disease after a pint of blood was removed from the body, the physician would remove more blood. Widely practiced by physicians, surgeons, and "barbers," bloodletting resulted in the deaths of millions of people. The barbaric and medically unsound practice of bloodletting had been invented fifteen centuries earlier by the ancient Greek physician Galen, who wrongly believed that four humours (blood, phlegm, black bile, and yellow bile) regulated the human body.

These same Medieval doctors concocted all sorts of expensive elixirs, potions, and tonics to allegedly cure serious ailments. In 1685, when English King Charles II fell ill from kidney disease, his royal doctors let his blood, cut off his hair, applied blistering agents on his scalp, and adhered plasters of pitch and pigeon dung on the bottom of his feet. They blew the herb hellebore up his nose to make him sneeze out the nonexistent humours from his brain, had him drink antimony and sulfate of zinc to induce vomiting to excise the humours, and gave him purgatives to cleanse his bowels of these humours. After the doctors administered an overabundance of tonics, herbs, and drugs, and let another twelve ounces of blood, King Charles II did what anyone receiving this daft medical treatment would do. He died.

As luck would have it, peasants could not afford the services of these university-trained quacks. Instead, they employed the less expensive services of local "wise women" who cleverly brewed homemade elixirs and devised ingenious herbal remedies, based on folklore, tradition, and common sense. These resourceful women ingeniously used honey to heal wounds and burns. They prescribed apple cider vinegar to relieve heartburn. They applied mustard plasters to decongest a chest cold—all for a mere pittance compared to the exorbitant fees that their eminent counterparts charged for far more lethal treatments.

Over the succeeding centuries, peasants passed these home remedies from generation to generation, and as medical science progressed, becoming more sound and sophisticated, home remedies fell by the wayside, replaced by pre-scription medicines, antibiotics, and drugs. Feeling sick? Just run out to the drugstore to buy a pill, ointment, or cherry-flavored syrup to remedy whatever ails you.

If you came down with a cold and your grandmother told you to put mustard on your chest and cover it with a wet washcloth to decongest it, you'd say, "C'mon grandma, get with the program! The drugstore sells decongestants that really work."

But a funny thing happened on the way to the Information Age. The costs of health care and health insurance skyrocketed. The number of Americans without health insurance climbed to 49.9 million in 2011, with nearly one out of four adult Americans uninsured, according to the U.S. Census Bureau. The average health insurance premium for family coverage more than doubled over the past decade to $13,770 a year, reported the Kaiser Family Foundation. In 2008 alone, the average American spent $7,538 on health-care costs, said the Organisation for Economic Co-operation and Development. And the average out-of-pocket health-care costs for a family of four with employer-sponsored health insurance ballooned from $3,634 in 2002 to $8,008 in 2011, proclaimed the Milliman Medical Index.

No wonder so many of us eagerly try inexpensive home remedies before call-ing a doctor or running to the drug store. In fact, generic prescription drugs now account for 67 percent of the prescriptions dispensed in the United States, according to the AARP Public Policy Institute, which attributes the growing popularity of generic drugs to the low cost. And as of 2007, approximately 38 percent of American adults used some form of complementary or alternative medicine, reported the National Institutes of Health. That's a whole lot of people willing to smear mustard on their chest.

When our youngest daughter Julia came down with the flu, did I race her to the doctor's office to be told "It's the flu" and get hit with an astronomical bill?

Instead, I pulled out the large bowl we ordinarily use to serve popcorn, filled it with boiling water, and added three Lipton Chamomile Tea bags. I placed a towel over my daughter's head to form a tent over the bowl, and told her to hold her face close to the steaming tea and breathe deeply for ten minutes. I put a box of Kleenex Tissues nearby. The chamomile steam broke up the congestion in her sinuses by liquefying the mucous, and Julia blew her nose repeatedly, clearing her head completely. The effect lasted two hours. Now, whenever she gets a stuffy nose, Julia immediately demands the chamomile tea treatment.

When our oldest daughter Ashley came down with a stomach virus that made her feel nauseous and fatigued, I handed her a box of Nabisco Ginger Snaps and a bottle of Gatorade. The ginger soothed the nausea and relieved the pain, and the electrolytes in the sports drink reenergized her.

Whenever my wife Debbie experiences back pain, I reach into the pantry and hand her a clean sock filled with Uncle Ben's Converted Brand Rice, tied shut with a knot. She heats the sock in the microwave oven for ninety seconds, lies on her stomach, and places the sock on her back. The rice-filled sock conforms to the shape of her back, stays warm for roughly thirty minutes, and provides soothing relief. We've had that sock in our pantry for more than six years, we've used it hundreds of times, and we've never had to replace the rice. Of course, socks come in pairs, so I stuffed three Wilson Tennis Balls into the other sock, tied a knot in the end, and when Debbie finishes with the rice-filled sock, I roll the tennis-ball-filled sock over her back, giving her a revivifying therapeutic massage.

As for myself, well, when I inadvertently grabbed the scalding hot handle of a pot while cooking, I shrieked like a banshee and then grabbed a nearby squeeze bottle of French's Mustard and slathered the bight yellow paste on my hand to stop the burning pain. Instant relief! And no blistering!

Turns out, grandma didn't need her head examined after all. In fact, loads of medical studies have proven (and continue to prove) what grandma knew all along. Those strange folklore remedies she avidly touted really do work—for less money and with far fewer side effects than cures offered by modern medicine. Yes, as French journalist Alphonse Karr wrote in 1849, "The more things change, the more they stay the same."

To share hundreds of home remedies with the American public, I wrote a book more than ten years ago called *Joey Green's Amazing Kitchen Cures*. Since that time, I've collected thousands more tips, and medical researchers have conducted a plethora of scientific studies corroborating heretofore anecdotal evidence. And so, I decided to write this book to provide you with the latest and most reliable kitchen cures using everyday brand-name products you probably already have in your house. This book covers many more ailments and contains more than twice as many remedies and tips as *Amazing Kitchen Cures*. You'll learn how to relieve a migraine with Dole Pineapple Chunks, alleviate hay fever with Heinz Apple Cider Vinegar, reduce caffeine withdrawal symptoms with Jif Peanut Butter, decrease arthritis pain with Jell-O, and relieve constipation with Aunt Jemima Original Syrup.

While putting this book together, I discovered that Heinz Baked Beanz lowers your risk of heart disease, Cool Whip soothes chapped lips, Jif Peanut Butter lowers your risk of diabetes, and Heinz Ketchup reduces the frequency and severity of asthma attacks. I literally jumped for joy.

I had to know more. I locked myself in the library, ecstatically unearthing medical studies that clearly demonstrate that eating Chicken of the Sea Tuna improves acne, drinking Welch's Grape Juice lowers cholesterol, and chewing Wrigley's Spearmint Gum reduces stress. I was tickled pink to find scientific evidence confirming that drinking Maxwell House Coffee reduces the risk of kidney stones, catching a whiff of McCormick Pure Vanilla Extract remedies erectile dysfunction, and drinking Ocean Spray Cranberry Juice Cocktail really does cure urinary tract infections.

But I didn't stop there. Each chapter of this book concludes with handy medical advice and more clever home remedies that, unlike the featured tips in each chapter, involve no products at all. Like how you can help soothe bronchitis by drinking water, why you should never take aspirin to relieve pain from a bruise, why sleep and rest combats a fever, how rubbing your belly can alleviate indigestion and bloating, and how you can relieve the symptoms of menopause by simply going for a walk.

The book you hold in your hands is the culmination of my obsessive journey into the world of home remedies. Now all I have to do is find a cure for my overzealousness. I just hope it's not bloodletting.

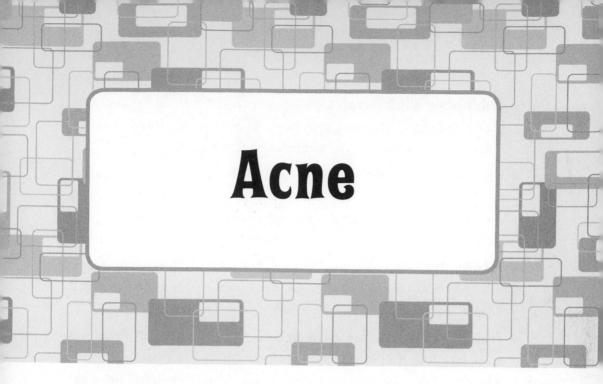

Acne

- **Bayer Aspirin.** To clear up a blemish, use a mortar and pestle to pulverize one Bayer Aspirin tablet into powder, add just enough water to make a paste, and apply it to the blemish (unless you're allergic to aspirin). The salicylic acid dries up pimples. You can also soothe an acne outbreak by taking one or two Bayer Aspirin (regular strength) tablets four times a day. Aspirin reduces inflammation. (Before taking aspirin regularly, consult a doctor.)

- **Chicken of the Sea Salmon, Chicken of the Sea Sardines,** or **Chicken of the Sea Tuna.** To bring acne under control, eat salmon, sardines, or tuna three times a week to add the fatty acids commonly known as omega-3 oils to your diet. These fatty acids help reduce inflammation, strengthen the immune system, and increase resistance to stress. A study published in 2008 in *Lipids in Health and Disease* showed that omega-3 fatty acids improved inflammatory acne lesions.

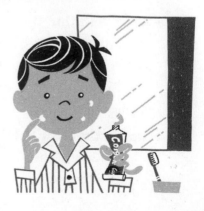

- **Colgate Regular Flavor Toothpaste.** To dry up pimples, apply a dab of Colgate Regular Flavor Toothpaste and let sit overnight.

- **Dickinson's Witch Hazel.** Saturate a cotton ball with Dickinson's Witch Hazel, and use it to cleanse your skin twice a day. A natural astringent, witch hazel helps dry pimples and reduce inflammation.

- **Dr. Teal's Epsom Salt.** To help clear up blackheads, mix one teaspoon Dr. Teal's Epsom Salt, three drops iodine, and one-half cup of water. Bring the solution to a boil, let cool, and using a cotton ball, apply the mixture to clean your pores. The solution removes dirt and excess oil from the pores.

- **Fels-Naptha Soap.** If your sebaceous glands are working overtime, wash excess oil from your skin and cleanse your pores with caustic Fels-Naptha Soap. Rinse thoroughly and dry.

- **Fruit of the Earth Aloe Vera Gel.** To heal pimples, apply Fruit of the Earth Aloe Vera Gel to the blemishes three times a day until they clear up. Aloe vera fights infection and heals most skin blemishes within five days.

- **Heinz Apple Cider Vinegar.** Pour one cup Heinz Apple Cider Vinegar into a large bowl and carefully add two cups of boiling water. Lean over the bowl and drape a towel like a tent over your head and the bowl. Inhale the rising steam for five to ten minutes. Twice a week, use this facial steam bath, followed by rinsing with a mixture of equal parts Heinz Apple Cider Vinegar and cold water to close the pores.

- **Heinz White Vinegar.** To help clear up acne pimples, use a cotton ball to apply Heinz White Vinegar to the blemishes. The acids in vinegar help flush out blocked pores and dry up blemishes.

- **Knox Gelatin.** To eliminate blackheads, dissolve one tablespoon Knox Gelatin in two tablespoons milk over low heat. Let cool, then use a cotton ball to apply the mixture to your face, avoiding the eyes. Wait thirty minutes, and then peel off the mask, exfoliating a thin layer of skin and removing blackheads with it.

- **Lipton Chamomile Tea.** To reduce acne inflammation, place two Lipton Chamomile Tea bags in one cup of boiling water, cover with a saucer, and steep for five minutes. Squeeze and remove the tea bags, and let the liquid cool to the touch. After cleansing your face, use a cotton ball to apply the tea to the blemishes. When applied topically, chamomile is an anti-inflammatory that can help soothe pain.

- **Lipton Green Tea.** Brew a cup of Lipton Green Tea, cover with a saucer, steep for ten minutes, and let cool. Then use a cotton ball to wash your face with the tea. Do this twice a day until the acne clears. Or dampen a Lipton Green Tea bag with warm water, and apply it to the affected area as a compress for ten minutes. The antimicrobial and antioxidant compounds in green tea help eliminate acne pimples, according to a 2009 study at the University of Miami.

- **Listerine.** Use a cotton ball to dab original formula Listerine antiseptic mouthwash on pimples. The antiseptic doubles as an astringent (which tightens the skin, reducing inflammation and relieving pain) and an anti-bacterial (which kills the bacteria causing the blemish).

- **McCormick Ground Nutmeg** and **SueBee Honey.** For a folk remedy to heal pimples, mix equal parts McCormick Ground Nutmeg and SueBee Honey, and apply the mixture to the pimple. Let sit for twenty minutes, and then wash thoroughly. Compounds in nutmeg exhibit strong antibacterial and antifungal properties, according to a 1999 study published in the *Journal of Natural Products*. Honey is hygroscopic. The antibacterial compounds in honey fight the infection and reduce the inflammation, and the hygroscopic properties help dry up the blemish.

- **Pepto-Bismol.** To dry up pimples, put a dab of Pepto-Bismol on the blemish. The salicylate reduces the inflammation and redness, and benzoic acid is an antifungal that fights the bacteria causing the pimples.

- **Phillips' Milk of Magnesia.** Using a cotton ball, apply Phillips' Milk of Magnesia to the entire face as a mask, let dry, and then wash clean with warm water, followed by cool water. Or apply a dab to pimples and let dry overnight. The alkalinity of the magnesia hydroxide absorbs oils from the skin and the antibacterial properties help kill bacteria. The trace amounts of zinc help heal the blemishes.

℞ STRANGE MEDICINE ℞

LET MY PIMPLES GO

● When the sebaceous glands in the skin produce too much sebum, the excess oil blocks the pores, causing acne pimples.

● Puberty, menstruation, pregnancy, perimenopause, or birth control pills cause hormone production to vary. The hormones, in turn, increase the production of sebum, triggering an acne outbreak.

● The two types of acne are acne vulgaris (whiteheads, blackheads, or red blemishes on the face, chest, shoulders, or back) and cystic acne (painful cysts or firm lumps).

● Emotional stress can also trigger an outbreak of acne pimples.

● Do not pick, pop, or squeeze pimples. Doing so can cause infection or scarring.

● Drugs containing corticosteroids, androgens, or lithium can cause acne.

● Dairy products and carbohydrate-rich foods—such as bread, bagels, and chips—may trigger acne.

● Contrary to popular belief, eating chocolate or greasy foods does not cause acne.

● Certain cosmetics or greasy or oily substances applied directly to the skin can provoke or aggravate acne.

● Every night while you sleep, you rub your face in your pillowcase for eight hours. If that pillowcase is dirty, you're rubbing your face in accumulated sebum oil, dirt, and dead skin cells that can block pores, causing blemishes. Changing your pillowcase and sheets at least once a week allows you to rest your face on a clean surface.

● **Quaker Oats.** To clear up acne, mix up a bowl of Quaker Oats according to the directions on the side of the canister, let cool, spread it on your face, cover with a clean, damp washcloth, and let sit for fifteen minutes. Wash clean. Repeat daily for two weeks. As an astringent, oatmeal cleans the pores, kills bacteria, and contains beneficial proteins.

- **ReaLemon.** Use a cotton ball to apply ReaLemon lemon juice to pimples to quicken healing. The acid in lemon juice works like an antiseptic to kill bacteria and clean pores.

- **SueBee Honey.** To improve acne, apply a dab of SueBee Honey to the blemishes twice a day. The antibacterial compounds in honey fight the infection and reduce the inflammation, and the hygroscopic properties help dry up the blemish.

Doctor's Orders

X marks the spot! If blemishes fail to respond to over-the-counter treatments or home remedies within three months, consult a dermatologist.

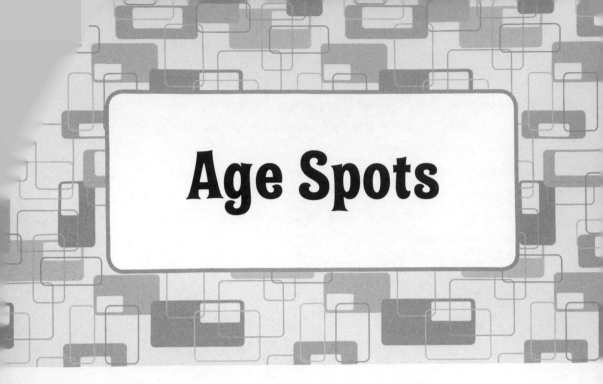

Age Spots

- **Castor Oil.** To fade age spots, rub Castor Oil onto the spots twice a day—once in the morning and again in the evening. Within a month, the age spots should start to fade.

- **Coppertone.** To prevent age spots, use a high-quality sunscreen like Coppertone with a sun protection factor (SPF) rating of at least 30 (ideally 40 to 45). Apply the sunscreen fifteen to thirty minutes before going outdoors, and once outside, reapply the sunscreen every two hours. Limiting your exposure to the sun or other forms of ultraviolet light helps prevent age spots from forming.

- **Dannon Yogurt** and **SueBee Honey.** To diminish age spots, blend equal parts Dannon Plain Nonfat Yogurt and SueBee Honey. Apply the mixture to the affected area, let sit for thirty minutes, and wash clean. Use daily until the homemade bleaching agent fades the age spots.

- **Fruit of the Earth Aloe Vera Gel.** Once or twice a day, apply Fruit of the Earth Aloe Vera Gel to the age spots and rub. Aloe contains chemicals that exfoliate dead skin and allow healthy new skin to grow in its place.

- **Gerber Peaches, SueBee Honey,** and **Quaker Oats.** To fade age spots, mix five ounces (one small container) Gerber Peaches, one tablespoon Sue-Bee Honey, and enough Quaker Oats to create a thick paste. Apply to the affected area, wait ten minutes, and then rinse well with cool water. Peaches contain large amounts of alpha-hydroxy acids, which gently exfoliate skin, accelerate cell renewal, and fade age spots.

- **ReaLemon.** To lighten age spots, use a cotton ball to rub some ReaLemon lemon juice on the spots twice daily. The acid in the lemon juice safely peels away the upper layer of skin, and in six to eight weeks, the age spots should start to lighten or fade completely.

- **Saco Buttermilk.** Apply Saco Buttermilk, the only brand of buttermilk containing natural emulsifiers, to the age spots on a daily basis. The lactic acid in buttermilk exfoliates the overly pigmented patches of skin.

- **SunGuard.** Clothes do not fully absorb the ultraviolet (UV) rays of the sun, which, over time, cause age spots. A typical white t-shirt, for example, has an ultraviolet protection factor (UPF) rating of 5 or less. To help stop UV rays from penetrating clothing, add SunGuard to your washing machine when laundering clothes. SunGuard infuses your clothes with a UV protectant that gives the fabric a UPF rating of 30, helping to prevent 96 percent of the sun's UV rays from reaching your skin. The protection lasts for up to twenty washings.

Doctor's Orders

Johnny-on-the-spot! If an age spot looks irregular or feels raised, or if you notice changes in the appearance of an age spot, consult a doctor to confirm it is not skin cancer.

☥ STRANGE MEDICINE ☥

PUT 'EM ON THE SPOT

● Exposure to ultraviolet (UV) light accelerates the production of melanin, the pigment in the epidermis that gives your skin its color, creating a tan to help protect deeper layers of skin from UV rays. After years of sun exposure, clusters of high concentrations of melanin produced in the skin create age spots. Besides sun exposure, aging sometimes causes excess production of melanin.

● Age spots, while sometimes considered unsightly, are generally harmless.

● Also known as liver spots, age spots are not caused by the liver or liver function. The name refers to the shape of the painless, flat, brown-black age spots.

● Common after age forty, age spots occur most frequently on areas with the greatest exposure to sun, primarily the face, backs of hands, forearms, and shoulders.

● To protect your skin from the sun, wear a wide-brimmed hat (providing more protection than a baseball cap) and clothes that cover your arms and legs. Actress Natalie Schafer, best known as Lovey Howell on the sitcom *Gilligan's Island,* wore a pair of white gloves whenever she went outside to avoid getting age spots on her hands.

● Susceptibility to age spots may be influenced by your genetic makeup.

● Age spots range from the size of a freckle to more than one-half inch in diameter.

● The easiest way to prevent age spots is to avoid the sun.

● Age spots can be faded by applying skin bleaching creams (containing hydroquinone, deoxyarbutin, glycolic acid, or kojic acid) or retinoids. These products may cause skin irritation. Consult a doctor before using any of these products.

● Dermatologists can remove age spots with cryotherapy (freezing the spots to destroy the extra pigment), laser treatments (to destroy the cells that produce melanin), or dermabrasion or chemical peels (to remove the outer layer of skin).

● Since exposure to UV light causes age spots, using commercial tanning lamps and tanning beds can contribute to the development of age spots.

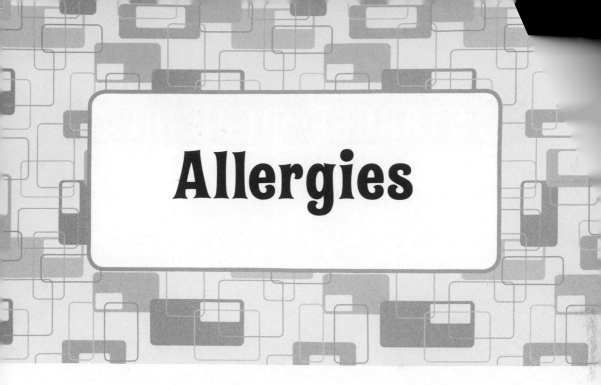

Allergies

- **Clorox Bleach.** To kill the mold in your home that may be causing an allergic reaction, mix three-quarter cup Clorox Bleach in one gallon of water, clean bathroom and kitchen surfaces with the solution, let sit for five minutes, and rinse thoroughly.

- **Gold's Horseradish** and **Nabisco Original Premium Saltine Crackers.** To decongest your chest, eat one teaspoon Gold's Horseradish spread on a Nabisco Original Premium Saltine Cracker. Horseradish is a scientifically proven decongestant.

- **Huggies Baby Wipes.** If you're allergic to your pet, have a family member wipe down your pet daily with some hypoallergenic, fragrance-free Huggies Baby Wipes to lessen dander and shedding.

- **Johnson's Baby Shampoo.** Have a family member or friend bathe your pet with Johnson's Baby Shampoo on a weekly basis to reduce shedding and decrease the amount of dander.

- **Kellogg's All-Bran, Kellogg's Special K,** or **Total.** To fortify your immune system against allergens to stop allergic reactions before they

℞ STRANGE MEDICINE ℞

DUST YOURSELF OFF

● Allergies result when your immune system overreacts to a harmless substance—such as pollen, pet dander, dust, or mold—interpreting it as a genuine threat.

● When you inhale an allergen—such as the aforementioned pollen, pet dander, dust, or mold—your body produces an antibody that detects the invader and then signals the immune system to neutralize it. The immune system releases histamine and other chemicals, which cause the runny nose, sneezing, itchy eyes, the sinus headache, and the scratchy throat.

● While allergies tend to mimic the symptoms of a cold, more itching and sneezing accompany an allergy.

● Other common allergens include peanuts, strawberries, bee venom, dust mites, latex, penicillin, and poison ivy.

● Taking an antihistamine treats the symptoms of an allergy, not the cause. Antihistamines cause drowsiness, and non-drowsy antihistamines may cause heart arrhythmias.

● Taking a detoxifying bath decreases the amount of infections, environmental toxins, and stress in your body, enabling your immune system to better cope with allergens. In the bathtub, immerse your entire body (with the exception of your head) in the hottest water you can tolerate (without inflicting any pain) for five minutes. Doctors believe the heat from the bath releases stored toxins from fat cells into the blood, allowing them to travel to the surface of the skin. Then wash the toxins off your skin with a

start, eat a bowl of Kellogg's All-Bran, Kellogg's Special K, or Total cereal every day to increase the amount of folate in your diet. A study at Johns Hopkins School of Medicine showed that people with high levels of this B vitamin in their bloodstream tend to have fewer of the antibodies that trigger allergy symptoms. One-half cup of Kellogg's All-Bran, Kellogg's Special K, or Total cereal contains 100 percent of the daily value of folate.

warm shower. (Do not take detoxifying baths if you suffer from multiple sclerosis or severe heart disease.)

● Air-conditioning your home and car alleviates allergy problems with pollen, mold, and dust mites by lowering the humidity, filtering the air, and sealing the environment.

● To clear allergens from your living space, use an air purifier with a HEPA filter.

● Vacuum and dust your home often to remove as much pollen and dust as possible, and change the air-conditioning filters once a month. You can also try to restrict your pet to rooms in your house with tile or wood floors and blinds, rather than rooms with carpeting and drapes, which retain dust and pollen.

● To reduce your exposure to household allergens, frequently wash bedding and stuffed animals in hot water, and replace carpeting with hard flooring.

● Contrary to popular belief, people who are allergic to cats are not allergic to the fur. They're allergic to *Fel d 1*, an element found in cat saliva and deposited on the skin and fur when the cat grooms itself. Fel d 1 becomes airborne through dander, the dried flakes of skin, saliva, and secretions that fall from the cat through petting or jumping.

● If you live with both a pet and an allergy, keep your bedroom permanently off-limits to the animal. Have a non-allergic member of the family do the dusting and vacuuming and clean the litter box. Have that same person groom the animal outdoors and bathe the animal on a weekly basis to decrease the amount of dander.

● **Kretschmer Wheat Germ.** Sprinkle a few tablespoons of Kretschmer Wheat Germ on meals or into a bowl of cereal or oatmeal every day. Vitamin E, a potent antioxidant, reduces the need for allergy medication and tames the part of the immune system that triggers allergic reactions. A one-ounce serving of wheat germ contains 4.53 milligrams of vitamin E, or 30 percent of the recommended daily allowance.

- **Lipton Tea, SueBee Honey,** and **ReaLemon.** To manage allergies, drink a cup of Lipton Tea with two teaspoons SueBee Honey and one teaspoon ReaLemon lemon juice first thing in the morning. The tea helps thin the mucus and stimulate the cilia, the small hairs in your nose that capture dust and pollen. Also, the flavonoids in the tea inhibit inflammation.

- **McCormick Thyme Leaves.** To relieve allergy symptoms, place one teaspoon McCormick Thyme Leaves in a glass jar, fill with two cups of boiling water, seal the lid shut, and let steep and cool for thirty minutes. Remove the lid and inhale the vapors. Thymol reduces inflammation in the bronchial tract and has antibacterial properties.

- **Morton Salt** and **Arm & Hammer Baking Soda.** To cleanse allergens from your nose, make a saline nose wash to rinse your nasal passages. Purify eight ounces of water by boiling for three minutes, let cool to room temperature, and dissolve one-quarter teaspoon Morton Salt and one-quarter teaspoon Arm & Hammer Baking Soda in the purified water. Use a bulb syringe or neti pot to rinse the inside of your nose.

- **Mr. Coffee Filters.** If you're experiencing a strong allergic reaction, hold a Mr. Coffee Filter over your nose and mouth as a dust mask and breathe normally. The coffee filter helps filter out allergans.

- **Planters Dry Roasted Almonds.** To help calm the part of the immune system that triggers allergic reactions and to help reduce the need for allergy medication, eat a handful of Planters Dry Roasted Almonds daily (unless, of course, you're allergic to almonds). A one-ounce handful of almonds provides 7.4 milligrams of vitamin E, or approximately 50 percent of the recommended daily allowance.

- **Purell Instant Hand Sanitizer.** If you're allergic to your dog or cat, wash your hands with Purell Instant Hand Sanitizer after touching your pet.

- **Scotch Packaging Tape.** Remove pet hair and dander from clothing and upholstery by wrapping a strip of Scotch Packaging Tape around your hand, adhesive side out, and patting your clothes and furniture.

- **Tabasco Pepper Sauce** and **Campbell's Tomato Juice.** To help clear congestion from the bronchial tract and calm the mucosa (the inner lining of the nasal passages), add ten to twenty drops Tabasco Pepper Sauce to a glass of Campbell's Tomato Juice, and drink this mixture several times a day. The capsaicin in the hot sauce numbs the mucosa, making it less susceptible to allergens and inflammation, and doubles as a decongestant.

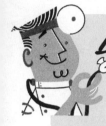

Doctor's Orders

Don't bite the dust! If your allergy produces welts, wheezing, or asthma, seek medical attention immediately. If an allergy attack fails to subside after a week of using over-the-counter medications, see your doctor.

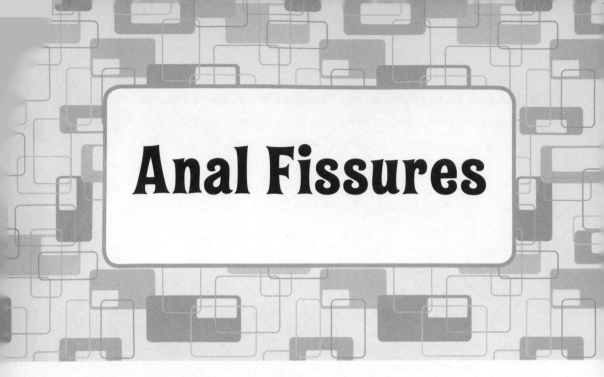

Anal Fissures

- **Arm & Hammer Baking Soda.** Mix one handful of Arm & Hammer Baking Soda in a bathtub filled with warm water and soak for fifteen minutes. The sodium bicarbonate soothes inflammation.

- **Dickinson's Witch Hazel** and **Stayfree Maxi Pads.** To soothe anal itching, chill a bottle of Dickinson's Witch Hazel in the refrigerator, saturate a Stayfree Maxi Pad with the cold witch hazel, and hold it against the affected area until the cold dissipates. Repeat if desired. The cold provides relief, and as a vasoconstrictor, the witch hazel shrinks swelling. Witch hazel is a main ingredient in Tucks medicated pads.

- **Huggies Baby Wipes.** To avoid irritating anal fissures after a bowel movement, clean yourself gently using pre-moistened Huggies Natural Care Baby Wipes. These convenient, hypoallergenic, fragrance-free, alcohol-free wipes also contain soothing aloe and vitamin E.

- **Kingsford's Corn Starch.** To soothe the itching and discomfort of an anal fissure, sprinkle Kingsford's Corn Starch on the affected area after every shower, bath, and bowel movement. The cornstarch reduces the friction that causes irritation.

- **Lipton Chamomile Tea** and **Stayfree Maxi Pads.** Place two Lipton Chamomile Tea bags in one cup of boiling water, cover with a saucer, and steep for five minutes. Squeeze and remove the tea bags, and let the liquid cool to the touch. Saturate a Stayfree Maxi Pad with the tea, and press it to the affected area. When applied topically, chamomile is an anti-inflammatory that can help soothe pain.

- **Lipton Tea Bags.** To sterilize and soothe an anal fissure, dampen a Lipton Tea Bag with warm water and apply it to the affected area. The tannin in the tea acts as an astringent, tightening the skin, reducing inflammation, and relieving pain.

- **Metamucil.** To prevent the hard stools that irritate anal fissures, take one serving of Metamucil (as instructed on the package label) in or with eight ounces of water once a day. Metamucil contains psyllium seed husk, a natural dietary fiber originating from the psyllium plant, which absorbs liquid,

℞ STRANGE MEDICINE ℞

BEHIND THE SCENES

- An anal fissure is a break or ulcer in the lining of the anal canal. Like hemorrhoids, anal fissures itch, bleed, and cause pain.

- Anal fissures are generally caused by a hard bowel movement or other trauma to the anal canal.

- Most anal fissures heal within a few weeks.

- Adopting a diet high in fiber—fruits, vegetables, and whole grains—prevents and relieves anal fissures by producing soft bowel movements.

- Drink eight 8-ounce glasses of water every day to keep your stools soft.

- Fight the impulse to scratch an anal fissure. Doing so can make the fissure worse.

bulking up your stool and allowing it to pass through your system more comfortably. (Metamucil generally produces a laxative effect in twelve to seventy-two hours.)

- **Quaker Oats** and **L'eggs Sheer Energy Panty Hose.** To relieve the itching and discomfort of an anal fissure, grind one cup uncooked Quaker Oats in a blender, pour a few tablespoons of the fine powder into the foot cut from a clean, used pair of L'eggs Sheer Energy Panty Hose, and tie a knot in the open end. Fill a bathtub with lukewarm water, pour the remaining powdered oats into the tub, and, while soaking for fifteen minutes, saturate the panty hose sachet with water, and gently press it against the affected area. The antioxidants in the oats reduce inflammation and soothe irritated inflamed skin.

- **Vaseline Petroleum Jelly.** To keep anal fissures from worsening, before each bowel movement, take a dab of Vaseline Petroleum Jelly on your finger and insert it approximately one-half inch into your rectum. The lubrication helps the stool pass without inflicting additional damage.

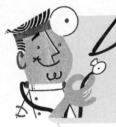

Doctor's Orders

Don't get left behind! If an anal fissure doesn't heal within two months or if you notice a discharge of mucus, consult a doctor to rule out cancer or an abscess.

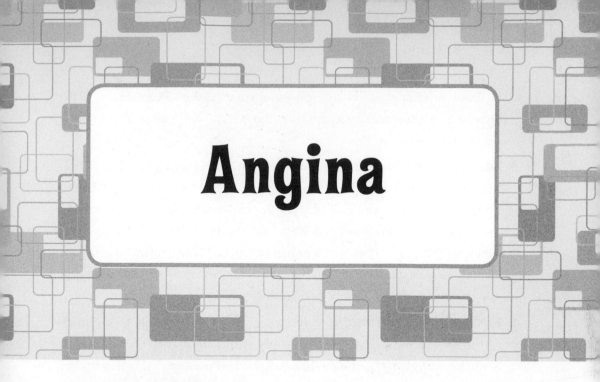

Angina

- **Heinz Baked Beanz.** To lower your risk of heart disease, eat Heinz Baked Beanz at least four times a week. One serving of baked beans provides more than half the recommended daily intake of folate and manganese, two nutrients important for heart health. A 2001 study published in the *Archives of Internal Medicine* showed that people who consume legumes four or more times a week had a 22 percent less chance of developing coronary heart disease than those who ate legumes less than once a week. The tomato sauce in Heinz Baked Beanz is also a rich source of lycopene, an antioxidant that lowers the risk of heart disease. The canning process actually increases the bio-availability of the lycopene. A 2003 study at the Brigham and Women's Hospital and Harvard Medical School found that women with the highest lycopene levels were up to 34 percent less likely to develop heart disease than women with lower levels.

- **Jif Peanut Butter.** Eating one tablespoon Jif Peanut Butter five times a week can reduce the risk of angina. The monounsaturated fat in peanut butter can help lower total cholesterol, triglycerides, and LDL (or "bad" cholesterol), and raise HDL (or "good" cholesterol), which lowers the risk of cardiovascular disease, according to numerous studies. Peanut butter also helps reduce inflammation in the body and boosts the health of blood vessels around the heart.

- **Kellogg's All-Bran.** To help prevent angina, eat one cup Kellogg's All-Bran every morning. Adding 20 to 35 grams of fiber to your diet every day helps remove excess cholesterol from the body and helps prevent ot from passing through the intestinal wall into the bloodstream. One cup of Kellogg's All-Bran contains 20 grams of fiber. A daily minimum of five servings of fruits and vegetables, three servings of whole-grain foods, and one serving of beans adds fiber to your body to lower cholesterol.

- **McCormick Garlic Powder.** Cook your food with as much McCormick Garlic Powder as possible. A 2008 study at the University of Adelaide in Australia showed that garlic can help lower blood pressure, and other studies have found that garlic reduces cholesterol, inhibits platelet aggregation, and increases antioxidant status.

- **McCormick Ground Ginger.** Add one teaspoon McCormick Ground Ginger to salads or use it in recipes. Ginger, containing the active ingredient gingerol, is scientifically proven to inhibit arterial inflammation, lower cholesterol, and hinder the formation of blood clots. (Do not use ginger if you have gallstones. Ginger can increase bile production.)

- **McCormick Ground Turmeric.** Take one tablespoon McCormick Ground Turmeric daily by simply sprinkling it on your food or using the spice in recipes for rice, casseroles, soups, and stews. Turmeric contains curcumin, an anti-inflammatory that inhibits arterial inflammation that may lead to or worsen angina. (Turmeric may increase the likelihood of bleeding when taken in combination with the blood thinner Coumadin or other anti-coagulant medications.)

- **Planters Dry Roasted Almonds, Planters Dry Roasted Cashews,** or **Planters Dry Roasted Peanuts.** Eating foods high in magnesium—like Planters Dry Roasted Almonds, Planters Dry Roasted Cashews, or Planters

℞ STRANGE MEDICINE ℞

HAVE A HEART

● Angina (medically known as angina pectoris) is a potentially life-threatening condition that feels like painful pressure in your chest, sometimes extending to your left shoulder blade and arm, possibly including your neck, jaw, or back—for anywhere from one to twenty minutes. The cause? Not enough blood and oxygen to the heart.

● Stress, alcohol, cigarettes, heavy meals, extreme temperatures, or physical exertion can trigger angina. The heart's demand for oxygen increases, which, coupled with arteries narrowed by plaque buildup, results in severe chest pain, signaling a future heart attack.

● Angina requires medical attention. To relieve the discomfort of angina, doctors generally prescribe nitroglycerine, which dilates the arteries, allowing more blood (and hence more oxygen) to reach the heart.

● Nutritional remedies that increase blood flow to the heart and give the heart muscle additional energy can eventually reduce angina attacks, decrease reliance on medication, and possibly eliminate angina completely.

● To prevent angina or reduce attacks, lower your cholesterol, which adheres to the inner walls of your arteries and reduces blood flow to the heart.

● A daily dose of 90 to 180 milligrams of coenzyme Q_{10} taken with or after meals can decrease angina attacks, lowering the need for nitroglycerine. Found in every cell of your body, coenzyme Q_{10} helps the body produce ATP (adenosine triphosphate), the chemical that provides energy for physiological processes such as the muscular contraction of the heart.

● Going for a walk for thirty minutes every day helps prevent heart disease.

● To prevent angina, stop smoking and keep away from second-hand smoke. The smoke deprives your body of oxygen, which can spur an attack.

● Limit the amount of coffee you drink. Drinking five or more cups of coffee a day increases your chances of an angina attack.

Dry Roasted Peanuts—can help keep the heart healthy and strong. One ounce of almonds provides 80 milligrams of magnesium, one ounce of cashews provides 75 milligrams, and one ounce of dry roasted peanuts provides 50 milligrams.

- **St. Joseph Aspirin.** To reduce the risk of blood clots, take one St. Joseph Aspirin every day. Developed for children, one St. Joseph Aspirin tablet contains 81 milligrams of aspirin (compared with 325 milligrams in a regular-strength adult aspirin tablet), thinning the blood without increasing the risk of bleeding. By thinning the blood, aspirin enables blood to flow through narrowed heart arteries and reduces the risk of a heart attack. (Consult with your doctor before starting any medicine regimen.)

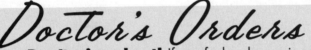

Doctor's Orders

Don't miss a beat! If you feel a change in your typical pattern of angina—such as more intense pain or shortness of breath—get to an emergency room immediately.

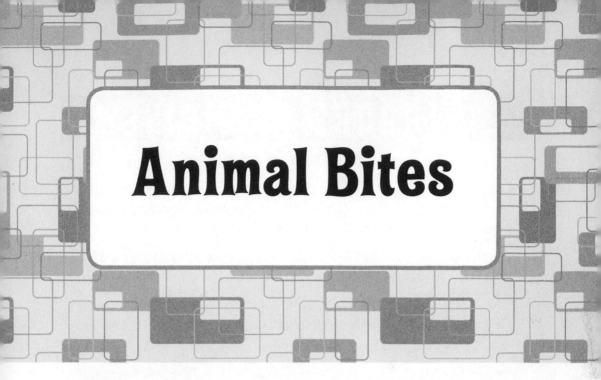

Animal Bites

- **Birds Eye Frozen Peas** and **Bounty Paper Towels.** If an animal bites you, use a plastic bag of Birds Eye Frozen Peas as an icepack to control the swelling and relieve the pain, and see a doctor immediately. If the bag of peas feels too cold, wrap the bag in a sheet of Bounty Paper Towels to create a layer of insulation to prevent frostbite. The sack of peas conforms to the contours of your body, and you can refreeze the peas for future ice-pack use—just label the bag for ice-pack use only. If you want to eat the peas, cook them after they thaw the first time, never after refreezing.

- **Dial Soap, Neosporin,** and **Band-Aid Bandages.** If an animal bites you, immediately wash the wound with Dial Antibacterial Soap and water for at least five minutes to remove any saliva and dirt (and accompanying bacteria), and rinse thoroughly under running water to remove any soap. Apply Neosporin antibiotic ointment, dress with a Band-Aid Bandage, and see a doctor immediately.

- **Hydrogen Peroxide.** To prevent infection from a dog or cat bite, pour Hydrogen Peroxide on the wound. Then wash with soap and water for at least five minutes.

℞ STRANGE MEDICINE ℞

BITING BACK

● If you are bitten by an animal, immediately and thoroughly wash the wound with plenty of soap and warm water (see Dial Soap tip on page 21). If washing the wound hurts, remind yourself that an infection will hurt much more.

● According to a review published in the *New England Journal of Medicine* in 1999, more than 130 disease-causing microbes have been isolated and identified from dog and cat bite wounds.

● When treating an animal bite, a doctor may prescribe antibiotics to prevent an infection from developing.

● If you are bitten by a wild or stray animal that could have rabies, you may need to begin an anti-rabies treatment.

● According to the Centers for Disease Control and Prevention, dogs bite approximately 4.7 million people in the United States every year. Roughly 800,000 of those people, half of them children, seek medical treatment for the bites.

● Dog bites kill between 15 and 20 Americans during a year.

● Five times more Americans die every year from being struck by lightning than from being bitten by a dog.

● If you're bitten by a dog or cat, contact the owner immediately for written proof that the animal's rabies shots are up to date.

● If you're bitten by an animal and your last tetanus booster shot was more than five years ago, get one immediately.

● To prevent animal bites, never pet, handle, or feed unknown animals; leave snakes alone; and watch your children closely around animals.

- **Listerine.** To disinfect an animal bite, pour original formula Listerine antiseptic mouthwash over the wound. Developed by Dr. Joseph Lawrence in 1857 as a safe and effective antiseptic for use in surgical procedures, Listerine is an astringent and antibacterial.

- **Pampers.** In a pinch, use a clean Pampers disposable diaper as a compress to stop an animal bite wound from bleeding.

- **Purell Instant Hand Sanitizer.** Applying Purell Instant Hand Sanitizer to an animal bite disinfects the wound and helps stop the bleeding. The ethyl alcohol in the gel is an antiseptic.

- **Smirnoff Vodka.** To prevent an animal bite from getting infected, pour Smirnoff Vodka over the wound. As an antiseptic, the alcohol in the vodka disinfects the wound.

- **Stayfree Maxi Pads.** To stop a deep animal bite from bleeding, apply direct pressure to the wound with a Stayfree Maxi Pad and raise the wound above heart level of the victim.

- **Vaseline Petroleum Jelly.** To expedite healing, rub a few dabs of Vaseline Petroleum Jelly over the bite wound. In 1859, Brooklyn chemist Robert Augustus Chesebrough learned from petroleum drilling workers in Titusville, Pennsylvania, that the jelly residue that gunked up oil drilling rods quickened healing when rubbed on a wound.

Doctor's Orders

Bite the bullet! If you get bit by an animal that might carry rabies—or any wild or domestic animal whose immunization status is unknown (such as a bat, raccoon, skunk, and fox)—see your doctor immediately. Animals carry diseases like cat scratch fever, rabies, and tetanus.

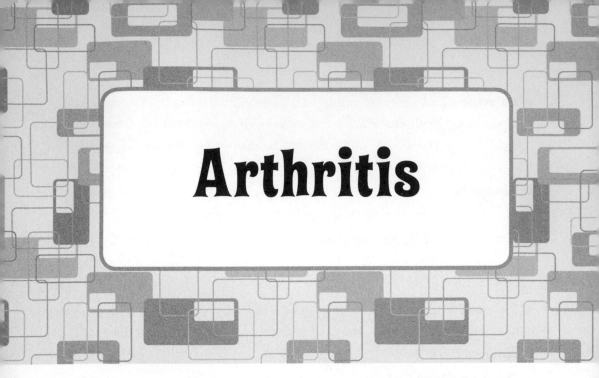

Arthritis

- **Birds Eye Frozen Peas** and **Bounty Paper Towels.** To relieve arthritis pain, cover a bag of Birds Eye Frozen Peas with a sheet of Bounty Paper Towels, and apply to the affected area for fifteen minutes to quell the burning sensation. The frozen peas act like small ice cubes, reducing the inflammation causing the pain, and the bag of peas conforms to the shape of your body. The paper towel creates a layer of insulation to prevent frostbite. Refreeze the bag of peas for future ice-pack use. Be sure to label the bag for ice-pack use only. If you want to eat the peas, cook them after they thaw the first time, never after refreezing.

- **Certo** and **Welch's Grape Juice.** To ease arthritis pain, mix one tablespoon Certo liquid fruit pectin—a plant extract used as a thickening agent to can jams and jellies—in eight ounces Welch's Grape Juice, and drink the mixture daily. The grape juice contains the powerful antioxidant resveratrol, and pectin binds cells together and monitors the flow of fluid in and out of the cells, according to a paper from London South Bank University. While no scientific studies show that pectin relieves arthritis pain, ample anecdotal evidence does.

- **Chicken of the Sea Salmon, Chicken of the Sea Sardines,** or **Chicken of the Sea Tuna.** Eating salmon, sardines, or tuna three times a week adds the fatty acids commonly known as omega-3 oils to your diet. All of these fish are rich in eicosapentaenoic acid (EPA) and docosahexaenoic acid (DHA), which help reverse some of the symptoms and complications of both osteoarthritis and rheumatoid arthritis. These fatty acids help reduce inflammation and pain, strengthen the immune system, and increase resistance to stress.

- **Colgate Regular Flavor Toothpaste.** To soothe arthritis pain, rub Colgate Regular Flavor Toothpaste into the affected area. The menthol in the mint, a common ingredient in salves developed to combat muscle aches, provides quick, temporary relief.

- **Dole Pineapple Juice.** Drinking one 8-ounce glass of Dole Pineapple Juice daily may relieve arthritis pain. Aside from being packed with vitamins and minerals, pineapple juice contains the plant enzyme bromelain, which appears to subdue joint inflammation.

- **Dr. Teal's Epsom Salt.** To soothe arthritis pain, fill the bathtub with warm water, add two cups Dr. Teal's Epsom Salt, and soak for fifteen minutes. The magnesium sulfate draws out carbon from the skin, reducing inflammation.

- **Jell-O.** To reduce arthritis pain, eat one serving of Jell-O brand gelatin every day. The amino acids purportedly stimulate production of collagen and provide nutritional support for cartilage structure, lessening pain. You should start noticing a significant improvement after three months.

- **Lakewood Black Cherry Juice.** To soothe arthritis pain, drink one 8-ounce glass of Lakewood Black Cherry Juice every day until the pain subsides. Black cherry juice is packed with anti-inflammatory antioxidants, and a 2011 study published in *Arthritis & Rheumatism* showed that drinking cherry juice provided relief for patients with arthritis of the knee.

- **Lipton Chamomile Tea** and **Stayfree Maxi Pads.** Place four Lipton Chamomile Tea bags in a cup, fill with boiling water, cover with a saucer, and steep for twenty minutes. Squeeze and remove the tea bags, and let the liquid cool to the touch. Saturate a Stayfree Maxi Pad with the tea, and place it over the affected joint. When applied topically, chamomile is an anti-inflammatory that can help soothe arthritis pain.

- **Lipton Ginger Tea.** To alleviate arthritis pain, place two Lipton Ginger Tea bags in a cup of boiling water, cover with a saucer, steep for ten minutes, and drink the tea. Do this three times a day. The compounds in ginger reduce inflammation and relieve pain—without the side effects of medication. (Do not drink ginger tea if you have gallstones. Ginger can increase bile production.)

- **Lipton Green Tea.** Reduce your chances of developing arthritis, slow its progression, and reduce pain by drinking four cups of Lipton Green Tea every day. The polyphenols in green tea may prevent arthritis and lessen the severity of symptoms, according to a 1999 study conducted at Case Western Reserve University.

- **McCormick Ground Cloves.** Prevent inflammation and slow the damage to cartilage and bone caused by arthritis by using one-half to one teaspoon McCormick Ground Cloves in your cooking every day. Cloves contain eugenol, an anti-inflammatory that, like Celebrex, impedes the release of the protein that triggers swelling. The antioxidants in cloves help decelerate the deterioration of cartilage and bone.

- **McCormick Ground Ginger.** Add one teaspoon McCormick Ground Ginger to salads or use it in recipes. Ginger, containing the active ingredient gingerol, is scientifically proven to reduce inflammation, mimicking non-steroidal anti-inflammatory drugs used to treat arthritis. (Do not use ginger if you have gallstones. Ginger can increase bile production.)

- **McCormick Ground Turmeric.** Take one tablespoon McCormick Ground Turmeric daily by simply sprinkling it on your food or using the spice in recipes. Turmeric contains curcumin, an anti-inflammatory that reduces the pain and inflammation of arthritis, just like nonsteroidal anti-inflammatory drugs such as aspirin, ibuprofen, and naproxen (but without the side effects). A 2010 study by endocrinologist Dr. Janet Funk at the University of Arizona College of Medicine showed that turmeric controls the formation of new blood vessels at the site of inflammation. (Turmeric may increase the likelihood of bleeding when taken in combination with the blood thinner Coumadin or other anticoagulant medications.)

- **McCormick Pure Vanilla Extract** and **Kleenex Tissues.** To reduce the stress exacerbating arthritis pain, put a few drops of McCormick Pure Vanilla Extract on a Kleenex Tissue and sniff it every so often. The aroma of vanilla triggers your pituitary gland and hypothalamus to produce endorphins, the neurotransmitters that produce a feeling of well-being. Studies show that the scent of vanilla significantly reduces stress, which in turn lowers pain sensitivity.

- **Tabasco Pepper Sauce** and **Crisco All-Vegetable Shortening.** To relieve arthritis pain, mix one-quarter teaspoon Tabasco Pepper Sauce with two tablespoons Crisco All-Vegetable Shortening, and apply the spicy homemade ointment to the affected areas up to five times a day for a week or two. The capsaicin in the Tabasco Pepper Sauce numbs the nerves that send pain signals to the brain. (Do not apply this salve on open sores and avoid contact with eyes and nose.)

- **Uncle Ben's Converted Brand Rice.** To relieve arthritis pain, fill a clean sock with Uncle Ben's Converted Brand Rice, tie a knot in the end, and heat in the microwave oven for ninety seconds. Making sure the sock isn't too hot, apply the heat pack to the sore, stiff joint. The rice-filled sock conforms to the shape of your body, stays warm for roughly thirty minutes, and provides soothing heat. The homemade heating pad is also reusable.

- **Vicks VapoRub.** To alleviate arthritis pain, rub Vicks VapoRub on the affected areas. The camphor, eucalyptol, and menthol in the balm reduce pain and inflammation.

LET'S BLOW THIS JOINT

- When the cartilage that forms a cushion between the ends of bones wears down, bones begin to rub against each other, causing pain and stiffness.

- Arthritis refers to more than one hundred different types of diseases, including osteoarthritis and rheumatoid arthritis. Osteoarthritis is a degenerative joint disease in which the cartilage covering the ends of bones in the joint deteriorates, causing pain and loss of movement as bone begins to rub against bone. Rheumatoid arthritis is an autoimmune disease in which the body's immune system attacks the joint lining.

- Other forms of arthritis include gout (usually affecting small joints), ankylosing spondylitis (affecting the spine), juvenile arthritis (any type occurring in children), systemic lupus erythematosus (typically causing inflammation and damage to joints and other connective tissues), scleroderma (a disease of the body's connective tissue), and fibromyalgia (widespread pain affecting the muscles and attachments to the bone).

- As of 2006, nearly 46 million Americans suffered from arthritis or chronic joint symptoms, according to the Arthritis Foundation.

- To attack the cause of arthritis (rather than the symptoms), adopt relaxation techniques and lifestyle changes to reduce stress; seek professional help to devise a diet (including nutritional supplements) to alleviate arthritis pain and reduce any excess weight; identify any food allergies or fungi, bacteria, or viruses that may be causing or amplifying the disease; and flush surfeit toxins from your body.

- To allow your body to metabolize fatty acids that reverse the symptoms of arthritis, avoid foods that contain hydrogenated oils, such as most cooking oils, margarine, peanut butter, junk food, and salad dressings.

- To prevent arthritis and reduce osteoarthritis pain, drink nine to twelve 8-ounce glasses of water daily. Hydration keeps your joints well lubricated.

- While too much exercise can make osteoarthritis pain worse, mild exercise (like walking for thirty minutes three times a week, riding a stationary bicycle, or swimming) can help reduce stiffness and pain, and improve the health of your joints.

- **Welch's Grape Juice, Mott's Apple Juice,** and **Heinz Apple Cider Vinegar.** Mix four cups Welch's Grape Juice, three cups Mott's Apple Juice, and one cup Heinz Apple Cider Vinegar in a two-quart pitcher or bottle. Drink one-half cup of this mixture daily to help reduce arthritis pain. Grape juice contains the powerful antioxidant resveratrol, apple juice reduces inflammation, and apple cider vinegar provides important nutrients, including potassium.

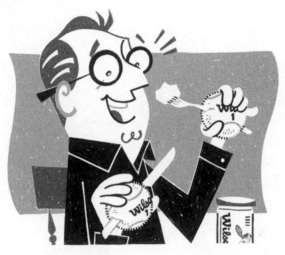

- **Wilson Tennis Balls.** To make a toothbrush or silverware easier to grip, use a razor blade or utility knife to carefully slice small slits in the opposite sides of a Wilson Tennis Ball, and then slip the handle of the toothbrush or utensil through the tennis ball. The bright yellow ball makes a convenient and practical grip.

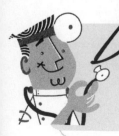

Doctor's Orders

Get a grip! If you feel pain, stiffness, and swelling in and around the joints, and have limited movement that lasts more than two weeks, see a doctor to determine the cause.

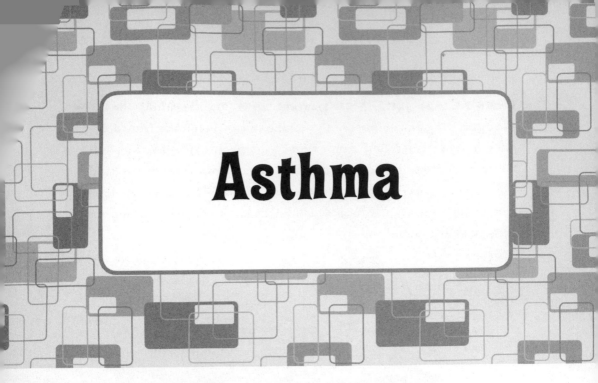

Asthma

- **Campbell's Tomato Juice.** To reduce the frequency of asthma attacks, drink an 8-ounce glass of Campbell's Tomato Juice every day. A 2008 study at Hunter Medical Research Institute in Newcastle, Australia, showed that consuming tomato juice, rich in the antioxidant lycopene, results in fewer asthma attacks by reducing the inflammation that causes asthma. One cup of tomato juice provides approximately 23 milligrams of lycopene.

- **Chicken of the Sea Salmon, Chicken of the Sea Sardines,** or **Chicken of the Sea Tuna.** The late-phase inflammatory reaction that can occur up to twenty-four hours after the initial acute inflammatory response and last for weeks can be averted by omega-3 fatty acids. Eating salmon, sardines, or tuna three or four times a week adds omega-3 oils to your diet. The eicosapentaenoic acid (EPA) and docosahexaenoic acid (DHA) in these fish reduce inflammation naturally. (People with asthma who are sensitive to aspirin or have a high risk of stroke should consult a doctor before adding fish to their diet.)

- **Coca-Cola.** After using your inhaler and calming your breathing, subdue an asthma attack by drinking a can of Coca-Cola. Chemically related to the asthma drug theophylline, caffeine helps open up constricted bronchial tubes—which swell during an asthma attack. If you feel the onset of an asthma attack and you don't have your inhaler with you, drink two 12-ounce cans of Coke. The caffeine can help dilate the bronchial passages in an emergency until you can get to your medicine or inhaler. In a 2010 study published in the *Cochrane Database of Systematic Reviews,* researchers found that caffeine produced modest improvements in airway function for up to four hours in people with asthma. (Do not rely solely on Coca-Cola to control asthma symptoms.)

- **Heinz Ketchup.** Using plenty of ketchup on your food helps reduce the frequency of asthma attacks. A 2008 study at Hunter Medical Research Institute in Newcastle, Australia, showed that consuming tomato products, rich in the antioxidant lycopene, reduces the inflammation that causes asthma. One tablespoon of ketchup provides 2.5 milligrams of lycopene. (Be aware that ketchup contains high amounts of sodium and added sugar.)

- **Hunt's Tomato Paste.** To reduce the frequency of asthma attacks, use plenty of Hunt's Tomato Paste in your cooking. A 2008 study at Hunter Medical Research Institute in Newcastle, Australia, showed that consuming tomato paste, rich in the antioxidant lycopene, results in fewer asthma attacks by reducing the inflammation that causes asthma.

- **Jif Peanut Butter.** Magnesium helps relax and keep the bronchial tract, the passageway to the lungs that becomes constricted during an asthma attack, open. While eating a wide range of legumes, nuts, whole grains, and vegetables will help you meet your daily dietary need for magnesium, you can quickly replace magnesium in your body by eating Jif Peanut Butter (straight from the jar or in a sandwich). Four tablespoons of peanut butter contain 100 milligrams of magnesium (or 25 percent of the recommended daily value).

☧ STRANGE MEDICINE ☧

A BREATH OF FRESH AIR

● During an asthma attack, an irritant or allergen causes the bronchi, the tubes that connect the trachea with the lungs, to spasm, swell, and produce mucus, clogging the airways and making breathing difficult.

● Asthma requires professional treatment from a doctor who tracks the effects of medication, asthma triggers (such as allergies), and diet.

● An asthma attack can be triggered by pollen, mold, dust mites, smoke, cold or dry air, stress, anger, or hormone levels.

● Staying calm during an asthma attack can help reduce the symptoms. Panicking makes the symptoms worse. Anxiety causes you to clench, restricting your airways even more flagrantly.

● Use a peak-flow meter, available at drug stores, to measure the speed of air leaving your lungs to detect the onset of an asthma attack.

● If you have asthma, don't smoke, and stay clear of secondhand smoke.

● When cooking, make sure the kitchen is well ventilated.

● To clear allergens from your living or work space, use an air purifier with a HEPA filter.

● The perfumed pages of a magazine can trigger an asthma attack.

● To help prevent an asthma attack, the moment you feel early signs of symptoms, use your inhaler.

● **Lipton Green Tea.** Drink one cup of strongly brewed Lipton Green Tea two to three times daily. Green tea contains theophylline, which opens the bronchial tubes.

● **Maxwell House Coffee.** After using your inhaler and calming your breathing (or in an emergency if you forget your inhaler), help quell an asthma attack by drinking a cup of Maxwell House Coffee. Similar to the asthma drug theophylline, caffeine helps dilate the constricted bronchial tubes. Drinking coffee can also reduce the frequency of asthma attacks. A 1988 study at the Central Institute of Statistics in Italy showed that people with asthma who drank two cups of coffee a day had 23 percent fewer asthma attacks than non-coffee drinkers. (Do not rely on Maxwell House Coffee to control asthma symptoms.)

- **McCormick Ground Turmeric.** To prevent or relieve inflammation of the bronchial tract, take one tablespoon McCormick Ground Turmeric daily by simply sprinkling it on your food, mixing it with a glass of warm milk, or using the spice in recipes for rice, casseroles, soups, and stews. Curcumin, an antioxidant in turmeric, reduces inflammation and also inhibits the body from producing prostaglandins, the compounds that help signal pain. (Be aware that turmeric may increase the likelihood of bleeding when taken in combination with the blood thinner Coumadin or other anticoagulant medications.)

- **Morton Salt.** To stop a sinus infection from making asthma worse, make a saline nose wash to rinse your nasal passages. Purify one cup of water by boiling for three minutes, let cool to room temperature, and dissolve one-half teaspoon Morton Salt in the purified water. Use a bulb syringe or neti pot to rinse each nostril to loosen mucus and reduce inflammation.

- **Mott's Apple Juice.** Drinking one glass of apple juice every day wards off asthma symptoms in children, according to a 2007 study by the National Heart and Lung Institute in the United Kingdom.

- **Planters Dry Roasted Almonds, Planters Dry Roasted Cashews,** or **Planters Dry Roasted Peanuts.** Eating foods high in magnesium—like Planters Dry Roasted Almonds, Planters Dry Roasted Cashews, or Planters Dry Roasted Peanuts—can help keep the bronchial tract relaxed and open. One ounce of almonds provides 80 milligrams of magnesium, one ounce of cashews provides 75 milligrams, and one ounce of dry roasted peanuts provides 50 milligrams.

- **Swiss Miss Hot Cocoa** and **McCormick Ground (Cayenne) Red Pepper.** If you don't have your inhaler at the start of an asthma attack, mix up a cup of Swiss Miss Hot Cocoa according to the directions, add a pinch of McCormick Ground (Cayenne) Red Pepper, and slowly sip the concoction. The caffeine in the hot chocolate helps dilate the constricted bronchial tubes, and cayenne contains anti-asthmatic compounds. (Do not rely on this spicy beverage to control asthma symptoms.)

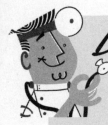

Doctor's Orders

Breathe easy! If you experience an asthma attack, immediately use the inhaler prescribed by your doctor and get away from whatever triggered the attack. If you continue having difficulty breathing, immediately call 911 or have someone take you to an emergency room.

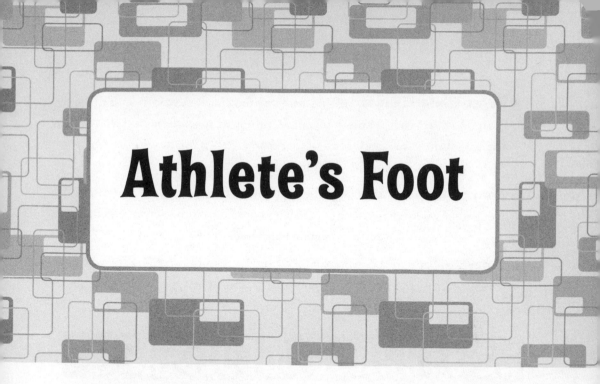

Athlete's Foot

- **Arm & Hammer Baking Soda.** For instant relief from athlete's foot, mix one tablespoon Arm & Hammer Baking Soda with enough water to make a paste, slather the mixture on the affected parts of your feet, and let sit for ten minutes. Rinse clean and dry thoroughly. The sodium bicarbonate anesthetizes the itching.

- **Colman's Mustard Powder.** Dissolve two tablespoons Colman's Mustard Powder in a basin of warm water, and soak your feet in the solution for fifteen minutes. The antifungal properties in mustard help eliminate the tinea pedis fungus on your feet.

- **Conair Hair Dryer.** After washing or soaking your feet and toweling them dry, blow-dry your feet with a Conair Hair Dryer set on low and held six inches away from each foot. Drying your feet completely eliminates the moisture that provides a breeding ground for the fungus.

- **Dannon Yogurt.** To soothe athlete's foot, apply Dannon Plain Nonfat Yogurt to the affected areas, let dry, then rinse clean, and dry thoroughly. The *Lactobacillus acidophilus* bacteria (probiotics) in the yogurt counteract tinea pedis, the fungus that has invaded your feet.

- **Heinz White Vinegar.** To kill athlete's foot, saturate a cotton ball with Heinz White Vinegar and dab your feet three or more times a day. To kill the fungus in your socks, soak the socks in a bucket filled with equal parts Heinz White Vinegar and water for thirty minutes.

- **Kingsford's Corn Starch.** After washing or treating your feet, dust your feet and powder the insides of your shoes with Kingsford's Corn Starch. The cornstarch absorbs moisture, denying bacteria a breeding ground.

- **Listerine.** Saturate a cotton ball (or fill a trigger-spray bottle) with original formula Listerine antiseptic mouthwash and apply it to your feet and

℞ STRANGE MEDICINE ℞

GETTING OFF ON THE RIGHT FOOT

- The fungus that causes athlete's foot—or tinea pedis—breeds on shower stall floors, bathroom floors, locker room floors, and pool decks.

- Wearing flip-flops when using public showers and other facilities can prevent the onset of athlete's foot.

- To cure athlete's foot, do not wear the same pair of shoes two days in a row (allow twenty-four hours for the shoes to dry out), and if your feet sweat, change your socks during the day.

- The tinea fungus also causes jock itch. If you have athlete's foot, wash your hands thoroughly after touching your feet to avoid infecting your crotch, and put on your socks before putting on your underwear.

- If you use medication or any antifungal solutions listed in this section to cure athlete's foot, continue applying the ointment or liquid for two weeks after the problem clears to make sure it doesn't return.

- Air out your shoes in the sun, allowing the heat to dry up all the moisture and kill any fungi.

between your toes. Let air dry. The thymol in Listerine kills the fungus. (Be aware that applying Listerine to your feet if you have broken skin or open sores will sting.)

- **Lysol.** After taking off your shoes, spray the inside with a blast of Lysol disinfectant, then let air dry. The disinfectant kills the fungus thriving in your shoes.

- **McCormick Thyme Leaves.** To alleviate athlete's foot, add two table-spoons McCormick Thyme Leaves to one cup of boiling water in a teacup, cover with a saucer, and let steep for ten minutes. Strain and let cool to the touch. Saturate a cotton ball with the thyme tea, and dab it on your feet and between your toes. Let air dry. The antifungal agents in the thymol kill the fungus causing your foot problem.

- **Morton Salt.** Dissolve one teaspoon Morton Salt for each cup of warm water you add to a basin, and soak your feet in the salty solution for ten min-utes every day until the athlete's foot vanishes. The salt water creates an inhos-pitable environment for the fungus, reduces perspiration, and softens the skin.

- **Ziploc Storage Bags.** To avoid making a mess when powdering your feet, place one-half cup of the powder in a gallon-size Ziploc Freezer Bag, insert your foot in the bag, seal the bag shut up to your leg, and shake.

Doctor's Orders

Don't put your foot in your mouth! If you've been suffering from athlete's foot for more than six months, see a doctor. You may require a prescription oral antifungal medication.

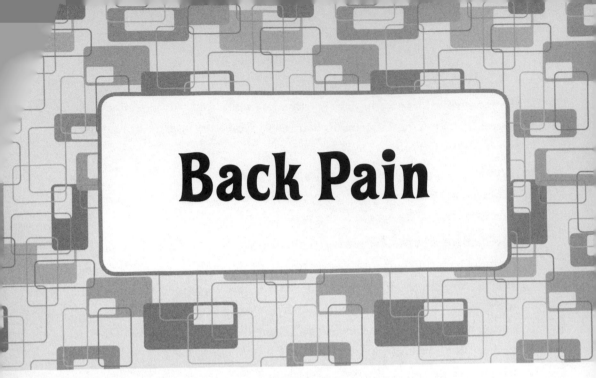

Back Pain

- **Birds Eye Frozen Peas** and **Bounty Paper Towels.** To tame a backache, cover a bag of Birds Eye Frozen Peas with a sheet of Bounty Paper Towels, and apply to the affected area for fifteen minutes every hour, starting within the first two hours of feeling pain. The frozen peas act like small ice cubes, reducing the inflammation causing the pain, and the bag of peas conforms to the shape of your back. The paper towel creates a layer of insulation to prevent frostbite. Refreeze the bag of peas for future ice-pack use. Be sure to label the bag for ice-pack use only. If you want to eat the peas, cook them after they thaw the first time, never after refreezing.

- **Bubble Wrap, Oral-B Dental Floss,** and **Scotch Packaging Tape.** Using a pair of scissors, cut a sheet of Bubble Wrap ten inches wide by fourteen feet long. Cut a piece of Oral-B Dental Floss forty inches long, center it along one of the ten-inch widths of Bubble Wrap, and starting at that end, roll up the sheet of Bubble Wrap into a tight cylinder. The resulting roll of Bubble Wrap will measure five inches in diameter and contain a length of dental floss threaded through the center. Secure the roll together with a few pieces of Scotch Packaging Tape. Position the roll horizontally to create lumbar support for your office chair and tie the ends of the dental floss together around the back of the chair to hold the roll in place. When you sit in the chair, the roll of Bubble Wrap should rest in the curve of your back, keeping your posture erect and your back pain-free.

- **McCormick Ground Turmeric.** To relieve back pain, take one tablespoon McCormick Ground Turmeric daily by simply sprinkling it on your food or using the spice in recipes for rice, casseroles, soups, and stews. Curcumin, an antioxidant in turmeric, reduces inflammation and also inhibits the body from producing prostaglandins, the compounds that help signal pain. (Turmeric may increase the likelihood of bleeding when taken in combination with the blood thinner Coumadin or other anticoagulant medications.)

- **McCormick Pure Vanilla Extract** and **Kleenex Tissues.** To reduce the stress exacerbating back pain, put a few drops of McCormick Pure Vanilla Extract on a Kleenex Tissue and sniff it every so often. The aroma of vanilla triggers your pituitary gland and hypothalamus to produce endorphins, the neurotransmitters that produce a feeling of well-being. Studies show that the scent of vanilla significantly reduces stress, which in turn lowers pain sensitivity.

- **Tabasco Pepper Sauce** and **Crisco All-Vegetable Shortening.** To relieve back pain, mix one-quarter teaspoon Tabasco Pepper Sauce with two tablespoons Crisco All-Vegetable Shortening, and apply the spicy homemade ointment to the affected areas up to five times a day. The capsaicin in the Tabasco Pepper Sauce relieves nerve pain. (Do not apply this salve on open sores and avoid contact with eyes and nose.)

- **Tums.** To relieve a sore back, eat one regular Tums tablet after breakfast and a second tablet after lunch. Your body can absorb only 500 to 600 milligrams of calcium at a time. A regular strength Tums tablet contains 500 milligrams of calcium carbonate. The calcium in Tums helps loosen and relax your tense back muscles. (If you've had calcium oxalate kidney stones, consult your doctor before taking Tums.)

℞ STRANGE MEDICINE ℞

BACK TO SQUARE ONE

● Back pain generally results from a strained muscle, a pulled ligament, or a herniated disk.

● Disks are cartilage-like pads that act as cushions between the vertebrae of your spine. A herniated disk is a disk that slips to one side or bulges, pressing against the root of a nerve and causing severe back pain.

● Most back pain gradually improves after seventy-two hours of home care, dissipating after anywhere from several days to several weeks.

● More than two days of bed rest to remedy back pain can cause more harm than good. A 1986 study at the University of Texas Health Science Center in San Antonio showed that patients with back pain who got out of bed after two days healed faster than those who stayed in bed for a week.

● To recover from back pain quickly, spend one or two days resting, then begin a mild exercise program, such as walking, riding a stationary bicycle, or swimming. Exercise increases circulation to your back, strengthens the muscles, and speeds healing.

● Stretching the back muscles expedites healing. Simply lie on your back, slowly bring your knees up to your chest, hold the position for ten seconds, and release. Repeat, and do this every few hours, if possible.

● For another helpful stretching exercise to relieve back pain, lie on your stomach, place the palms of your hands flat on the floor next to your ears, and lift your head and shoulders off the floor, arching your back.

● To ease back pain at night, sleep with a pillow between your legs if you sleep on your side, or, under your knees if you sleep on your back. Bending your knees relaxes your hamstring muscles, relieving pressure on your lower back.

● To prevent back pain, make sure you use a firm mattress that doesn't sag or have springs popping up into your back. To firm up a sagging mattress, place a sheet of ¾-inch plywood between the mattress and the box spring.

- **Uncle Ben's Converted Brand Rice.** After relieving the inflammation for the first day or two with the Birds Eye Frozen Peas tip on page 38, fill a clean sock with Uncle Ben's Converted Brand Rice, tie a knot in the end, and heat in the microwave oven for ninety seconds. Making sure the sock isn't too hot, apply the heat pack to the affected area. The rice-filled sock conforms to the shape of your back and stays warm for roughly thirty minutes, allowing the soothing warmth to increase circulation to the area. The homemade heating pad is also reusable.

- **Vicks VapoRub.** To alleviate back pain, rub Vicks VapoRub into your back muscles. The camphor and menthol in the balm reduce pain and inflammation.

- **Wilson Tennis Balls.** Insert three Wilson Tennis Balls into a sock, tie a knot in the open end of the sock, and have a partner roll the sock over your back for a soothing massage.

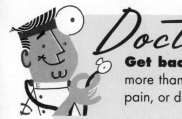

Doctor's Orders

Get back! If your back pain radiates down your leg, lasts for more than two weeks, or is accompanied by fever, cramps, chest pain, or difficulty breathing, consult a doctor.

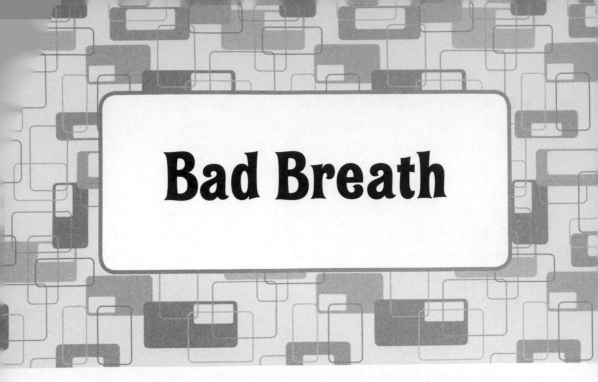

Bad Breath

- **Arm & Hammer Baking Soda.** Wet your toothbrush with water, dip it in a box of Arm & Hammer Baking Soda, and brush your teeth and tongue with the mildly abrasive powder. The sodium bicarbonate lowers the acidity in your mouth, making your mouth a hostile environment for odor-causing bacteria.

- **CharcoCaps Activated Charcoal.** To eliminate bad breath, take one 200- to 500-milligram CharcoCaps Activated Charcoal capsule. The charcoal absorbs toxins and other irritants in the digestive track, carrying them out of the body, leaving your breath fresh. (Don't confuse activated charcoal with charcoal briquettes. Activated charcoal is a charcoal that has been processed with oxygen to be extremely porous and absorb odors or other substances.) If the problem doesn't go away after ten days, consult your dentist.

- **Dannon Yogurt.** Eating a cup of Dannon Yogurt quells bad breath. The live bacteria in yogurt, specifically *Streptococcus thermophilus* and *Lactobacillus bulgaricus* (probiotics), seem to stymie the odor-producing anaerobic bacteria that grow on the tongue and in the mouth.

- **Life Savers Pep-O-Mints.** Suck on Life Savers Pep-O-Mints to freshen your breath temporarily. The volatile oils in peppermint kill odor-causing bacteria and increase saliva production, keeping the mouth moist. Unfortunately, the candy works only for a short time because the bacteria feed on the sugar.

- **McCormick Anise Seed.** Place a pinch of McCormick Anise Seed in your mouth, chew thoroughly, and swallow. Anise helps kill the bacteria in your mouth, and leaves your breath smelling like licorice. (Avoid consuming anise during pregnancy.)

- **McCormick Fennel Seed.** To freshen your breath, chew five to ten McCormick Fennel Seeds thoroughly after eating a meal and then swallow the seeds. The oils in the fennel aid the digestive process and deodorize your digestive track.

- **McCormick Whole Cloves.** To rid yourself of bad breath, bite into a McCormick Whole Clove, swish it around in your mouth for a minute or two, and discard it. The eugenol in the clove kills bacteria and simultaneously sweetens your breath.

- **Trident.** To relieve bad breath, chew a stick of Trident Sugarless Spearmint Gum. The spearmint freshens your breath. (Regular mint-flavored gums freshen your breath only temporarily because the bacteria feed on the sugar.)

- **Visa.** To remove odor-causing bacteria festering on your tongue, use a clean, expired Visa credit card to scrape your tongue from back to front ten to fifteen times.

- **Wrigley's Big Red Cinnamon Gum.** To reduce the bacteria that cause bad breath, chew a stick of Wrigley's Big Red Cinnamon Gum for twenty minutes. A 2011 study at the University of Illinois at Chicago showed that the cinnamic aldehyde in the gum reduces the amount of oral bacteria in your saliva by 50 percent, killing 40 percent of the types of oral bacteria linked to bad breath.

℞ STRANGE MEDICINE ℞

DON'T HOLD YOUR BREATH

● Brushing and flossing your teeth regularly eliminates most of the bacteria that causes halitosis, commonly called bad breath.

● To keep your breath fresh, drink at least eight 8-ounce glasses of water every day. The water washes away the food debris on which odor-causing bacteria flourish, and the liquid keeps your mouth moist, making it a hostile environment for bacteria.

● Bad breath can be a sign of periodontal (gum) disease or a side effect of a sinus infection or abscessed tooth.

● Garlic, onions, peppers, pastrami, salami, pepperoni, or Camembert, Roquefort, or blue cheese give you bad breath because the oils linger in your mouth for up to twenty-four hours, regardless of how much you brush your teeth or rinse with mouthwash.

● Smoking tobacco or drinking too many cups of coffee results in bad breath.

● Gargling with mouthwash keeps your breath fresh for approximately twenty minutes. The alcohol in the mouthwash causes dry mouth, which encourages odor-causing bacteria to breed.

● Skipping meals makes your mouth dry, creating the perfect environment for the bacteria that cause bad breath to proliferate.

● Many medications—including antihistamines and decongestants—cause dry mouth, which makes your mouth a breeding ground for odor-causing bacteria.

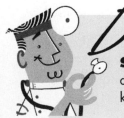

Doctor's Orders

Save your breath! If you can't get rid of your bad breath, see a doctor to make sure it isn't being caused by gingivitis, diabetes, kidney failure, or cancer.

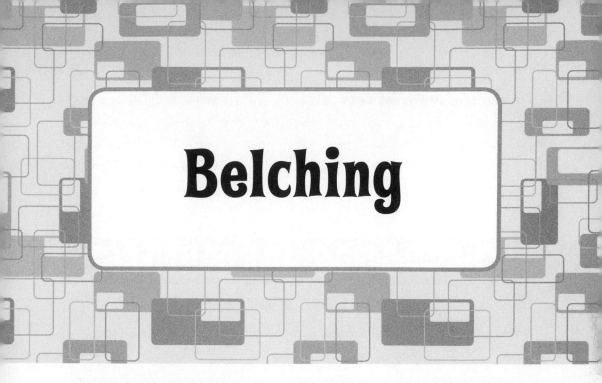

Belching

- **Dole Pineapple Juice.** To prevent belching, drink Dole Pineapple Juice during meals. The digestive enzyme bromelain, found in pineapple, helps prevent gas and bloating.

- **French's Mustard.** To prevent belching after meals, a half hour before eating, eat one teaspoon French's Mustard (or mix the mustard in one-half cup of water and drink the mixture).

- **Lipton Ginger Tea.** To relieve and prevent belching, sip a cup of Lipton Ginger Tea with each meal. Ginger stimulates digestion. (Do not drink ginger tea if you have gallstones. Ginger can increase bile production.)

- **Lipton Peppermint Tea.** To quell belching, pour one cup of boiling water over two Lipton Peppermint Tea bags in a cup, cover with a saucer (to prevent the medicinal peppermint oil from evaporating), let steep for ten minutes, and drink. The peppermint soothes digestion, calms stomach muscles, and clears up the gas.

- **McCormick Anise Seed.** Place a pinch of McCormick Anise Seed in your mouth, chew thoroughly, and swallow. The carminative agents in the anise help purge gas from your system to relieve belching. (Avoid anise during pregnancy.)

● **McCormick Fennel Seed.** Chew five to ten McCormick Fennel Seeds thoroughly after eating a meal and then swallow the seeds. Or make fennel tea by placing a tea infuser filled with one tablespoon McCormick Fennel Seed in a teacup, adding boiling water, covering with a saucer, and steeping for ten minutes. As an antispasmodic, fennel aids the digestive process,

℞ STRANGE MEDICINE ℞

FULL OF HOT AIR

● Belching results from accumulated air in the stomach. To reduce the built-up pressure, the body belches.

● The average person unconsciously swallows roughly ten cups of air and other gases during a typical day—merely by eating, drinking, and gulping.

● Excessive belching may signal that the digestive system isn't producing sufficient amounts of stomach acid and digestive enzymes.

● If you belch repeatedly throughout the day, you have a condition called aerophagia, which means you're unconsciously and constantly swallowing air. To overcome aerophagia, recognize that swallowing air is the cause of your constant belching, become aware of yourself in the present and observe yourself swallowing air, and force yourself to stop it.

● To avoid swallowing excessive air, eat slowly, chew with your mouth closed, and don't talk with your mouth full.

● Chewing gum, drinking through a straw, or eating foods pumped full of air (like ice cream or whipped cream) increase the amount of air you swallow.

● Wearing a skirt, girdle, or pair of pants that fit tightly around your waist can cause belching by squeezing out ingested air. Instead, wear loose clothes.

● Drinking carbonated soft drinks or beer adds excess gas to your stomach, and drinking coffee or eating fried foods causes the lower esophageal sphincter (the valve at the base of the esophagus) to relax, allowing air and gas to travel back out of your mouth.

dispersing gas from the intestinal tract. In India, fennel seeds are served after meals like after-dinner mints.

- **McCormick Ground Cardamom.** Add one teaspoon McCormick Ground Cardamom to eight ounces of water, boil for ten minutes, and drink the hot tea. Cardamom increases the production of digestive fluids in the stomach and also may help reduce muscle spasms in the stomach.

Doctor's Orders

Come up for air! If you belch constantly and experience abdominal discomfort, see a gastroenterologist to determine if you're suffering from an ulcer, gastroesophageal reflux disease, or any other stomach disorder.

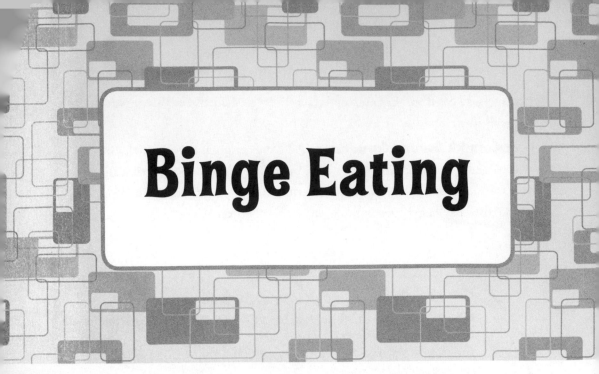

Binge Eating

- **Hershey's Chocolate Bar.** Carry a Hershey's Chocolate Bar with you at all times and eat only one square of chocolate after each meal, concentrating fully on the experience and savoring the taste with your undivided attention. Learning to enjoy a small amount of a forbidden food without any guilt and not treating it as a prelude to a chocolate binge helps you truly comprehend the difference between hunger and satisfaction.

- **Kellogg's All-Bran.** To reduce your desire to binge, eat one-half cup Kellogg's All-Bran for breakfast every day, sweetened with blueberries, strawberries, or sliced banana. A 1992 study at Vanderbilt University concluded that eating breakfast every morning helps reduce dietary fat and minimize impulsive snacking. One-half cup of Kellogg's All-Bran also contains 10 grams of fiber, which fills you up.

- **Quaker Oats.** To help fill your stomach and impede the need to binge, start each day with a bowl of Quaker Oats oatmeal. With only 150 calories in a one-cup serving, oatmeal makes you feel full longer, minimizing the urge to snack.

℞ STRANGE MEDICINE ℞

FOOD FOR THOUGHT

● People generally binge eat to counterbalance a diet, alleviate stress and anxiety, or suppress feelings of loneliness, depression, or anger.

● People use food as a substance to act out, repress, or avoid feelings. People—generally women—deny themselves food on a strict, low-fat diet and then binge eat to rebel against the deprivation, punish themselves, and numb their feelings of guilt.

● In 2007, researchers at Harvard published a survey that showed binge eating to be the most common eating disorder, affecting 2.8 percent of adults—compared to 1 percent for bulimia and 0.6 percent for anorexia. Approximately 10 to 15 percent of the obese population suffers from binge eating.

● To minimize cravings for food, drink at least eight 8-ounce glasses of water every day. Drinking water not only keeps your body hydrated and functioning properly, but the water fills your stomach, reducing hunger pangs.

● Eating three substantial meals a day and a small wholesome afternoon snack prevents you from binging to recover from a feeling of starvation. If you skip breakfast and have a small lunch, you'll inevitably consume a huge dinner because you're famished.

● Going for a walk for twenty minutes a day eliminates your craving for food, reducing the stress that may trigger an eating-binge.

● Use positive affirmations. If you're repeating negative thoughts in your head ("I'm too fat," "I do terrible things," "I have an awful personality"), your self-hatred may be the cause of your binge eating. Instead, replace those thoughts with positive self-acceptance affirmations, such as, "I accept my body for the way it is," "I accept myself even though I make mistakes," or "I accept how I feel right now."

● Rather than denying yourself foods you crave, eat a smaller portion of a lower-fat food. If you yearn for a bowl of ice cream, treat yourself to a scoop of low-fat frozen yogurt instead.

- **Tabasco Pepper Sauce.** To slow down your eating, sprinkle Tabasco Pepper Sauce on your food. The spicy tang forces you to eat at a regular pace and consume smaller portions. The capsaicin in the hot sauce also suppresses your appetite and prompts your body to briefly burn more calories, lessening your potential weight gain.

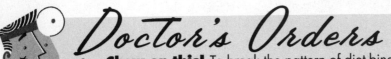

Doctor's Orders

Chew on this! To break the pattern of diet-binge eating or if you binge eat 2,000 calories (a full day's worth of food) for a snack at least twice a week for several months, seek a therapist who specializes in eating disorders or a support group.

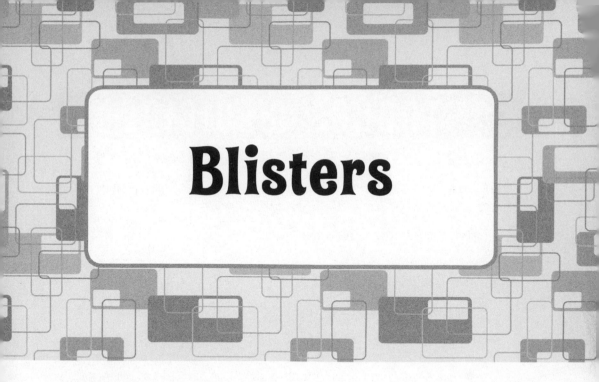

Blisters

Healing

- **Fruit of the Earth Aloe Vera Gel** and **Band-Aid Bandages.** To soothe and help heal a blister, smear Fruit of the Earth Aloe Vera Gel on the affected area and then cover it with a Band-Aid Bandage. As 100 percent pure aloe vera gel, Fruit of the Earth Aloe Vera Gel does not contain any alcohol, which can dry the blister rather than keep it properly moist.

- **Lipton Chamomile Tea** and **Arm & Hammer Baking Soda.** To soothe and disinfect a blister, pour one cup of boiling water over two Lipton Chamomile Tea bags in a cup, cover with a saucer, let steep for ten minutes, and let cool to the touch. Dissolve one-half teaspoon Arm & Hammer Baking Soda in the brew, and soak the blister in the solution (or apply with a washcloth).

- **Listerine.** To dry out a blister, use a cotton ball to apply original formula Listerine antiseptic mouthwash to the site three times a day. As an astringent, Listerine causes the blistered skin tissues to contract.

- **McCormick Rosemary Leaves, McCormick Thyme Leaves,** and **Stay-free Maxi Pads.** To prevent a blister from getting infected, place one teaspoon McCormick Rosemary Leaves and one teaspoon McCormick

℞ STRANGE MEDICINE ℞

GETTING RUBBED THE WRONG WAY

● A blister results when too much friction ruptures cell tissue. The subsequent release of plasma fills a pocket between the layers of skin with clear fluid.

● Popping a blister increases the risk of infection.

● If you leave a blister intact, the area under the cushion of fluid forms new skin, and blistered white skin forms a scab and falls off.

● Placing a washcloth dampened with cool water on the affected area soothes the pain.

● To drain a blister, first disinfect the area around the blister by washing with an antibacterial soap or pouring rubbing alcohol over the spot. Sterilize a needle by holding it over a lit match for a few seconds (or dipping it in rubbing alcohol), let cool, and then gently pierce the blister. Press the blister gently with a cotton ball or gauze pad to absorb the fluid. Leave the white skin on the blister, apply an antibiotic ointment, and cover with a protective adhesive bandage. Before going to bed, remove the bandage to let the blister breathe. In the morning, wash the blister with an antibacterial soap and put on a new bandage.

● To prevent blisters on your feet, buy your shoes in the afternoon, when your feet are most swollen, and consider insoles, which add protective cushioning. Be sure you buy a pair of shoes with plenty of room in the toe area. From the tip of the shoe, your longest toe should have space measuring the width of your thumb.

● Wearing socks with your shoes prevents blisters on the back of your heels.

● To avoid getting blisters on your hands, wear work gloves when doing manual labor or gardening and wear the appropriate sports gloves when playing golf or tennis.

Thyme Leaves in one cup of boiling water, cover with a saucer, and let steep for ten minutes. Let cool to room temperature, strain, saturate a Stayfree Maxi Pad with the liquid, and press it against the blister for twenty minutes. Do this once or twice a day until the blister heals. Rosemary and thyme are antibacterials.

- **Morton Salt.** To speed healing, mix two ounces Morton Salt and one ounce of cold water, apply the solution to a washcloth, and press it against the blister for one hour. Salt water expedites healing.

- **Preparation H.** To speed healing, smear a dab of Preparation H on the blister. The hemorrhoid cream relieves the burning sensation.

- **Vaseline Petroleum Jelly.** To help a blister heal more rapidly and reduce further friction, rub a few dabs of Vaseline Petroleum Jelly over the affected area. In 1859, Brooklyn chemist Robert Augustus Chesebrough learned from petroleum drilling workers in Titusville, Pennsylvania, that the jelly residue that gunked up oil drilling rods quickened healing when rubbed on a wound or burn.

Preventing

- **Johnson's Baby Powder.** To reduce the risk of getting blisters on your hands, rub some Johnson's Baby Powder into your hands. The talc allows your hands to glide better, reducing the friction that causes blisters.

- **Kingsford's Corn Starch.** To prevent blisters on your feet, dust your feet with Kingsford's Corn Starch before putting on your socks and shoes. The cornstarch absorbs the perspiration from your feet, reducing friction and the likelihood of blisters.

- **Vaseline Petroleum Jelly.** Rub a thin coat of Vaseline Petroleum Jelly over your feet to prevent the friction that causes blisters. If your shoes don't fit snuggly, the lubricant allows your feet to glide better, reducing the risk of a blister.

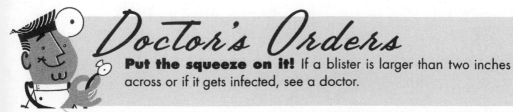

Doctor's Orders

Put the squeeze on it! If a blister is larger than two inches across or if it gets infected, see a doctor.

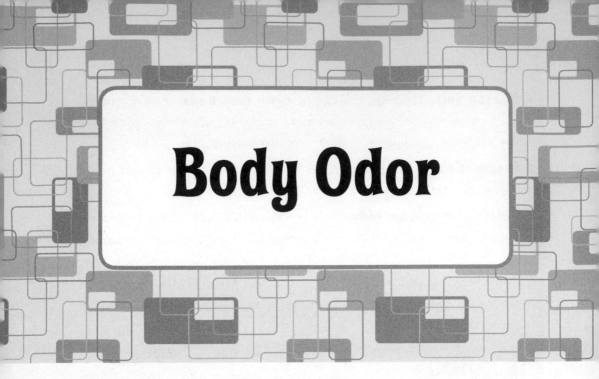

Body Odor

- **Arm & Hammer Baking Soda.** To deodorize your body the same way you would deodorize your refrigerator, add a handful of Arm & Hammer Baking Soda to the water in your bathtub, and soak for ten minutes. The mild antiseptic kills bacteria, and the alkalinity of the baking soda neutralizes the acidity of your skin, making your skin an inhospitable environment for the bacteria the cause body odor.

- **Campbell's Tomato Juice.** Add two cups Campbell's Tomato Juice to the warm water in your bathtub, and soak in the solution for fifteen minutes. The acids in the tomato juice neutralize any smells.

- **Dannon Yogurt.** Eating a cup of Dannon Nonfat Yogurt daily reduces the malign bacteria in the intestine that can cause fierce body odor. Dannon Nonfat Yogurt contains the beneficial bacteria *Lactobacillus acidophilus* (probiotics), which help minimize the proliferation of bad bacteria and sustain the health of the intestines.

- **Desitin.** Rub a dab of Desitin, the baby rash ointment, under each arm. The zinc oxide in the salve kills bacteria.

- **Dickinson's Witch Hazel** and **Stayfree Maxi Pads.** To subdue body odor, saturate a Stayfree Maxi Pad with Dickinson's Witch Hazel, and apply the astringent to your skin. Witch hazel dries and deodorizes the skin.

- **Heinz Apple Cider Vinegar.** Use a cotton ball to apply Heinz Apple Cider Vinegar under your arms. The acetic acid in the vinegar kills bacteria and simultaneously raises the pH of your skin, making your skin an inhospitable environment for the bacteria that cause body odor.

- **Jell-O.** To prevent your underarms from perspiring, mix up a box of your favorite flavor of Jell-O with two cups of warm water, fill a trigger-spray bottle with the gelatin solution, and mist your underarms with it. Like an antiperspirant, the gel plugs up the sweat glands.

- **Kingsford's Corn Starch, Stayfree Maxi Pads,** and **Ziploc Storage Bags.** Pour one-half cup Kingsford's Corn Starch into a Ziploc Storage Bag. Peel the adhesive strip from the back of a Stayfree Maxi Pad, fold the pad in half against the adhesive strip to form a two-ply powder puff, dip it in the bag, and use it to powder cornstarch under your arms. The cornstarch absorbs moisture. Seal the pad inside the bag for future use.

- **Lipton Chamomile Tea.** Stress causes your sweat glands to perspire. If you're feeling anxious, pour one cup of boiling water over two Lipton Chamomile Tea bags in a cup, cover with a saucer, let steep for ten minutes, and then drink the tea. Chamomile subdues tension, calming down your sweat glands. A 2009 study at the University of Pennsylvania showed that taking chamomile reduces the symptoms of generalized anxiety disorder by 50 percent. (Coumarin, an anticoagulant in chamomile, may increase the likelihood of bleeding when taken in combination with the blood thinner Coumadin or other anticoagulant medications.)

- **Listerine.** To prevent body odor, after showering use a cotton ball to apply original formula Listerine antiseptic mouthwash under your arms. Let dry, and then apply your regular deodorant or antiperspirant. The thymol, eucalyptol, and menthol in the mouthwash kill the bacteria that cause body odor.

☥ STRANGE MEDICINE ☥

STINKING TO HIGH HEAVEN

● The apocrine glands in your armpits and groin produce sweat that odor-causing bacteria adore.

● Unlike the apocrine glands, sweat glands produce clear, clean, odorless perspiration.

● Antiperspirants contain chemicals that clog the pores, preventing perspiration from escaping the body and drying the wetness. Rather than inhibiting perspiration, deodorants contain chemicals that kill odor-causing bacteria.

● In your digestive system, toxins from processed food, environmental chemicals, or medications can pass through the thin membrane of the intestine, enter the bloodstream, and exit the body through your perspiration, creating foul body odor.

● If you still smell after taking a shower or bathing, change your clothes more frequently. The fabrics absorb your odiferous perspiration.

● Your clothes and hair absorb odors from cooking foods, like garlic, onions, and various strong spices. The smell of cigarette smoke and fuel also infuses clothing and hair.

● Cotton clothes and other natural fabrics absorb perspiration quickly, which then evaporates. Synthetic fabrics don't do the job as well.

● Shaving the hair from your underarms reduces body odor by eliminating an environment where odor-causing bacteria breed and coat with pungent secretions.

● Your sweat glands secrete the extracts from oils—and the accompanying smell—from cumin, curry, garlic, onion, and fish for hours after you eat them.

● **McCormick Ground Sage.** To reduce perspiration and kill the bacteria causing body odor, place a tea infuser filled with two teaspoons McCormick Ground Sage in a teacup, add boiling water, cover with a saucer, and steep for ten minutes. Let cool to room temperature and apply with a washcloth to your body (excluding your face and genitals). Sage doubles as an antibacterial and antiperspirant.

- **Purell Instant Hand Sanitizer.** Rub a dollop of Purell Instant Hand Sanitizer into your underarms. The alcohol in the gel kills the bacteria responsible for emitting the odor.

- **ReaLemon.** Add one-half teaspoon ReaLemon lemon juice to a ten-ounce glass of water, and drink ten glasses a day. Drinking plenty of water daily enables the body to expel odor-causing toxins and the lemon juice stimulates liver detoxification.

- **ReaLemon.** Saturate a cotton ball with ReaLemon lemon juice and apply it under your arms, to the soles of your feet, and between your toes. The acidity of the lemon juice raises the pH of your skin, making it an inhospitable environment for the bacteria that cause body odor.

- **Smirnoff Vodka.** Use a cotton ball to apply Smirnoff Vodka under your arms. The alcohol kills the odor-causing bacteria.

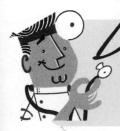

Doctor's Orders

That stinks! Profuse sweating and excessive odor could signal a thyroid problem or low blood sugar. Consult your doctor to rule out these problems or a more serious disease like diabetes.

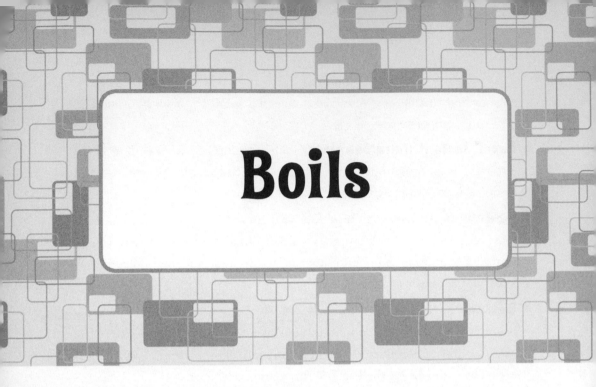

Boils

- **Clearasil.** To help dry out a boil and kill the *Staphylococcus aureus* bacteria causing it, apply Clearasil to the boil twice a day. The benzoyl peroxide combats the bacteria and dries the area.

- **Dial Soap.** If you have a history of boils, switch to Dial Antibacterial Soap. Triclosan, the antibacterial ingredient in the soap, kills the bacteria that cause boils.

- **Dr. Teal's Epsom Salt.** To shrink a boil, fill the bathtub with warm water, add two cups Dr. Teal's Epsom Salt, and soak for fifteen minutes. The Epsom Salt draws out fluid from the skin, reducing inflammation.

- **Hydrogen Peroxide** and **Neosporin.** When the boil bursts, to avoid spreading the infection, pour Hydrogen Peroxide over the boil, let it bubble for five minutes, pat dry, and apply Neosporin antibiotic ointment.

- **Kingsford's Corn Starch.** In spots where chafing or moisture prompts boils, dust the area with Kingsford's Corn Starch, which reduces friction and absorbs dampness.

- **Lipton Tea Bags.** To soothe a boil and help it drain, use a Lipton Tea Bag dampened with warm water as a compress against the protrusion for five minutes. The antibacterial tannin in the tea can kill the *Staphylococcus aureus* bacteria that usually cause the skin infection. The tannin also soothes the inflammation and relieves pain.

- **Listerine.** Wipe the boil with original formula Listerine antiseptic mouthwash to keep it clean and disinfected. Developed by Dr. Joseph Lawrence in 1857 as a safe and effective antiseptic for use in surgical procedures, Listerine is an astringent and antibacterial. The thymol in the mouthwash kills bacteria.

℞ STRANGE MEDICINE ℞

IT ALL BOILS DOWN TO THIS

- A boil is a bacterial infection of a sweat gland or hair follicle caused by dead skin cells or other debris blocking a pore or follicle. White blood cells die fighting the bacterial infection, creating pus, redness, and swelling.

- Perennial boils may be caused by gastrointestinal bacteria that entered the bloodstream or from eating too much sugar.

- A boil typically comes to a head and bursts on its own within two weeks.

- Never press or lance a boil to pop it open. Doing so can spread the infection and cause scarring.

- Placing a washcloth dampened with hot water on the boil for twenty minutes twice a day brings blood to the affected area, which can kill the bacteria causing the boil. After applying hot compresses for several days, apply a washcloth dampened with hot water for ten minutes, followed by a washcloth dampened with ice-cold water for ten minutes. Repeat twice more, and do this twice a day. Alternating hot and cold should draw out the pus.

- **McCormick Ground Turmeric.** To soothe a boil, mix four tablespoons McCormick Ground Turmeric with enough water to make a paste, and apply to the boil. Curcumin, an antioxidant in turmeric, reduces inflammation, and studies show that curcumin also inhibits the *Staphylococcus aureus* bacteria that generally cause boils.

- **McCormick Thyme Leaves** and **Stayfree Maxi Pads.** To help drain a boil or disinfect a ruptured boil, place a tea infuser filled with one teaspoon McCormick Thyme Leaves in a cup, fill with boiling water, cover with a saucer, and let steep for ten minutes. Let cool to the touch, and then saturate a Stayfree Maxi Pad with the tea and use as a compress. The thymol in thyme is a natural antiseptic.

- **Stayfree Maxi Pads.** Saturate a Stayfree Maxi Pad with warm water and press it against the boil for twenty minutes several times a day. The heat promotes circulation, bringing more white blood cells to combat the infection, and the compress helps the boil drain.

- **SueBee Honey.** When the boil bursts, apply a thick coat of SueBee Honey. Honey is hygroscopic, meaning it absorbs liquid from the boil and kills bacteria, sealing out contaminants. The honey dries to form a unique bandage.

Doctor's Orders

Don't get all boiled up! If a boil is bigger than a dime or does not diminish after a few days, see a doctor, who may prescribe antibiotics, draining, or a steroid injection.

Breast Discomfort

- **Birds Eye Frozen Peas** and **Bounty Paper Towels.** To soothe breast tenderness or pain, cover a bag of Birds Eye Frozen Peas with a sheet of Bounty Paper Towels, and place it on each breast for ten minutes. The frozen peas act like small ice cubes, providing quick relief, and the bag of peas conforms to the shape of your breast. The paper towel creates a layer of insulation to prevent frostbite. Refreeze the bag of peas for future ice-pack use. Be sure to label the bag for ice-pack use only. If you want to eat the peas, cook them after they thaw the first time, never after refreezing the bag.

- **Castor Oil, Saran Wrap, Arm & Hammer Baking Soda,** and **Ziploc Storage Bags.** Applying a castor oil pack to your breasts three times during the week before your period can reduce inflammation and eliminate breast pain. Fold a soft flannel cloth in half once or twice and dampen it with Castor Oil. Lie down, place the saturated cloth over your breasts, place a sheet of Saran Wrap over the cloth, and place a hot-water bottle or heating pad on top of the plastic sheet. Fold a bath towel lengthwise, place it over the hot-water bottle or heating pad, and tuck the ends of the bath towel under your body to hold everything in place snuggly for one hour. When finished, dissolve two teaspoons Arm & Hammer Baking Soda in one quart of warm water, and cleanse your skin with the solution. Store the castor oil-soaked flannel cloth in a Ziploc Storage Bag and refrigerate. Repeat the treatment for two to three months.

- **Dr. Teal's Epsom Salt.** To relieve breast pain, fill the bathtub with warm water and add two cups Dr. Teal's Epsom Salt. Soak for twenty minutes, during which time the magnesium in the Epsom Salt passes into the body through osmosis and eases soreness. The calming effect of the bath also reduces stress, inhibiting the adrenal glands from producing epinephrine, a substance that interferes with the body's ability to convert fatty acids into gamma linoleic acid, which leads to breast pain.

- **Jif Peanut Butter.** Magnesium helps decrease breast soreness, particularly if you consume 200 to 400 milligrams of magnesium every day, starting two weeks before the onset of your period. While eating a wide range of legumes, nuts, whole grains, and vegetables will help you meet your daily dietary need for magnesium, you can quickly replace magnesium in your body by eating Jif Peanut Butter (straight from the jar or in a sandwich). Four tablespoons of peanut butter contain 100 milligrams of magnesium (or 25 percent of the daily value).

- **Planters Dry Roasted Almonds.** To reduce breast discomfort, eat a handful of Planters Dry Roasted Almonds every day. Consuming 200 to 400 milligrams of magnesium every day, starting two weeks before the onset of your period can minimize breast soreness. One ounce of dry roasted almonds provides 80 milligrams of magnesium.

- **Quaker Oats.** To lessen breast tenderness, eat a bowl of Quaker Oats oatmeal for breakfast every day. Consuming plenty of fiber—20 to 25 grams a day—reduces breast tenderness. Oats contain the mild sedative gramine, the fiber absorbs excess estrogen, and the complex carbohydrates seem to increase serotonin levels in the brain, relieving stress.

℞ STRANGE MEDICINE ℞

GETTING IT OFF YOUR CHEST

● During the menstrual cycle (typically during the week before your period), fluctuating levels of hormones—estrogen and progesterone—cause tissue growth and fluid build-up in the breasts. The expanding tissue stretches nerves, causing breast pain.

● Once called fibrocystic breast disease, cyclical breast tenderness is now considered a side effect of menstruation.

● Half of all women under age fifty experience breast tenderness.

● Prescription medicines (including birth control pills) can trigger breast tenderness.

● To alleviate breast discomfort, wear a sports bra rather than an underwire bra. Also, consider wearing a bra to sleep at night.

● Massaging the breasts in a circular motion helps direct accumulated fluid from the breasts into the lymph passageways, relieving the pain and discomfort.

● Exercising for thirty minutes three times a week decreases the production of the stress hormones in your body that contribute to breast pain.

● Reduce the amount of hydrogenated oils you eat. The hydrogenated fats in margarine and junk foods lessen your body's ability to convert fatty acids into gamma linoleic acid, a key to preventing breast pain.

● **Silk Soymilk.** To minimize breast tenderness, add more soy foods to your diet, such as one 8-ounce glass of Silk Soymilk once a day. A 2000 study at Western General Hospital in Scotland showed that drinking 34 milligrams of soy protein daily had a mild analgesic effect on cyclical breast pain. One 8-ounce glass of soymilk contains 6 grams of soy protein.

- **Uncle Ben's Converted Brand Rice.** To relieve breast discomfort, fill a clean sock with Uncle Ben's Converted Brand Rice, tie a knot in the end, and heat in the microwave oven for sixty seconds. Making sure the sock isn't too hot, apply the heat pack to your breast. The rice-filled sock conforms to the shape of your body, stays warm for roughly twenty minutes, and provides soothing heat. The homemade heating pad is also reusable.

Doctor's Orders

Make a clean breast of it! If you experience breast pain monthly or notice a lump or any thickening, see a doctor to rule out breast cancer.

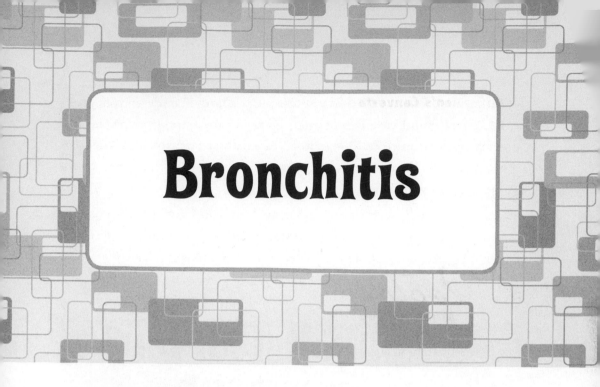

Bronchitis

- **French's Mustard.** Spread French's Mustard on your chest and cover with a washcloth dampened with warm water. Let sit for one hour (unless the mustard plaster becomes too hot). Repeat every four hours. The penetrating warmth from the plaster thins the mucus in your bronchi.

- **Gold's Horseradish** and **Nabisco Original Premium Saltine Crackers.** Eat one teaspoon Gold's Horseradish spread on a Nabisco Original Premium Saltine Cracker. Horseradish helps dissipate congested mucus in your bronchi so you can cough it out.

- **Life Savers Pep-O-Mints.** To help calm a cough and moisten the throat, suck on a Life Savers Pep-O-Mint candy. The volatile oils in peppermint increase saliva production, soothing your throat, and ease the cough.

- **Lipton Chamomile Tea.** To clear congestion from the bronchial tract, fill a large bowl with boiling water, and add three Lipton Chamomile Tea bags. Wearing a towel over your head to form a tent over the bowl, hold your face close to the steaming tea for ten minutes. Keep a box of tissues nearby to blow your nose repeatedly.

- **McCormick Garlic Powder.** Use McCormick Garlic Powder in your cook-ing, or once a day, eat a slice of lightly buttered bread sprinkled with one-half teaspoon McCormick Garlic Powder. As a natural expectorant, garlic helps break apart blocks of mucus in your bronchi, enabling you to cough it out.

- **McCormick Thyme Leaves.** To relieve bronchitis, place a tea infuser filled with two teaspoons McCormick Thyme Leaves in a cup, fill with boiling water, cover with a saucer, and let steep for ten minutes. Drink the resulting tea. The flavonoids in thyme reduce inflammation and relax the tracheal and ileal muscles.

℞ STRANGE MEDICINE ℞

WASTING YOUR BREATH

- Typically caused by a viral infection (though sometimes by bacteria), bronchitis is inflammation of the lining of the bronchial passages, the tubes that connect the trachea to the lungs.

- Antibiotics usually won't cure bronchitis, because viruses, responsible for 95 percent of bronchitis cases, do not react to antibiotics.

- Acute bronchitis typically lasts seven to ten days.

- When suffering from acute bronchitis, avoid milk and other dairy products, which produce extra mucus.

- Drinking eight 8-ounce glasses of water a day helps thin mucus.

- If you smoke, stop. Smoking makes bronchitis worse, and quitting significantly raises your chances of getting rid of the ailment. Second-hand smoke also causes and prolongs bronchitis.

- Using a vaporizer (or a humidifier) helps moisten the mucous membranes, making it easier for you to clear phlegm from the bronchi.

- **Morton Salt** and **Arm & Hammer Baking Soda.** To loosen mucus and reduce inflammation, make a saline nose wash to rinse your nasal passages. Purify eight ounces of water by boiling for three minutes, let cool to room temperature, and dissolve one-quarter teaspoon Morton Salt and one-quarter teaspoon Arm & Hammer Baking Soda in the purified water. Use a bulb syringe or neti pot to rinse each nostril.

- **Tabasco Pepper Sauce** and **Campbell's Tomato Juice.** To help clear congestion from the bronchial tract, add ten to twenty drops Tabasco Pepper Sauce to a glass of Campbell's Tomato Juice, and drink this mixture several times a day. The capsaicin in Tabasco Pepper Sauce helps break apart mucus clumped in your bronchi, enabling you to cough it out.

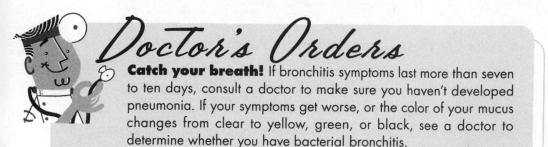

Doctor's Orders

Catch your breath! If bronchitis symptoms last more than seven to ten days, consult a doctor to make sure you haven't developed pneumonia. If your symptoms get worse, or the color of your mucus changes from clear to yellow, green, or black, see a doctor to determine whether you have bacterial bronchitis.

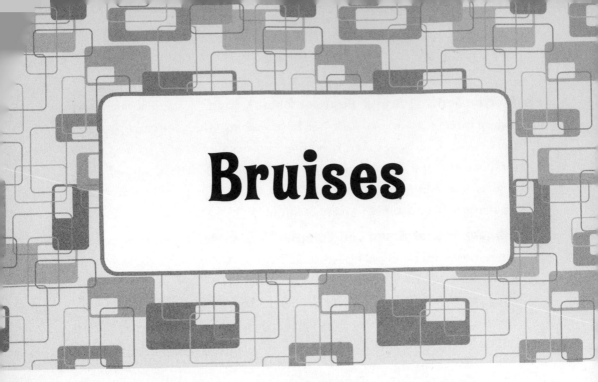

Bruises

- **Birds Eye Frozen Peas** and **Bounty Paper Towels.** To stop the bleeding under the skin and help reduce the swelling, cover a bag of Birds Eye Frozen Peas with a sheet of Bounty Paper Towels, and apply to the affected area. The frozen peas act like small ice cubes, reducing the inflammation causing the pain, and the bag of peas conforms to the shape of your body. The paper towel creates a layer of insulation to prevent frostbite. Refreeze the bag of peas for future ice-pack use. Be sure to label the bag for ice-pack use only. If you want to eat the peas, cook them after they thaw the first time, never after refreezing.

- **Castor Oil.** To speed the healing of a black eye, gently massage a few drops of Castor Oil into the shiner (without getting the oil in your eye). Castor oil reduces the swelling, lessens the discoloration, and relieves the pain.

- **Dickinson's Witch Hazel** and **Bounty Paper Towels.** To help a bruise heal quickly, saturate a sheet of Bounty Paper Towels with Dickinson's Witch Hazel, and press the wet paper towel to the bruise. The astringent witch hazel doubles as a vasoconstrictor, shrinking inflamed blood vessels to speed healing.

℞ STRANGE MEDICINE ℞

CRUISIN' FOR A BRUISIN'

● When a fall or bump breaks the blood vessels beneath the surface of your skin, the blood vessels bleed into surrounding tissue, turning the surface of your skin purple or blue.

● To relieve a bruise quickly, place a washcloth dampened with hot water on the bruised area for three minutes, then remove it and apply a washcloth dampened with ice-cold water for three minutes. Repeat the cycle four times. Alternating hot and cold brings blood to the area and then sends it away, bringing fresh nutrients and purging waste products.

● When blood leaks out of the capillaries under your skin and seeps into the surrounding tissue, the bruised skin appears black and blue. As the bruise heals, the colors change to purple, green, and yellow.

● A bruise typically disappears without any treatment in anywhere from ten days to two weeks.

● To minimize discoloration when you get a bruise, elevate the affected body part above heart level to reduce blood flow to the spot.

● Don't take aspirin, Advil, or Aleve to relieve the pain from a bruise. Aspirin, ibuprofen, and naproxen all thin the blood, which will increase the amount of blood that leaks from the capillaries, making the bruise larger. If you need a pain reliever, take Tylenol. The acetaminophen won't enlarge the bruise.

● Bruising easily could be a sign of a vitamin C or vitamin K deficiency. Vitamin C helps strengthen blood vessels, and vitamin K helps blood to clot. To get more vitamin C, eat more citrus fruit and leafy green vegetables, and to get more vitamin K, eat more alfalfa sprouts, broccoli, Brussels sprouts, and other leafy green vegetables.

● **Domino Sugar.** To prevent a bruise from forming, the moment you bang yourself, wet your fingertips with water, dip them in Domino Sugar, and massage the bruise firmly and swiftly. The sugar crystals seem to prevent the blood vessels from bleeding under the skin, containing the bruise.

- **Heinz Apple Cider Vinegar** and **Bounty Paper Towels.** To heal a bruise using an old folk remedy, mix equal parts Heinz Apple Cider Vinegar and warm water, saturate a sheet of Bounty Paper Towels with the pungent liquid, and apply it to the bruise. The vinegar compress works as an anti-inflammatory and likely improves circulation to speed healing.

- **McCormick Arrowroot.** To stop a bruise from discoloring the skin, immediately upon injuring yourself, mix one tablespoon McCormick Arrowroot with enough water to make a paste, slather it on the affected area, and let dry.

- **McCormick Oregano Leaves** and **L'eggs Sheer Energy Panty Hose.** Reduce the inflammation and soothe the pain of a bruise by placing one heaping tablespoon McCormick Oregano Leaves in one cup of boiling water, covering with a saucer, and steeping for ten minutes. Scoop out the oregano leaves and place them inside the foot cut from a clean, used pair of L'eggs Sheer Energy Panty Hose, and tie a knot in the open end. Press the poultice against the bruise for fifteen minutes, occasionally rewetting it with the oregano tea. The oregano oil helps heal the bruise.

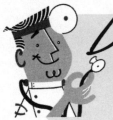

Doctor's Orders

Black and blue? If you bruise easily and frequently, or if bruises appear for no apparent reason, consult a doctor to rule out hemophilia, leukemia, or aplastic anemia.

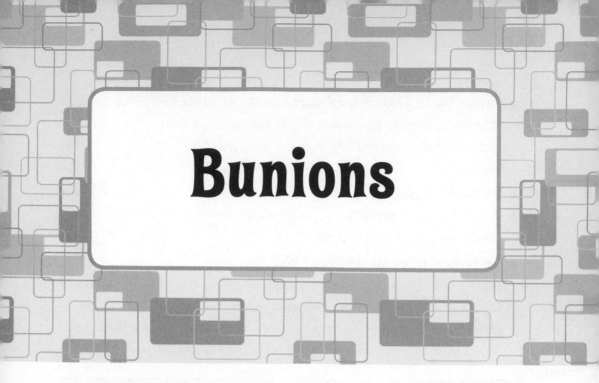

Bunions

- **Bayer Aspirin.** To soothe inflamed bunions, use a mortar and pestle to crush four Bayer Aspirin tablets into powder, dissolve the powder in a basin filled with warm water, and soak your feet for fifteen minutes. (Do not use this technique if you are allergic to aspirin or if any skin irritation results.)

- **Birds Eye Frozen Peas** and **Bounty Paper Towels.** To relieve bunion pain, cover a bag of Birds Eye Frozen Peas with a sheet of Bounty Paper Towels, and apply to the affected area three times a day. The frozen peas act like small ice cubes, reducing the inflammation causing the pain, and the bag of peas conforms to the shape of your toe. The paper towel creates a layer of insulation to prevent frostbite. Refreeze the bag of peas for future ice-pack use. Be sure to label the bag for ice-pack use only. If you want to eat the peas, cook them after they thaw the first time, never after refreezing.

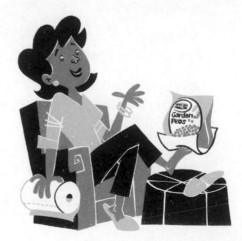

- **Castor Oil** and **Band-Aid Bandages.** To reduce bunion inflammation, after soaking your feet (using the Bayer Aspirin tip on page 71 or the Dr. Teal's Epsom Salt tip below), rub Castor Oil on your bunion. Cover the oiled bunion with a Band–Aid Bandage to keep the oil in place.

- **Dr. Teal's Epsom Salt.** To soothe painful bunions, dissolve a handful of Dr. Teal's Epsom Salt in a basin filled with warm water and soak your foot in the solution for twenty minutes.

- **Uncle Ben's Converted Brand Rice.** To reduce the swelling and relieve the pain of a bunion, fill a clean sock with Uncle Ben's Converted Brand Rice, tie a knot in the end, and heat in the microwave oven for ninety seconds. Making sure the sock isn't too hot, apply the heat pack to the affected

STRANGE MEDICINE

MAKING YOUR TOES CURL

- A bunion—a red, swollen, painful knob of overgrown bone on the outside of the joint of the big toe—is caused by wearing shoes that scrunch the toes.

- Bunions can be removed only with surgery through a simple outpatient procedure.

- Approximately 140,000 Americans have a bunion surgically removed each year.

- Women are ten times more likely than men to get bunions, and tight, high-heeled shoes worsen the pain.

- People with flat feet or low arches are most prone to developing bunions. Wearing a specially made insole, prescribed by a podiatrist, can prevent you from developing bunions.

- The most effective way to treat a bunion is by switching to roomier shoes with custom-made shoe inserts.

- Massaging across the bunion can help relieve bunion pain.

toe. The rice-filled sock conforms to the shape of your toe and stays warm for roughly thirty minutes, allowing the soothing warmth to increase circulation to the area, breaking up the inflammation. The homemade heating pad is also reusable.

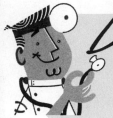

Doctor's Orders

Stay on your toes! If a bunion causes excruciating pain or threatens to deform your toes, consult a doctor to discuss possible non-surgical and surgical treatment options.

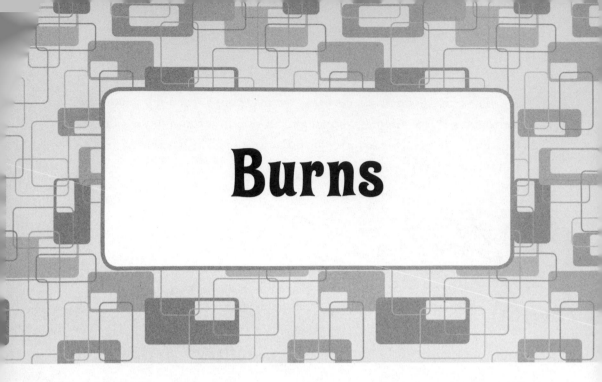

Burns

- **Arm & Hammer Baking Soda.** Mix one tablespoon Arm & Hammer Baking Soda with enough water to make a thick paste and apply it to the burn. The sodium bicarbonate soothes inflammation, relieving the pain.

- **Bayer Aspirin.** Taking two Bayer Aspirin tablets every four hours helps relieve the pain and inflammation of a mild burn.

- **Colgate Regular Flavor Toothpaste.** To soothe a burn, apply Colgate Regular Flavor Toothpaste as an ointment to the affected area. The glycerin in the toothpaste provides a soothing cooling sensation and fast, temporary relief from the searing pain.

- **Dannon Yogurt.** To relieve the pain of a minor burn, smear Dannon Plain Nonfat Yogurt over the affected area and let sit for fifteen minutes.

- **French's Mustard.** If you burn yourself while cooking, grab French's Mustard and slather it on the burn to stop the stinging and prevent blistering. Let the mustard dry on the skin. Short-order cooks have used this mustard remedy for centuries.

- **Fruit of the Earth Aloe Vera Gel.** To soothe a minor burn, apply a thick coat of Fruit of the Earth Aloe Vera Gel to the affected area. Aloe vera gel moisturizes the burn, bringing instant relief. As 100 percent pure aloe vera gel, Fruit of the Earth Aloe Vera Gel does not contain any alcohol, which can dry the burn rather than keep it properly moist.

- **Heinz White Vinegar** and **Bounty Paper Towels.** Saturate a sheet of Bounty Paper Towels with Heinz White Vinegar and wrap it around the burned skin. Let sit until the paper towel dries. The acetic acid in the vinegar helps relieve the pain and inflammation.

- **Kikkoman Soy Sauce.** After running lukewarm water over a minor burn, apply Kikkoman Soy Sauce to the affected area. No one knows why it works, but soy sauce relieves burning pain.

- **Kingsford's Corn Starch.** To relieve a burn, mix one-half cup Kingsford's Corn Starch with enough water to make a paste, and apply it to the affected area.

- **Lipton Chamomile Tea** and **Arm & Hammer Baking Soda.** To soothe and disinfect a blister from a burn, pour one cup of boiling water over two Lipton Chamomile Tea bags in a cup, cover with a saucer, let steep for ten minutes, and then let cool to the touch. Dissolve one-half teaspoon Arm & Hammer Baking Soda in the brew, and soak the blister in the solution (or apply with a washcloth).

- **Lipton Green Tea** and **Stayfree Maxi Pads.** To soothe a burn, brew a strong cup of Lipton Green Tea and let it cool. Saturate a Stayfree Maxi Pad with the liquid and apply it as a compress on the burn. The tannins in green tea soothe and strengthen the skin and reduce inflammation.

- **Lipton Tea Bags.** Saturate a Lipton Tea Bag with cool water, squeeze out the excess water, and press it to the burn. The tannin in the tea reduces the inflammation and relieves the pain.

- **Listerine.** To dry out a blister from a burn, use a cotton ball to apply original formula Listerine antiseptic mouthwash to the site three times a day. As an astringent, Listerine causes the blistered skin tissues to contract.

- **Morton Salt.** To speed healing of a blister from a burn, mix two ounces

Morton Salt and one ounce of cold water, apply the solution to a washcloth, and press it against the blister for one hour. Salt water expedites healing.

- **Nestlé Carnation Nonfat Dry Milk.** Mix one-half cup Nestlé Carnation Nonfat Dry Milk powder with enough water to make a thick paste, and spread it on the burned skin. The protein from the milk anesthetizes the pain.

- **Preparation H.** To soothe burning pain and speed healing, smear a dab of Preparation H on the affected area. The hemorrhoid cream relieves the burning sensation.

- **Quaker Oats** and **L'eggs Sheer Energy Panty Hose.** To relieve a burn, grind one cup uncooked Quaker Oats in a blender, pour the fine powder into the foot cut from a clean, used pair of L'eggs Sheer Energy Panty Hose,

℞ STRANGE MEDICINE ℞

IN THE HEAT OF THE MOMENT

- To stop the skin from burning, immediately flush the burn with lukewarm water until the burning sensation dissipates.

- After cooling and cleaning the burn, wrap it in a clean, thick gauze pad, or if necessary, strips torn from a clean bed sheet.

- Never soothe a burn with butter. Butter seals the heat in your tissue, worsening the pain and scarring.

- A first-degree burn is red, painful, and looks like a sunburn.

- A second-degree burn is a painful blister and may ooze.

- A third-degree burn looks charred and white (or the color of cream) and is usually painless because the nerve endings are deadened. Third-degree burns always require medical attention.

and tie a knot in the open end. Saturate the sachet with cool water, and press it against the burn.

- **SueBee Honey.** To speed healing of a minor burn and prevent infection, coat the affected area with SueBee Honey. Honey is hygroscopic, meaning it absorbs moisture from burns, making the wound an inhospitable environment for bacteria and sealing out any possible contaminants. A 2009 study published in the *Indian Journal of Plastic Surgery* showed that treating a burn with honey also lessened pain, provided rapid sterilization, and reduced scarring.

- **Vaseline Petroleum Jelly.** To help a burn heal more rapidly, rub a few dabs of Vaseline Petroleum Jelly into the affected area. In 1859, Brooklyn chemist Robert Augustus Chesebrough learned from petroleum drilling workers in Titusville, Pennsylvania, that the jelly residue that gunked up oil drilling rods quickened healing when rubbed on a burn.

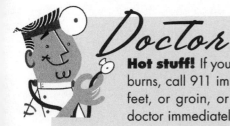

Doctor's Orders

Hot stuff! If you have severe second-degree burns or third-degree burns, call 911 immediately. For any burn on the face, eyes, hands, feet, or groin, or any burn larger than a half-dollar coin, see a doctor immediately.

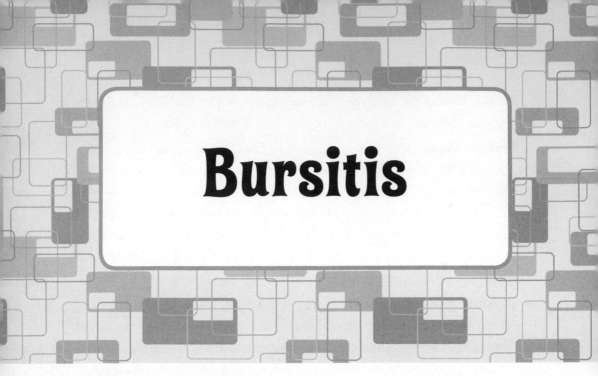

Bursitis

- **Birds Eye Frozen Peas** and **Bounty Paper Towels.** To relieve bursitis pain, cover a bag of Birds Eye Frozen Peas with a sheet of Bounty Paper Towels, and use the bag to gently massage around the affected joint for five to ten minutes to numb the area. Repeat every two hours for the first day, and then reduce the treatment to three times a day. The frozen peas act like small ice cubes, reducing the inflammation causing the pain, and the bag of peas conforms to the shape of your body. The paper towel creates a layer of insulation to prevent frostbite. Refreeze the bag of peas for future ice-pack use. Be sure to label the bag for ice-pack use only. If you want to eat the peas, cook them after they thaw the first time, never after refreezing the bag.

- **Chicken of the Sea Salmon, Chicken of the Sea Sardines,** or **Chicken of the Sea Tuna.** To help prevent bursitis from flaring up, eat salmon, sardines, or tuna twice a week. All of these fish add the fatty acids commonly known as omega-3 oils to your diet, reducing inflammation and pain, strengthening the immune system, and increasing resistance to stress, which helps avert an outbreak of bursitis.

- **Dr. Teal's Epsom Salt.** To ease bursitis pain, fill the bathtub with warm water, add two cups Dr. Teal's Epsom Salt, and soak for twenty minutes. The magnesium in the Epsom Salt passes into the body through osmosis and relieves muscle and joint aches.

- **Lakewood Black Cherry Juice.** To soothe bursitis pain, drink two 8-ounce glasses of Lakewood Black Cherry Juice every day until the pain subsides. Black cherry juice is packed with anti-inflammatory antioxidants, and a 2009 study at Oregon Health & Science University in Portland showed that people who drank tart cherry juice while training for a long-distance run reported significantly less pain after exercise than those who did not drink cherry juice.

- **Lipton Ginger Tea.** To alleviate bursitis pain, place two Lipton Ginger Tea bags in a cup of boiling water, cover with a saucer, steep for ten minutes, and drink the resulting tea. Do this three times a day until the bursitis pain disappears. The compounds in ginger reduce inflammation and relieve pain. (Do not drink ginger tea if you have gallstones. Ginger can increase bile production.)

- **McCormick Ground (Cayenne) Red Pepper** and **Vaseline Petroleum Jelly.** Mix one-half teaspoon McCormick Ground (Cayenne) Red Pepper and two teaspoons Vaseline Petroleum Jelly, and apply the spicy salve to the affected joint. The homemade balm brings soothing warmth to relieve the pain. (Do not apply on open sores.)

- **McCormick Ground Turmeric.** To relieve the pain and inflammation of bursitis, take one tablespoon McCormick Ground Turmeric daily by simply sprinkling it on your food or using the spice in recipes for rice, casseroles, soups, and stews. Curcumin, an antioxidant in turmeric, reduces inflammation and also inhibits the body from producing prostaglandins, the compounds that help signal pain. (Turmeric may increase the likelihood of bleeding when taken in combination with the blood thinner Coumadin or other anticoagulant medications.)

℞ STRANGE MEDICINE ℞

CUSHIONING THE BLOW

● Bursitis is inflammation of a bursa, a sac filled with fluid that provides cushioning between a muscle and the end of a bone at a joint. The typical cause? Repetitive motions or sudden overuse of the joint.

● The human body houses more than 150 bursae in the joints.

● Bursitis usually occurs at the shoulders, elbows, hips, knees, heels, and the first joint of the big toes.

● The best way to treat bursitis is to rest the affected joint and protect it from any further trauma.

● Bursitis pain typically starts with four to five days of acute pain, which subsides and dissipates within a few weeks. Unfortunately, recurrences are common.

● Bursitis occurs more commonly with increased age.

● Currently, there is no known cure for bursitis.

● To relieve the pain, doctors frequently recommend physical therapy or exercises, injecting a corticosteroid drug into the bursa to relieve inflammation, or surgically draining the inflamed bursa.

● Once the acute pain dissipates, exercise the joint gently to maintain range of motion.

● **SueBee Honey** and **Heinz Apple Cider Vinegar.** Mix two tablespoons SueBee Honey and two tablespoons Heinz Apple Cider Vinegar in an eight-ounce glass of water, and drink the solution once or twice daily to help relieve bursitis pain.

● **Tabasco Pepper Sauce** and **Crisco All-Vegetable Shortening.** To numb bursitis pain, mix one-quarter teaspoon Tabasco Pepper Sauce with two tablespoons Crisco All-Vegetable Shortening, and apply the spicy homemade ointment to the affected area up to five times a day for a week or two. The capsaicin in the Tabasco Pepper Sauce numbs the nerves that send pain signals to the brain. (Do not apply this salve on open sores and avoid contact with eyes and nose.)

- **Uncle Ben's Converted Brand Rice.** After applying the cold treatment for three days with the Birds Eye Frozen Peas tip on page 78, fill a clean sock with Uncle Ben's Converted Brand Rice, tie a knot in the end, and heat in the microwave oven for ninety seconds. Making sure the sock isn't too hot, apply the heat pack to the affected joint. The rice-filled sock conforms to the shape of your body and stays warm for roughly thirty minutes, allowing the soothing warmth to increase circulation to the joint, expediting healing. The homemade heating pad is also reusable.

- **Vicks VapoRub.** To relieve bursitis pain, rub some Vicks VapoRub on the affected area whenever the need arises. The menthol in this salve relieves pain when applied topically.

Doctor's Orders

Don't get bent out of shape! If rest, ice, and taking a pain reliever don't soothe bursitis pain, see a doctor to determine the cause of the pain and suggest proper treatment.

Caffeine Withdrawal

- **Bayer Aspirin.** Caffeine expands blood vessels, allowing more oxygen to get to the brain. If you cease taking caffeine, those same blood vessels contract to their regular size, causing headache pain. To relieve a headache caused by caffeine withdrawal, take Bayer Aspirin as directed on the label. Unlike many other brands of aspirin, Bayer Aspirin does not contain any caffeine; however, if you feel a small dose of caffeine will help improve blood flow, take Bayer AM Extra Strength, an aspirin that contains 65 milligrams of caffeine. A typical nine-ounce cup of coffee contains 150 milligrams of caffeine.

- **Jif Peanut Butter.** Caffeine acts as a diuretic to flush magnesium from your body. Since magnesium normally helps your body produce energy, a deficiency of magnesium may make you anxious and irritable. While eating a wide range of legumes, nuts, whole grains, and vegetables will help you meet your daily dietary need for magnesium, you can quickly replace magnesium in your body by eating Jif Peanut Butter (straight from the jar or in a sandwich). Four tablespoons of peanut butter contain 100 milligrams of magnesium (or 25 percent of the daily value).

- **Lipton Peppermint Tea.** To soothe the headache that often accompanies caffeine withdrawal, drink a cup of caffeine-free Lipton Peppermint Tea. Peppermint tea relieves headache pain.

- **Maxwell House Decaffeinated Coffee.** To soothe a headache caused by caffeine withdrawal, drink a cup of Maxwell House Decaffeinated Coffee, giving your body a low dose of 5 milligrams of caffeine, which helps increase blood flow to the brain.

- **McCormick Cardamom Seed.** To stop the craving for coffee during the withdrawal period, suck on McCormick Cardamom Seeds throughout the day. Cardamom, a spice that originated in India, mimics the effects of coffee in the brain, reducing your desire for coffee.

- **Minute Maid Orange Juice.** Caffeine raises blood sugar levels and disrupts the blood sugar–regulating effect of insulin, the hormone produced in the pancreas. If you stop drinking caffeine products, you can offset the resulting lull in your energy by raising your blood sugar level. Drinking an eight-ounce glass of Minute Maid Orange Juice boosts your blood sugar, reviving your energy. An eight-ounce serving of Minute Maid Orange Juice contains 22 grams of natural sugar.

- **Planters Dry Roasted Almonds, Planters Dry Roasted Cashews,** or **Planters Dry Roasted Peanuts.** Since caffeine depletes magnesium from the body, consuming foods high in magnesium—like Planters Dry Roasted Almonds, Planters Dry Roasted Cashews, or Planters Dry Roasted Peanuts—can provide some relief from caffeine withdrawal symptoms. One ounce of almonds provides 80 milligrams of magnesium, one ounce of cashews provides 75 milligrams, and one ounce of dry roasted peanuts provides 50 milligrams.

- **Swiss Miss Hot Cocoa.** To wean yourself off caffeinated coffee, drink Swiss Miss Hot Cocoa instead. A six-ounce cup of coffee contains 100 milligrams of caffeine, but a six-ounce cup of Swiss Miss Hot Cocoa contains only 6 milligrams, making hot chocolate an excellent hot beverage substitute.

℞ STRANGE MEDICINE ℞

WAKE UP AND SMELL THE COFFEE

● Rather than going cold turkey, wean yourself off caffeine gradually by reducing the amount of caffeine you drink by 25 percent each week to avoid (or significantly minimize) the withdrawal symptoms. During the first week, fill the first quarter of your cup with decaffeinated coffee, tea, or cola, and then fill the rest of the cup with your regular caffeinated beverage. During the second week, fill the cup halfway with the decaffeinated beverage and fill the rest of the way with your regular beverage. For the third week, fill your cup three-quarters full with decaf to one-quarter of regular. In other words, if you've been drinking four cups of coffee a day, by the third week you'll be down to one cup of caffeinated coffee a day. At the end of the third week, fill the cup completely with the decaffeinated beverage. If you brew your own coffee at home, instead of making two separate pots of coffee, blend the caffeinated and decaffeinated coffee together before brewing.

● Caffeine withdrawal symptoms—throbbing headaches, drowsiness, fatigue, difficulty concentrating, decreased motivation, irritability, anxiety, and/or depression—range from mild to extreme and typically start anywhere from twelve to twenty-four hours after a person stops consuming caffeine. Symptoms tend to peak up to forty-eight hours later and frequently last anywhere from two days to a week. Other symptoms may include muscle stiffness, hot or cold sensations, and nausea.

● Before you stop consuming the major sources of caffeine (coffee, tea, or cola), eliminate the smaller sources of caffeine from your life (soft drinks, chocolate, and some over-the-counter pain relievers) by switching to caffeine-free varieties.

● Other simple ways to taper off caffeine are to reduce your consumption of coffee by one cup a day or to stop drinking coffee after a certain time of day, substituting decaffeinated or non-caffeinated beverages instead.

● Tea drinkers can lower their caffeine consumption by brewing tea for less time, slowly allowing the body to adjust to less caffeine.

● Instead of relying on coffee to wake you up in the morning, take a warm shower and end with a quick blast of cold water to jolt yourself awake.

● Exercise reduces caffeine withdrawal symptoms. Instead of drinking a caffeinated beverage, take a ten-minute walk or do some pushups or sit-ups to get your blood pumping and reinvigorate yourself.

● Keep well hydrated during the day by drinking several glasses of water or non-caffeinated beverages. Quenching your thirst with healthy liquids will help prevent you from reaching for a can of soda or a cup of coffee or tea.

● Reassure yourself that the pangs of caffeine withdrawal will eventually end—usually within a few days, at which point, your body will stop craving caffeine.

● Americans drink nearly 500 million cups of caffeinated coffee daily.

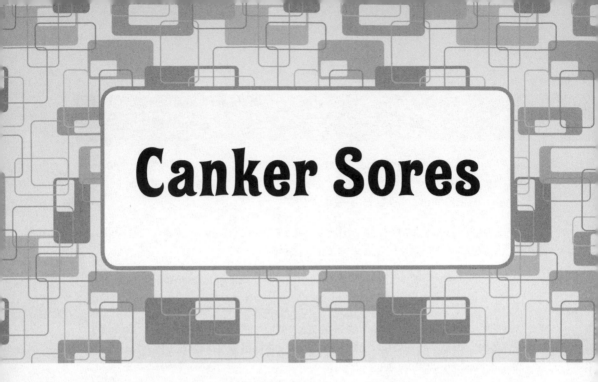

Canker Sores

- **Arm & Hammer Baking Soda.** To tame a canker sore, dissolve one teaspoon Arm & Hammer Baking Soda in four ounces of warm water, rinse your mouth with the solution, and spit out. The alkalinity of the baking soda helps kill the bacteria in your mouth, neutralize the acids etching away at the sore, and soothe the pain.

- **Dannon Yogurt.** To prevent canker sores or ease the pain of an existing canker sore and speed healing, eat a cup of Dannon Plain Nonfat Yogurt once or twice a day. The beneficial *Lactobacillus acidophilus* (probiotics) in yogurt reduce the number of harmful bacteria in your mouth. Yogurt also contains high amounts of lysine, an amino acid that seems to fight canker sores.

- **Fruit of the Earth Aloe Vera Gel** and **Q-Tips Cotton Swabs.** To relieve the pain of a canker sore, dab some Fruit of the Earth Aloe Vera Gel with a Q-Tips Cotton Swab as often as needed. Aloe gel helps heal damaged skin.

- **Hydrogen Peroxide.** Mix one ounce Hydrogen Peroxide and three ounces of water, rinse your mouth with the solution, and spit out. Do this several times a day. The hydrogen peroxide kills the bacteria festering in the canker sore and simultaneously reduces the acidity of your saliva, relieving the pain.

- **Lipton Tea Bags.** To soothe a canker sore and speed healing, press a Lipton Tea Bag dampened with warm water against the spot for five to ten minutes. The tannin in the tea soothes inflammation and relieves pain, and the alkalinity neutralizes acids.

- **McCormick Ground Sage.** To kill the bacterium or virus that may be causing the canker sore and reduce inflammation, place a tea infuser filled with two teaspoons McCormick Ground Sage in a teacup, add boiling water, cover with a saucer, and steep for ten minutes. Let cool to room temperature and rinse your mouth with the sage tea several times a day.

℞ STRANGE MEDICINE ℞

DOWN IN THE MOUTH

- Canker sores appear as white rings around a red, ulcerated circle on the inside of your cheeks, lips, or the loose part of your gums.

- Canker sores should not be confused with cold sores, which appear on the outside of your lips or the hard part of your gums and are caused by the herpes virus.

- Although no one knows for certain what causes canker sores (known medically as aphthous stomatitis ulcers), possible triggers include spicy or acidic foods; toothpastes and mouth rinses containing sodium lauryl sulfate; a deficiency of vitamin B_{12}, zinc, folic acid, or iron; food sensitivities; *Helicobacter pylori* (the same bacteria that cause peptic ulcers); hormonal fluctuations during menstruation; or physical, mental, or emotional stress.

- Women get canker sores more frequently than men do.

- A canker sore generally lasts from a few days to two weeks.

- To help a canker sore heal, avoid spicy or salty foods, which irritate the lesion, and refrain from eating any food with sharp edges, which can poke and tear the ulcer.

- Placing an ice cube directly against the canker sore relieves the pain and helps reduce the swelling.

- **Mylanta.** To cure a canker sore, swish some Mylanta around in your mouth to give the lesion a protective coat, and then spit out.

- **Orajel.** To numb the pain of a canker sore, dab on Orajel. The benzocaine in the ointment anesthetizes the spot, instantly blocking the pain.

- **Pepto-Bismol.** Swish one teaspoon Pepto-Bismol around in your mouth for a few minutes, concentrating on the sore, and then spit out. The bismuth subsalicylate helps temporarily neutralize the acids and digestive enzymes in your mouth causing the pain.

- **Phillips' Milk of Magnesia.** Place one teaspoon Phillips' Milk of Magnesia in your mouth, swish it around for one or two minutes (soaking the canker sore), and spit out. Do this several times a day. Milk of magnesia is a soothing agent that appears to speed healing.

- **Requa Activated Charcoal.** To stop a canker sore before it starts, at the onset of the sore, press a Requa Activated Charcoal tablet against the area until the tingling sensations cease (roughly fifteen to twenty minutes). The charcoal will likely dye the treated area black, temporarily.

- **Saco Buttermilk.** Drinking Saco Buttermilk and then swishing around a mouthful helps heal canker sores. Buttermilk contains the amino acid lysine, which soothes the ulcers.

- **Tums.** Place a regular Tums tablet in your mouth and using your tongue, press it against the canker sore. The calcium carbonate in the Tums tablet neutralizes the acids in your mouth, bringing fast, temporary relief to the sore. (If you've had calcium oxalate kidney stones, consult your doctor before taking Tums.)

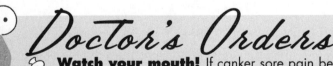

Doctor's Orders

Watch your mouth! If canker sore pain becomes unbearable, you get more than four canker sores at one time, or a sore lasts longer than two weeks, see your dentist.

Carpal Tunnel Syndrome

- **Birds Eye Frozen Peas** and **Bounty Paper Towels.** To relieve the inflammation causing the pain in your wrist and hand, cover a bag of Birds Eye Frozen Peas with a sheet of Bounty Paper Towels, and place the bag on the affected spot for twenty minutes. Repeat once an hour as needed. The frozen peas act like small ice cubes, soothing and numbing the pain, and the bag of peas conforms to the shape of your wrist and hand. The paper towel creates a layer of insulation to prevent frostbite. Refreeze the bag of peas for future ice-pack use. Be sure to label the bag for ice-pack use only. If you want to eat the peas, cook them after they thaw the first time, never after refreezing.

- **Bubble Wrap** and **Scotch Packaging Tape.** Make a tool or utensil easier to grip by wrapping it in a few layers of Bubble Wrap, secured in place with a strip of Scotch Packaging Tape.

- **Castor Oil, Saran Wrap,** and **Ziploc Storage Bags.** Applying a castor oil pack to your wrist every other night can reduce inflammation and eliminate the pain of carpal tunnel syndrome. Fold a soft flannel cloth in half once or twice and saturate it with Castor Oil. Wrap the saturated cloth around your wrist, place a sheet of Saran Wrap over the cloth, and place a hot-water bottle or heating pad around the plastic sheet for fifteen minutes. Store the castor oil-soaked flannel cloth in a Ziploc Storage Bag and refrigerate. Repeat the treatment for one week.

- **Chicken of the Sea Salmon, Chicken of the Sea Sardines,** or **Chicken of the Sea Tuna.** Eat salmon, sardines, or tuna three or four times a week to add omega-3 fatty acids to your diet. Omega-3 oils reduce inflammation and pain, strengthen the immune system, and increase resistance to stress. Also, one serving of Chicken of the Sea Chunk Light Tuna provides nearly 60 percent of the daily requirement for vitamin B_6. Some studies link a deficiency of vitamin B_6 to carpal tunnel syndrome, while others do not.

- **McCormick Ground (Cayenne) Red Pepper** and **Vaseline Petroleum Jelly.** Mix one-half teaspoon McCormick Ground (Cayenne) Red Pepper and two teaspoons Vaseline Petroleum Jelly, and apply the spicy salve to the wrist. The homemade balm brings soothing warmth to relieve the pain.

- **Tabasco Pepper Sauce and Crisco All-Vegetable Shortening.** To relieve carpal tunnel syndrome pain, mix one-quarter teaspoon Tabasco Pepper Sauce with two tablespoons Crisco All-Vegetable Shortening, and apply the spicy homemade ointment to the wrist up to five times a day for a week or two. The capsaicin in the Tabasco Pepper Sauce numbs the nerves that send pain signals to the brain. (Do not apply this salve on open sores and avoid contact with eyes and nose.)

- **Uncle Ben's Converted Brand Rice.** After reducing the inflammation with the Birds Eye Frozen Peas tip on page 89, fill a clean sock with Uncle Ben's Converted Brand Rice, tie a knot in the end, and heat in the microwave oven for one to two minutes. Making sure the sock isn't too hot, apply the heat pack against your aching wrist or hand. The rice-filled sock conforms to the shape of your appendage, allowing the warmth to relax the muscles.

- **Wilson Tennis Balls.** To make a toothbrush or silverware easier to grip, use a razor blade or utility knife to carefully slice small slits in the opposite sides of a Wilson Tennis Ball, and then slip the handle of the toothbrush or utensil through the tennis ball. The bright yellow ball makes a convenient grip.

℞ STRANGE MEDICINE ℞

GETTING OUT OF HAND

● Carpal tunnel syndrome, caused by a pinched nerve in the wrist, affects the hand and arm, and starts with numbness, tingling, pain, and loss of strength and flexibility—gradually increasing in severity.

● The way you perform repetitive movements with your hands and wrists—combined with the anatomy of your wrist and underlying health problems—is generally responsible for carpal tunnel syndrome.

● The carpal tunnel is a narrow passageway (roughly the diameter of a nickel) located in your wrist and surrounded by bones and ligaments. A main nerve to your hand runs through the tunnel, and if the surrounding tendons swell and compress the nerve, carpal tunnel syndrome results.

● With proper treatment, most people with carpal tunnel syndrome recover completely, regaining normal use of their wrists and hands.

● For temporary relief from carpal tunnel syndrome, rotate your wrists, stretch your palms and fingers, take frequent breaks from any activity requiring repetitive hand action, and wear a wrist splint (available at the drug store) to bed.

● To prevent carpal tunnel syndrome from working at the computer, adjust your chair so that your arms bend at a 90-degree angle with your forearms parallel to the floor when you type. Also, keep your hands in the air, allowing your fingertips to dance across the keyboard without letting your palms rest on the desktop. And sit upright with your shoulders held back.

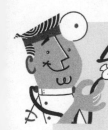

Doctor's Orders

Hand it over! If you experience any pain, cracks, or crunches in your hand or wrist, consult a doctor to rule out osteoarthritis, diabetes, or thyroid problems, and to prevent untreated carpal tunnel syndrome from leaving you with permanent pain.

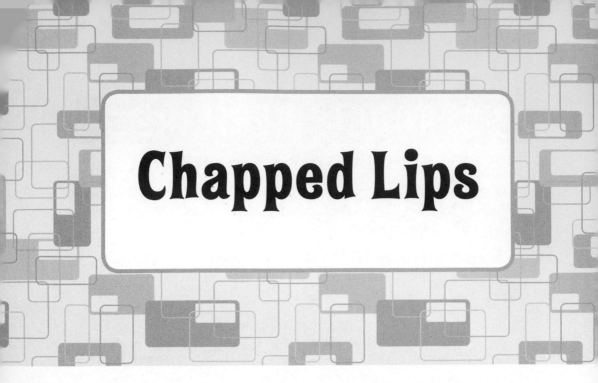

Chapped Lips

- **Bag Balm.** Applying a dab of Bag Balm, the salve developed in Vermont to soothe cows' udders, relieves chapped lips. The combination of lanolin and petrolatum moisturizes and protects the skin cells.

- **Chicken of the Sea Salmon, Chicken of the Sea Sardines,** or **Chicken of the Sea Tuna.** If your lips are perpetually dry and chapped, eat salmon, sardines, or tuna three times a week to add the fatty acids commonly known as omega-3 oils to your diet. These fatty acids enable your cells to absorb the calcium they need, which prevents the sensitive epithelial tissue in your lips from flaking and peeling.

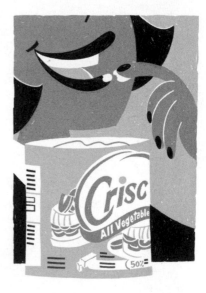

- **Crisco All-Vegetable Shortening.** To soothe and moisturize chapped lips, apply a dab of Crisco All-Vegetable Shortening. Made from soybean oil and cottonseed oil, the shortening softens and protects dry lips.

- **Desitin.** To prevent or heal chapped lips, rub a dab of Desitin, the baby rash ointment, on your lips (particularly at night if you drool in your sleep). The zinc oxide heals the skin and forms a barrier to protect the lips from saliva.

- **Jif Peanut Butter.** Magnesium helps your body process the calcium it needs to keep your lips healthy. While eating a wide range of legumes, nuts, whole grains, and vegetables will help you meet your daily dietary need for magnesium, you can quickly replace magnesium in your body by eating Jif Peanut Butter (straight from the jar or in a sandwich). Four tablespoons of

℞ STRANGE MEDICINE ℞

LIP SERVICE

- If your lips are constantly dry, make sure you're staying hydrated. Drink eight 8-ounce glasses of water daily, and if that doesn't work, drink twelve 8-ounce glasses a day, or more, if necessary. Drinking water keeps your lips (and entire body) properly hydrated, preventing chapped lips from getting worse and expediting healing.

- Chapped lips can be triggered by sunburn, windburn, licking your lips too often, cold weather, fever, or an allergic reaction.

- Wearing lip balm with a sun protection factor (SPF) of 15 or more protects your lips from getting dried out by the sun.

- Lips do not contain any oil glands to keep them moist, and they have very little melanin—the pigment that provides some protection from the sun.

- Licking your lips actually dries them out. The digestive enzymes in your saliva dry out the tissue.

- In a pinch, rub your finger along the side of your nose, and then rub the natural oil that you pick up on your fingertip along your lips.

- Running a humidifier in your bedroom during the dry, winter months provides the moisture necessary to prevent chapped lips and dry skin.

peanut butter contain 100 milligrams of magnesium (or 25 percent of the daily value).

- **Lipton Decaffeinated Tea.** To hydrate your lips, fill a thirty-two-ounce insulated hot-drink thermos with brewed Lipton Decaffeinated Tea, and take one or two sips every ten to fifteen minutes throughout the day. The hot water gently widens your capillaries, allowing the moisture to reach the tissues.

- **Planters Dry Roasted Almonds, Planters Dry Roasted Cashews,** or **Planters Dry Roasted Peanuts.** Eating foods high in magnesium—like Planters Dry Roasted Almonds, Planters Dry Roasted Cashews, or Planters Dry Roasted Peanuts—helps your body process the calcium it needs to keep your lips healthy. One ounce of almonds provides 80 milligrams of magnesium, one ounce of cashews provides 75 milligrams, and one ounce of dry roasted peanuts provides 50 milligrams.

- **Star Olive Oil.** In a pinch, a dab of Star Olive Oil smeared on chapped lips relieves the dryness and moisturizes the skin.

- **SueBee Honey.** To heal chapped lips, apply a thin coat of SueBee Honey and avoid licking it off. Honey moisturizes skin. (Do not apply honey to the lips of infants less than one year of age. Honey often carries a benign strain of *C. botulinum,* and an infant's immune system requires twelve months to develop to fight off disease and infection.)

- **Vaseline Petroleum Jelly.** Rubbing a dab of Vaseline Petroleum Jelly into rough, scaly, dry lips moisturizes them and speeds healing.

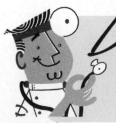

Doctor's Orders

Read my lips! If chapped lips linger for more than three weeks, consult a dermatologist to rule out a yeast infection, an allergic reaction, or actinic cheilitis.

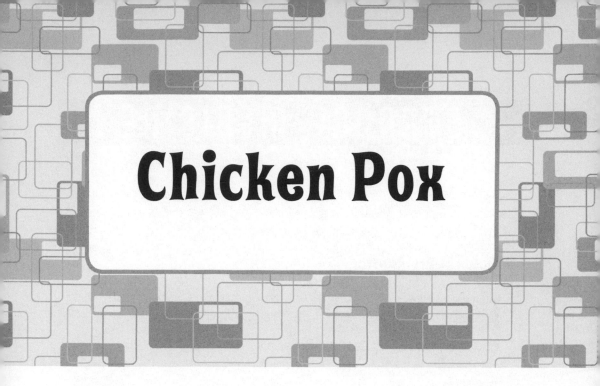

Chicken Pox

- **Desitin.** To soothe and dry up chicken pox blisters, apply a dab of Desitin, the diaper rash remedy, to the affected area. Zinc oxide, the active ingredient in Desitin, is an astringent that reduces blood supply to the skin.

- **Jell-O.** If you have chicken pox in your mouth, eat bland foods like Jell-O to soothe and avoid irritating the blisters.

- **Kiwi Shoe Whitener.** To soothe chicken pox in a pinch, apply Kiwi liquid white shoe polish to the rash. The pipe clay and zinc oxide in the shoe polish soothe the skin.

- **Lipton Tea.** To speed the healing of chicken pox, drink Lipton Tea during the outbreak stage of the disease. The orange pekoe tea expedites the eruption of the sores, and the faster the sores erupt, the sooner they begin healing.

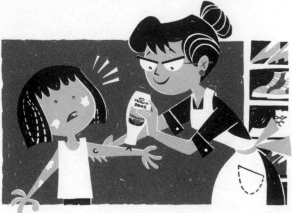

℞ STRANGE MEDICINE ℞

STARTING FROM SCRATCH

● Chicken pox starts with a rash of raised, red, itchy bumps (papules) appearing for several days on the face, scalp, chest, and back. These bumps turn into small, fluid-filled blisters (vesicles) that eventually burst and crust into scabs, which heal after several days. You may also experience fever, headache, a dry cough, loss of appetite, and general discomfort.

● Once infected with the chicken pox virus, you're contagious from up to forty-eight hours before the initial rash appears until all the blisters crust over.

● Scratching and bursting the blisters (before they do so on their own) causes permanent pockmarks in the skin.

● A case of chicken pox generally clears up within ten days to two weeks.

● The severity of chicken pox varies from a few blisters to hundreds of them.

● Adults experience an outbreak of chicken pox with greater severity and a greater risk of complications than children do.

● Chicken pox is highly contagious. People who have been vaccinated against chicken pox or have had chicken pox in the past are usually immune to the virus.

● While chicken pox is usually a mild disease, in severe cases, the rash can cover the entire body, and lesions may form in the throat, eyes, urethra, anus, and vagina.

● To prevent chicken pox safely and effectively, get the chicken pox vaccine.

● Never use an anti-itch hydrocortisone cream like Cortaid on chicken pox. The steroids can cause a bacterial infection and make the pox worse.

● **Morton Salt.** To soothe any chicken pox sores in the mouth, dissolve one teaspoon Morton Salt in an eight-ounce glass of warm water, and gargle with the solution. Salt water anesthetizes the pain and helps the lesions heal faster.

- **Phillips' Milk of Magnesia.** To soothe and dry the itchy pox, use a cotton ball to dab Phillips' Milk of Magnesia on the spots.

- **Popsicle.** If you have chicken pox in your mouth, soothe them by sucking on your favorite flavor Popsicle.

- **Quaker Oats** and **L'eggs Sheer Energy Panty Hose.** To relieve the itching and discomfort of chicken pox, grind one cup uncooked Quaker Oats in a blender, pour a few tablespoons of the fine powder into the foot cut from a clean, used pair of L'eggs Sheer Energy Panty Hose, and tie a knot in the open end. Fill a bathtub with lukewarm water, pour the remaining powdered oats into the tub, and while soaking for fifteen minutes, saturate the panty hose sachet with water, and gently pat it over the pox. The antioxidants in the oats reduce inflammation.

- **Vaseline Petroleum Jelly** and **Q-Tips Cotton Swabs.** To speed the healing of the scabbed sores, use a Q-Tips Cotton Swab to coat the scabs with a dab of Vaseline Petroleum Jelly. Use a fresh cotton swab each time you dip into the jar of petroleum jelly to avoid transmitting the virus from any open sores into the jelly. The lubricant also prevents the scabs from cracking and bleeding.

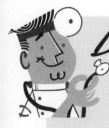

Doctor's Orders

Don't chicken out! If you have chicken pox and develop a worsening cough, a fever that lasts for several days, a fever higher than 103 degrees Fahrenheit, a severe headache, redness around one or more blisters, a stiff neck, dizziness, or if you start vomiting repeatedly or having convulsions, call your doctor immediately.

Cholesterol Control

- **Chicken of the Sea Salmon, Chicken of the Sea Sardines,** or **Chicken of the Sea Tuna.** Eat salmon, sardines, or tuna three times a week to add omega-3 fatty acids to your diet. The omega-3 oils actually lower your low-density lipoprotein (LDL), or "bad" cholesterol levels. The omega-3 fatty acids in fish can also reduce your blood pressure and lower your risk of developing blood clots.

- **Heinz Apple Cider Vinegar.** Take two teaspoons Heinz Apple Cider Vinegar daily in a glass of water or juice to lower your cholesterol. A 2011 study in Japan, published in the *Journal of Agricultural and Food Chemistry,* showed that apple cider vinegar lowered triglycerides and cholesterol in rats.

- **Heinz Baked Beanz.** To lower your cholesterol, eat one-half cup Heinz Baked Beanz daily. A 2007 study at Arizona State University-Polytechnic showed that eating one-half cup of baked beans daily as part of a healthy diet significantly lowers total cholesterol concentrations by 5.6 percent and "bad" (LDL) cholesterol by 5.4 percent. The high levels of soluble fiber in baked beans seem to reduce the absorption of cholesterol from the small intestine.

- **Hershey's Special Dark Chocolate Bar.** To lower your cholesterol, eat two ounces Hershey's Special Dark Chocolate Bar every day. A 2012 study at San Diego State University showed that eating dark chocolate lowers blood sugar levels and "bad" (LDL) cholesterol levels, while simultaneously raising "good" (HDL) cholesterol levels. (Before you start eating two ounces of chocolate daily, be aware that chocolate is high in saturated fats and calories.)

- **Jif Peanut Butter.** Eating one tablespoon Jif Peanut Butter five times a week can reduce cholesterol. The monounsaturated fat in peanut butter can help lower total cholesterol, triglycerides, and LDL (or "bad" cholesterol), and raise HDL (or "good" cholesterol), according to numerous studies. Peanut butter also helps reduce inflammation in the body and boosts the health of blood vessels around the heart.

- **Kellogg's All-Bran.** One cup of Kellogg's All-Bran contains 20 grams of fiber. Adding fiber to your diet helps remove excess cholesterol from the body and helps prevent it from passing through the intestinal wall into the bloodstream.

- **McCormick Ground Cinnamon.** To lower your cholesterol, sprinkle one-half teaspoon McCormick Ground Cinnamon on your cereal, oatmeal, yogurt, or other foods once a day. A 2003 study published in *Diabetes Care* showed that consuming roughly one-half teaspoon of cinnamon per day leads to dramatic improvements in blood sugar, overall cholesterol, LDL-cholesterol, and triglycerides in people with type 2 diabetes.

- **Metamucil.** To add fiber to your diet—reducing the absorption of cholesterol into your bloodstream—take one serving of Metamucil (as instructed on the package label) in or with eight ounces of water at each meal. Metamucil contains psyllium seed husk, a natural dietary fiber originating from the psyllium plant, which, when taken three times daily, can reduce LDL ("bad" cholesterol) by 7 percent.

- **Minute Maid Orange Juice.** Drinking three 8-ounce glasses of Minute Maid Orange Juice every day can raise your HDL ("good" cholesterol) levels by 21 percent and lower your overall ratio of LDL ("bad" cholesterol) to HDL by 16 percent, according to a 2000 study published in the *American Journal of Clinical Nutrition*.

- **Mott's Applesauce.** To lower your cholesterol, eat plenty of Mott's Applesauce. The pectin in applesauce binds to cholesterol in the digestive system, preventing it from entering the bloodstream, where it adheres to artery walls. A 1987 study at the University of Florida showed that eating three tablespoons of pectin daily lowered LDL ("bad" cholesterol) levels by 10.8 percent and the ratio of LDL to HDL ("good" cholesterol) by 9.8 percent.

- **Ocean Spray Cranberry Juice Cocktail.** Drinking three glasses of Ocean Spray Cranberry Juice Cocktail every day can raise your HDL ("good" cholesterol) levels up to 10 percent after three months, according to a 2006 study published in the *British Journal of Nutrition*.

- **Planters Walnuts** or **Planters Dry Roasted Almonds.** To lower your cholesterol, eat a handful of Planters Walnuts or Planters Dry Roasted Almonds every day. Rich in polyunsaturated fatty acids, walnuts and almonds help lower your "bad" (LDL) cholesterol levels, according to a 2009 study at Harvard University and a 2002 study published in the *Journal of Nutrition*.

- **Quaker Oats.** To lower your LDL ("bad" cholesterol) by 12 to 24 percent, eat one-and-a-half cups Quaker Oats oatmeal every day. Rich in soluble fiber, oatmeal reduces the absorption of cholesterol into your bloodstream. Five to 10 grams or more of soluble fiber a day decreases both your total and LDL cholesterol.

- **Star Olive Oil.** Using two tablespoons Star Extra Virgin Olive Oil a day in place of other oils can lower your "bad" (LDL) cholesterol in just one week, leaving your "good" (HDL) cholesterol untouched or even raising it. To substitute olive oil for foods with higher saturated fats in your diet, mix it with vinegar as a salad dressing, sauté vegetables in it, use it in place of margarine, or add it to a marinade.

℞ STRANGE MEDICINE ℞

A STICKY SITUATION

● Cholesterol, a waxy substance found in the fats in your blood, helps the body build healthy new cells, protect nerves, and create hormones, but high cholesterol can increase your risk of heart disease.

● Excess cholesterol adheres to the inner walls of arteries, and eventually the buildup narrows the arteries, restricting the flow of blood and preventing your heart from getting sufficient oxygen-rich blood. This increases the risk of heart attack and stroke.

● While high cholesterol can be genetically inherited, you can help reduce your cholesterol levels through diet, regular exercise, and proper medication.

● Serum cholesterol is the total amount of cholesterol in your bloodstream. Ideally, your serum cholesterol level should be under 200 and not above 240. Low-density lipoprotein (LDL) is the "bad" cholesterol that clogs arteries. High-density lipoprotein (HDL) is the "good" cholesterol that removes LDL from your artery walls and brings it to your liver.

● You're more likely to have high cholesterol if you smoke; eat foods high in cholesterol, saturated fat, and trans fats; are obese; lack exercise; or have high blood pressure, diabetes, or a family history of heart disease.

● To lower cholesterol, go for a thirty-minute walk every day. Exercise helps boost your body's HDL (or "good" cholesterol) levels while lowering your LDL (or "bad" cholesterol) levels, decreasing your risk of heart disease and stroke.

● A daily minimum of five servings of fruits and vegetables, three servings of whole-grain foods, and one serving of beans adds fiber to your body to lower cholesterol.

● Contrary to popular belief, eating garlic does not lower cholesterol. A 2007 study at Stanford University published in the *Archives of Internal Medicine* showed that garlic containing allicin, which has been shown to inhibit cholesterol synthesis in the test tube, had no significant effects on LDL cholesterol concentrations or triglyceride levels.

- **Welch's Grape Juice.** To lower your cholesterol, drink one-half cup Welch's Concord Grape Juice every day. A 2006 study published in the *American Journal of Clinical Nutrition* showed that drinking one-half cup of grape juice can raise your "good" (HDL) cholesterol levels while simultaneously lowering "bad" (LDL) cholesterol levels after only three weeks.

- **Wesson Canola Oil.** When compared to olive oil, replacing the saturated fat in your diet with canola oil results in lower LDL cholesterol levels. Rich in alpha-linolenic acid, canola oil is lower in both monounsaturated fat and saturated fat than olive oil. Like other vegetable oils, canola oil does have 125 calories per tablespoon.

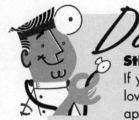

Doctor's Orders

Stick with it! Your doctor regularly tests your cholesterol levels. If your levels are high, your doctor will prescribe a statin drug to lower your cholesterol. If you don't have a regular doctor, make an appointment for a physical.

Chronic Fatigue Syndrome

- **Heinz Baked Beanz.** To keep your energy level well balanced, eat one-half cup Heinz Baked Beanz. Baked beans slow the release of blood sugar into your bloodstream, giving your body and brain a steady source of fuel, keeping you even-keeled and uniformly energized. Also, the high amounts of antioxidants in baked beans mop up the free radicals in your body that cause oxidative stress, which plays a significant role in chronic fatigue syndrome.

- **Jif Peanut Butter.** If you suffer from chronic fatigue syndrome, magnesium can boost your energy level, improve your emotional state, and reduce pain, according to a 1991 study published in the *Lancet*. While eating a wide range of legumes, nuts, whole grains, and vegetables will help you meet your daily dietary need for magnesium, you can quickly replace magnesium in your body by eating Jif Peanut Butter (straight from the jar or in a sandwich). Four tablespoons of peanut butter contain 100 milligrams of magnesium (or 25 percent of the daily value).

- **Planters Dry Roasted Almonds, Planters Dry Roasted Cashews,** or **Planters Dry Roasted Peanuts.** Eating foods high in magnesium—like

℞ STRANGE MEDICINE ℞

SICK AND TIRED

● Chronic fatigue syndrome feels like a combination of a flu and extreme fatigue that refuses to go away and whose causes seem inexplicable. Symptoms include fever, sore throat, muscular aches and pains, and severe fatigue that fails to improve with rest.

● To overcome chronic fatigue syndrome, reduce the stress in your life (by giving yourself time to relax), improve your sleeping habits (by going to bed and getting up at the same time each day), pace yourself (by keeping your schedule balanced), and exercise gently (until you begin to perspire).

● Avoiding caffeine, alcohol, and nicotine can help reduce the symptoms of chronic fatigue syndrome.

● Chronic fatigue syndrome is caused when the mitochondria, the microscopic organelles that produce energy in the form of adenosine triphosphate (ATP), function inefficiently, supplying insufficient amounts of ATP.

Planters Dry Roasted Almonds, Planters Dry Roasted Cashews, or Planters Dry Roasted Peanuts—can offset chronic fatigue syndrome. Studies show that many people who suffer from chronic fatigue syndrome have magnesium deficiencies. One ounce of almonds provides 80 milligrams of magnesium, one ounce of cashews provides 75 milligrams, and one ounce of dry roasted peanuts provides 50 milligrams.

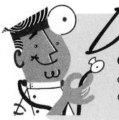

Doctor's Orders

Give it a rest! If you experience persistent or extreme fatigue, consult a doctor to determine the cause, which can range from diabetes or anemia to a viral infection or psychological disorder.

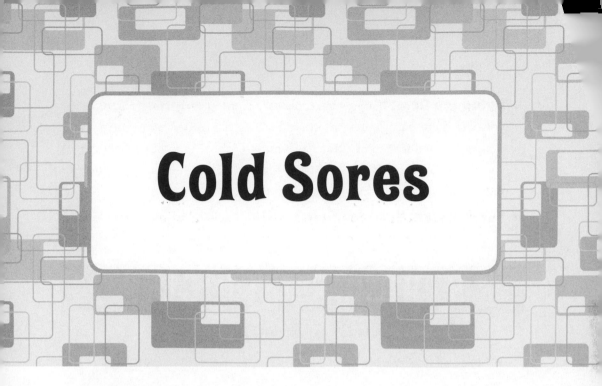

Cold Sores

- **Bayer Aspirin.** To relieve the pain and speed the healing of a cold sore, take one regular-strength Bayer Aspirin tablet daily. A 1998 study published in the *Annals of Internal Medicine* showed that 125 milligrams of aspirin a day can reduce the duration of an oral herpes outbreak by half. (One regular-strength Bayer Aspirin tablet contains 325 milligrams of aspirin.)

- **Dannon Yogurt.** To prevent the outbreak of chronic cold sores or speed healing during an outbreak, eat two to three cups of Dannon Nonfat Yogurt daily. The *Lactobacillus acidophilus* bacteria (probiotics) in the yogurt help fight off the herpes virus. Yogurt also contains high amounts of lysine, an amino acid that inhibits the virus.

- **Fruit of the Earth Aloe Vera Gel.** To relieve the pain and inflammation of a cold sore, dab some Fruit of the Earth Aloe Vera Gel on the sore several times a day. Aloe vera gel helps heal and moisturize damaged skin.

- **Kingsford's Corn Starch.** To soothe a cold sore, mix one teaspoon Kingsford's Corn Starch with enough water to make a paste, and apply it to the sore. Repeat whenever needed. The absorbent cornstarch helps dry out the sore.

- **Lipton Tea Bags.** To prevent a cold sore from materializing, the moment you feel it emerging, press a Lipton Tea Bag dampened with warm water against the spot for ten minutes. The tannin in the tea soothes inflammation and dries the skin. If the cold sore does break out, repeat frequently to reduce the cold sore's severity and duration.

- **Purell Instant Hand Sanitizer.** If you accidentally touch your cold sore,

℞ STRANGE MEDICINE ℞

TOUCHING A SORE SPOT

- A cold sore is a tiny white blister around your lips or the corners of your mouth.

- Cold sores are oral herpes, an infection caused by the herpes simplex virus type 1. HSV-1 is transmitted through oral secretions or sores on the skin and can be spread through kissing or sharing objects such as toothbrushes or eating utensils.

- A cold sore typically begins with a tingling sensation on a spot on your lip. Within the next forty-eight hours, a blister appears on the spot, and over a few days, it swells, bursts, oozes fluid, and crusts. Cold sores generally clear up within a week to ten days.

- Cold sore outbreaks can be triggered by stress, sunlight, menstruation, and fatigue.

- Foods containing lysine help heal cold sores, while foods containing arginine bring on and exacerbate cold sores.

- Foods rich in arginine include beer, chocolate, cola, gelatin, nuts, peas, and whole-grain cereals.

- Wearing lip balm with a sun protection factor (SPF) of 15 or more can reduce the frequency of cold sores.

- Cold sores are contagious. To avoid spreading the virus, refrain from touching the cold sore, kissing anyone, or sharing drinking glasses or eating utensils.

- The prescription medication acyclovir can stop a cold sore by fighting HSV-1.

wash your hands immediately with Purell Instant Hand Sanitizer to prevent spreading the highly contagious virus to another spot on your body or to another person.

- **Saco Buttermilk.** Drinking Saco Buttermilk helps heal and prevent cold sores. Buttermilk contains the amino acid lysine, which impedes the virus.

- **Vaseline Petroleum Jelly** and **Q-Tips Cotton Swabs.** Once a cold sore dries up and scabs, use a Q-Tips Cotton Swab to dab some Vaseline Petroleum Jelly on the lesion. The lubricant prevents the cold sore from cracking and bleeding. Use a fresh cotton swab each time you dip into the jar of petroleum jelly to avoid transmitting the virus from the open sore into the jelly.

- **Ziploc Storage Bags.** To prevent a cold sore from forming, as soon as you feel the tingling or throbbing sensation that signals an oncoming cold sore, place an ice cube in a Ziploc Storage Bag, wrap a paper napkin around the bag, and hold it against the affected spot until you feel discomfort from the ice. Take a short break, and then reapply the ice. Repeat for fifteen to thirty minutes. Cold impedes viruses and the ice can stop the cold sore in its tracks.

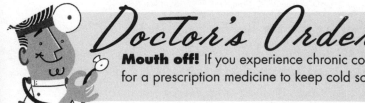

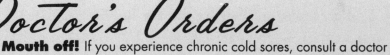

Doctor's Orders

Mouth off! If you experience chronic cold sores, consult a doctor for a prescription medicine to keep cold sores under control.

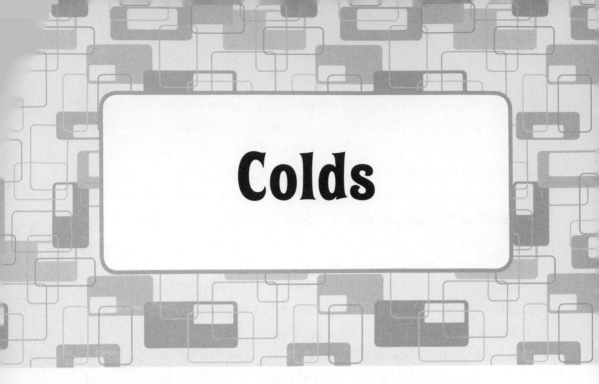

Colds

- **Campbell's Chicken Noodle Soup.** To soothe cold symptoms and make yourself feel nurtured, have a bowl of Campbell's Chicken Noodle Soup. Scientific studies verify that chicken soup, nicknamed "Jewish penicillin," stops specific white blood cells called neutrophils from causing the inflammation that triggers the body to produce large amounts of mucus.

- **Colman's Mustard Powder** and **SueBee Honey.** To loosen congestion in your chest, mix one-quarter teaspoon Colman's Mustard Powder and two tablespoons SueBee Honey, and swallow the mixture. (Do not feed honey to infants less than one year of age. Honey often carries a benign strain of *C. botulinum,* and an infant's immune system requires twelve months to develop to fight off disease and infection.)

- **Conair Hair Dryer.** To help kill the virus giving you the cold symptoms, set a Conair Hair Dryer on warm, hold the nozzle eighteen inches from your face, and inhale the warm air through your nose for twenty minutes. A 1989 study conducted at Harvard Hospital in Salisbury, England, demonstrated that patients with colds who breathed heated humidified air reduced their symptoms in half.

- **French's Mustard.** Spread French's Mustard on your chest and cover with a washcloth dampened with warm water. Let sit for fifteen minutes and wash clean. The penetrating warmth from the mustard plaster thins the mucus in your chest.

- **Gold's Horseradish** and **Nabisco Original Premium Saltine Crackers.** To break through congestion, eat one teaspoon Gold's Horseradish spread on a Nabisco Original Premium Saltine Cracker. Horseradish is a scientifically proven decongestant.

- **Lipton Chamomile Tea.** To clear congestion from your nose and sinuses, fill a large bowl with boiling water and add three Lipton Chamomile Tea bags. Wearing a towel over your head to form a tent over the bowl, hold your face close to the steaming tea for ten minutes. Keep a box of tissues nearby to blow your nose repeatedly.

- **Lipton Ginger Tea.** To alleviate cold symptoms, drink a cup of strongly brewed Lipton Ginger Tea every two or three hours. Ginger relieves nasal congestion and reduces sore throat pain. (Do not drink ginger tea if you have gallstones. Ginger can increase bile production.)

- **McCormick Garlic Powder.** To strengthen your immune system and fight a virus, mix one teaspoon McCormick Garlic Powder with applesauce, honey, or yogurt, and eat the tangy food. Garlic doubles as an antibiotic. (Do not feed honey to infants less than one year of age. Honey often carries a benign strain of *C. botulinum,* and an infant's immune system requires twelve months to develop to fight off disease and infection.)

- **McCormick Thyme Leaves** and **Lipton Peppermint Tea.** To decongest your sinuses, place three teaspoons McCormick Thyme Leaves and three Lipton Peppermint Tea bags into a large bowl and carefully add two cups of boiling water. Lean over the bowl and drape a towel like a tent over your head and the bowl. Inhale the rising steam for ten minutes, keeping your face roughly ten inches above the surface of the water. Repeat whenever needed. Thyme doubles as an antiseptic, and peppermint contains mint, a natural decongestant.

- **Morton Salt.** To relieve the sore throat that accompanies a cold, dissolve one teaspoon Morton Salt in an eight-ounce glass of warm water, and gargle with the solution. Salt water soothes the pain and washes out secretions.

- **Morton Salt** and **Arm & Hammer Baking Soda.** To clear clogged sinuses, make a saline nose wash to rinse mucus from your nasal passages. Purify eight ounces of water by boiling for three minutes, let cool to room

℞ STRANGE MEDICINE ℞

NOTHING TO SNEEZE AT

- A runny nose, sore throat, and sneezing are common symptoms of a cold. A fever, headache, hacking cough, muscle aches, and extreme fatigue rarely accompany a cold, but are symptoms of the flu. Unlike colds, the flu is rarely associated with sneezing.

- More than two hundred different types of viruses cause the common cold, an infection of the upper respiratory system.

- Antibiotics don't work against colds because they only kill bacteria.

- Getting plenty of rest helps cure a cold, enabling your body to focus all its energy on battling the virus.

- Colds are transmitted by a virus spewed into the air when an infected person coughs, sneezes, or blows his nose carelessly.

- Contrary to popular belief, you cannot catch a cold from merely going outside in the cold or getting your hair wet. A viral infection is solely responsible for a cold.

- To flush impurities from your system and keep yourself well hydrated during your bout with a cold, drink eight 8-ounce glasses of water, juice, or other clear fluids daily.

- The older you get, the less likely you are to fall prey to a cold. Every time you catch a cold, your body produces antibodies to fight that particular strain, giving you immunity from future infections from that virus.

temperature, and dissolve one-quarter teaspoon Morton Salt and one-quarter teaspoon Arm & Hammer Baking Soda in the purified water. Use a bulb syringe or neti pot to rinse the inside of your nose.

- **SueBee Honey** and **ReaLemon.** To assuage a sore throat brought on by a cold, dissolve three teaspoons SueBee Honey and one-teaspoon ReaLemon lemon juice in a cup of boiled water and drink. As a mild antiseptic, honey soothes the irritation, and the astringent lemon juice reduces the inflammation. (Do not feed honey to infants less than one year of age. Honey often carries a benign strain of *C. botulinum,* and an infant's immune system requires twelve months to develop to fight off disease and infection.)

- **Tabasco Pepper Sauce.** To soothe sore throat pain caused by a cold, mix ten drops Tabasco Pepper Sauce in a glass of water, and gargle with the spicy solution. The capsicum in the Tabasco Pepper Sauce numbs the throat.

- **Tabasco Pepper Sauce** and **Campbell's Tomato Juice.** To help clear sinuses and raise your body temperature to fight off the virus, add ten to twenty drops Tabasco Pepper Sauce to a glass of Campbell's Tomato Juice, and drink this mixture several times a day. The hot sauce doubles as a decongestant.

- **Vicks VapoRub.** For another way to decongest your sinuses, fill a large bowl with two cups of boiling water and add one teaspoon Vicks VapoRub. Lean over the bowl and drape a hand towel like a tent over your head and the bowl. Inhale the rising steam for ten minutes, keeping your face roughly ten inches above the surface of the water. Repeat whenever needed. The menthol is a natural decongestant.

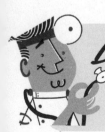

Doctor's Orders

Come in from the cold! If your cold doesn't get better within two weeks or if your cough brings up green or bloody mucus, see a doctor for proper treatment.

Conjunctivitis

- **Chicken of the Sea Salmon, Chicken of the Sea Sardines,** or **Chicken of the Sea Tuna.** To reduce the puffiness of conjunctivitis, eat a four-ounce serving of salmon, sardines, or tuna three times a week to add omega-3 fatty acids to your diet. The omega-3 oils in fish reduce inflammation.

- **Johnson's Baby Shampoo.** To clean away the crusty secretions, mix one-half teaspoon Johnson's Baby Shampoo and one ounce of warm water, and using a cotton ball dipped in the solution, wipe the affected eye.

- **Lipton Chamomile Tea.** To reduce the puffiness and redness of conjunctivitis, soak a Lipton Chamomile Tea bag in warm water for three minutes, squeeze out the excess liquid, lie down, and place the warm tea bag over your affected eye for five minutes. Use this treatment four times a day. The soothing chamomile compress reduces inflammation.

- **Lipton Tea Bags.** Place a Lipton Tea Bag dampened with warm water over the affected eye for five to ten minutes. The tannin in the tea eases the swelling. Do this several times a day (with a fresh tea bag each time).

- **Maxwell House Coffee** and **Stayfree Maxi Pads.** To treat pink eye, brew a pot of Maxwell House Coffee, let cool to the touch, saturate a

Stayfree Maxi Pad with the coffee, and place over closed eyes for five minutes. The acidity seems to relieve the symptoms, and as a vasoconstrictor, caffeine applied topically seems to reduce swelling.

● **McCormick Fennel Seed** and **Stayfree Maxi Pads.** To fight the conjunctivitis infection, place a tea infuser filled with one tablespoon McCormick Fennel Seed in a teacup, add boiling water, cover with a saucer, and

℞ STRANGE MEDICINE ℞

TICKLED PINK

● Popularly known as pink eye, conjunctivitis is a highly contagious inflammation of the conjunctiva, the mucous membrane that lines the inner eyelid and eyeball. The eye becomes red, teary, and swollen. It may also itch and produce a yellow discharge.

● The three types of conjunctivitis are allergic, bacterial, and viral. Allergic and viral conjunctivitis can be treated with home remedies, but bacterial conjunctivitis requires antibiotics.

● You can relieve the swelling and pain of conjunctivitis by dampening a washcloth with warm water and applying it to your eyes as a compress for ten minutes several times a day (using a fresh washcloth each time).

● Do not touch your eyes if you have conjunctivitis to avoid spreading the infection.

● Every day you have conjunctivitis, throw any towels, washcloths, sheets, or pillowcases that came into contact with your face into the washing machine to avoid spreading the infection to others.

● Sleeping for a full eight hours every night helps replenish the eye's moisture, relieves the pain, and speeds healing.

● To avoid infecting others, after eating at home, wash your own dishes and utensils, or place them in the dishwasher yourself.

● Refrain from wearing makeup or contact lenses while you have conjunctivitis to avoid infecting or reinfecting either eye.

steep for ten minutes. Let cool to the touch, saturate a Stayfree Maxi Pad with the fennel tea, and place over closed eyes for five minutes.

- **Morton Salt.** To make a saline solution to wash the affected eye, dissolve one teaspoon Morton Salt in two cups of water, bring to a rolling boil for three minutes, and let cool. Apply the eyewash with a sterilized eyedropper or eyecup.

- **Purell Instant Hand Sanitizer.** If you accidentally touch your eyes, wash your hands immediately with Purell Instant Hand Sanitizer to prevent spreading the conjunctivitis to your other eye or to another person.

- **SueBee Honey.** Dissolve three tablespoons SueBee Honey in two cups of boiling water, and let cool to room temperature. Saturate a cotton ball with the solution and wash the crust and pus from one eye, then use a second cotton ball dipped in the solution to wash the other eye. Do this three or four times a day. A 2004 study published in the *Journal of Medicinal Food* showed that applying honey to the eyes reduces pus discharge, inflammation, and redness—possibly due to honey's antimicrobial benefits.

Doctor's Orders

Get back in the pink! If pink eye does not respond to home remedies within a week, see a doctor. If you wake up in the morning with your eyes caked with discharge, consult a doctor to determine if you have bacterial conjunctivitis requiring antibiotics.

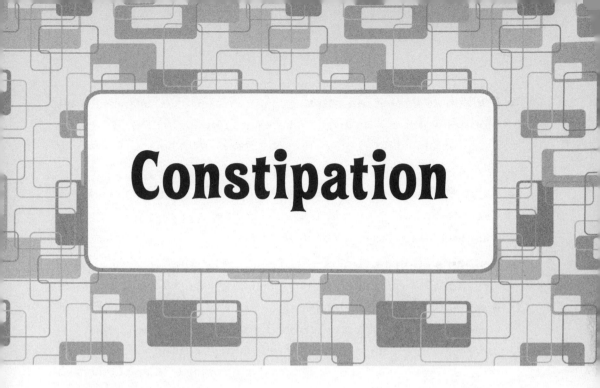

Constipation

- **Castor Oil.** To relieve constipation, take one to two teaspoons Castor Oil without any food, and allow six to twelve hours for the laxative to work. The glycerol and ricinoleic acid in Castor Oil stimulates the intestinal mucosa, causing a laxative effect. (Do not take Castor Oil during pregnancy or if you have abdominal pain.)

- **Coca-Cola.** Drinking a can of Coke can help relieve constipation. The caffeine in the Real Thing is a mild laxative.

- **Dr. Teal's Epsom Salt.** To relieve constipation, dissolve two to four level teaspoons Dr. Teal's Epsom Salt in an eight-ounce glass of water, and drink the solution. This concoction typically produces a bowel movement between thirty minutes and six hours. (If you have kidney disease, take prescription medicine, or have a magnesium-restricted diet, consult a doctor before ingesting Epsom Salt as a laxative.)

- **Fruit of the Earth Aloe Vera Gel.** Take one or two tablespoons Fruit of the Earth Aloe Vera Gel three times a day to ease constipation. Fruit of the Earth Aloe Vera Gel is 100 percent pure aloe gel and edible. Aloe lubricates the intestines, helping the bowels move more easily.

- **Grandma's Robust Molasses.** Taking two teaspoons Grandma's Robust Molasses works as a laxative to relieve constipation. In 1897, Dr. Henry Illoway discussed the laxative effect of molasses in his book *Constipation in Adults and Children.*

- **Heinz Baked Beanz.** To prevent constipation, eat one-half cup Heinz Baked Beanz every day. The fiber in baked beans absorbs water, making your stools softer, larger, and more regular.

- **Kellogg's All-Bran.** To prevent and relieve constipation, eat one cup Kellogg's All-Bran every morning. One cup of Kellogg's All-Bran contains 20 grams of fiber, and consuming 20 to 35 grams of fiber daily helps prevent constipation. Fiber absorbs water, making your stools softer, larger, and more regular. A daily minimum of five servings of fruits and vegetables, three servings of whole-grain foods, and one serving of beans puts enough fiber in your diet to prevent constipation.

- **Maxell House Coffee.** Drinking a cup of Maxwell House Coffee can relieve constipation. The caffeine in coffee doubles as a laxative by stimulating the colon.

- **McCormick Sesame Seed.** To speed things along, run one tablespoon McCormick Sesame Seed through a clean coffee grinder and sprinkle the powder on cereal or other foods. The oil from the seeds lubricates the intestines, helping dry stools glide through easier.

- **Metamucil.** To alleviate constipation, take one serving of Metamucil (as instructed on the package label) in or with eight ounces of water. Metamucil contains psyllium seed husk, a natural dietary fiber originating from the psyllium plant, which absorbs liquid, bulking up your stool and allowing it to pass through your system more comfortably. (Metamucil generally produces a laxative effect in twelve to seventy-two hours.)

- **Quaker Oats.** To relieve and prevent constipation, eat a bowl of Quaker Oats oatmeal every morning. The soluble fiber beta-glucan in the oats helps soften stools.

- **Sun-Maid Raisins.** Eating a small box of Sun-Maid Raisins every day helps speed along digestion and prevent constipation. The high fiber content and tartaric acid in raisins yield a laxative effect.

℞ STRANGE MEDICINE ℞

BEHIND SCHEDULE

- Constipation is simply the refusal of your digestive system to defecate. When you do move your bowels, after much straining and discomfort, your stools are hard, dark, and dry.

- The National Institutes of Health claims that normal human beings defecate anywhere from three times a day to three times a week. Alternative doctors, however, insist that healthy humans should excrete one soft bowel movement each day.

- Constant use of laxatives actually weakens the bowel muscles, causing defecation to be difficult without the aid of a laxative, making this over-the-counter medication rather addictive.

- Eating a high-fiber diet—20 to 35 grams a day—and drinking plenty of water (eight 8-ounce glasses a day) relieves constipation. The fiber absorbs water, creating soft bowel movements.

- Constipation can result from lack of exercise. To remedy this situation, simply walk for thirty minutes daily. Exercise helps speed food through the bowel.

- Various medications—such as antacids, antidepressants, antihistamines, blood-pressure drugs, calcium supplements, and diuretics—can cause constipation.

- When you feel the urge to defecate, abide by it. Otherwise, trying to contain your bowel movement can actually cause constipation.

- Never force a bowel movement. By doing so, you risk giving yourself painful hemorrhoids or anal fissures, which tend to narrow the anal canal, aggravating constipation.

- **Sunsweet Prune Juice.** To relieve constipation, mix twelve ounces Sunsweet Prune Juice and twelve ounces of water, and drink the solution once a day. When you have a bowel movement, reduce the prune juice solution by half for another day or two. Then cease the treatment.

Doctor's Orders

Make your move! If you fail to overcome constipation within three weeks of adding more fiber and water to your diet, consult a doctor to rule out diabetes, hyperthyroidism, irritable bowel syndrome, or colorectal cancer.

Corns and Calluses

- **Aunt Jemima Original Syrup.** Apply Aunt Jemima Original Syrup to the corn or callus and wrap with gauze. The corn syrup in the Aunt Jemima Original Syrup softens the hardened skin.

- **Bayer Aspirin, Heinz Apple Cider Vinegar,** and **Band-Aid Bandages.** To soften a corn or callus, use a mortar and pestle to crush six Bayer Aspirin tablets, and add just enough Heinz Apple Cider Vinegar to make a thick paste. Rub the paste into the corn or callus, and cover with a Band-Aid Bandage to hold the paste in place. Let sit for ten minutes, remove the bandage, and gently rub the callus (not the corn) with a pumice stone. The salicylic acid helps peel away the skin cells from the corn or callus.

- **Castor Oil** and **Q-Tips Cotton Swabs.** To help a corn heal, apply a non-medicated, doughnut-shaped pad around the corn (to protect the corn from rubbing against the inside of the shoe), use a Q-Tips Cotton Swab to coat the corn with Castor Oil, and put a small piece of adhesive tape over the corn to hold the oil in place. The castor oil moisturizes the corn all day long and promotes healing. Continue the treatment (changing the Castor Oil and adhesive tape daily) until the corn disappears.

- **Dr. Teal's Epsom Salt.** To soften a corn or callus, dissolve a handful of Dr. Teal's Epsom Salt in a basin filled with warm water, and soak your foot in the solution for twenty minutes.

- **Fruit of the Earth Aloe Vera Gel** and **Band-Aid Bandages.** To soften a callus, apply Fruit of the Earth Aloe Vera Gel to the spot before going to bed and cover with a Band-Aid Bandage. The aloe gel keeps the callus moist, enabling you to rub it off with a pumice stone in the morning.

℞ STRANGE MEDICINE ℞

KEEPING YOUR FEET ON THE GROUND

- A corn is a bump of thick, hard, dead skin usually found on your toes. A callus is a layer of thick, hard, dead skin generally found on the bottom of your feet.

- Wearing tight shoes causes both corns and calluses. To prevent or slow a callus or corn, stop wearing the shoes that are literally rubbing your feet the wrong way.

- Use a pumice stone to rub off the top layers of a callus—gently, without going too deep. Never try to grind off a callus in one sitting. Instead, soak the callus using one of the methods listed in this section and sand it down with a pumice stone a little bit each day. Never use a pumice stone on a corn. Doing so makes the corn more painful.

- Never attempt to cut off a corn or callus with a razor blade or other sharp implement.

- Switching to roomier shoes or adding an insole cushion to your shoes can prevent corns and calluses.

- Placing toe separators (little pieces of foam available at the drug store) between your toes can prevent corns by keeping your toes from rubbing against each other.

- When buying shoes, make sure your toes have ample room. From the tip of your longest toe to the tip of the shoe there should be enough space for the width of your thumb. And the width of the shoe should not squeeze your toes or the ball of your foot too tightly.

- **Heinz Apple Cider Vinegar** and **Dawn Dishwashing Liquid.** To remove calluses, add one cup Heinz Apple Cider Vinegar and one-half teaspoon Dawn Dishwashing Liquid to a basin of warm water. Soak your feet for twenty to thirty minutes. After the soapy vinegar solution softens the calluses, rub gently with a pumice stone for easy removal.

- **Lubriderm** and **Band-Aid Bandages.** To soften and heal the hardened skin of a corn or callus, apply Lubriderm to the affected area twice a day and cover with a Band-Aid Bandage to prevent the moisturizer from rubbing off. Keeping the corn or callus continually moisturized enables healing.

- **ReaLemon** and **Band-Aid Bandages.** To soften corns or calluses, saturate the gauze padding of a Band-Aid Bandage with ReaLemon lemon juice, and wrap it around the corn or callus. Change the dressing daily. The acid in the lemon juice softens the dead skin.

- **Star Olive Oil** and **Morton Salt.** To exfoliate dead skin from a corn or callus, mix equal parts Star Olive Oil and Morton Salt, apply the gritty mixture to your corn or callus when taking a shower, rub well, rinse clean, and dry thoroughly.

- **Wonder Bread, Heinz Apple Cider Vinegar,** and **Saran Wrap.** Saturate a slice of stale Wonder Bread with Heinz Apple Cider Vinegar, apply it to the corn or callus, and secure it in place with a sheet of Saran Wrap. Cover with a sock, and go to bed. By morning, the acetic acid in the vinegar should dissolve the corn or callus.

Doctor's Orders

Stand on your own two feet! If you experience chronic pain from a corn or callus, consult your doctor.

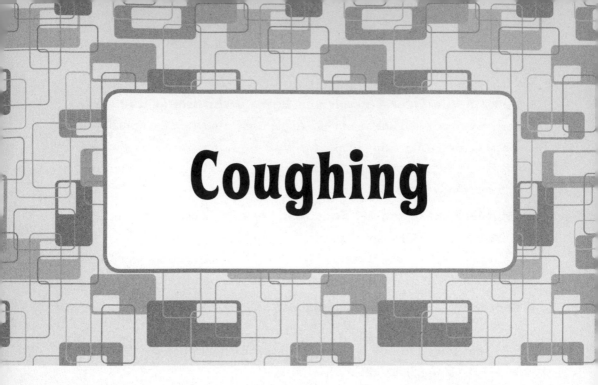

Coughing

- **Campbell's Chicken Noodle Soup** and **Tabasco Pepper Sauce.** Add one teaspoon Tabasco Pepper Sauce to a cup of Campbell's Chicken Noodle Soup, mix well, and eat. The hot soup and the capsaicin in the Tabasco Pepper Sauce help break up congestion in your chest and act as natural expectorants to clear the mucus.

- **French's Mustard.** To loosen congestion in your chest, spread French's Mustard on your chest and cover with a washcloth dampened with warm water. Let sit for fifteen minutes and wash clean. The penetrating warmth from the mustard plaster thins the mucus in your chest.

- **Life Savers Pep-O-Mint.** To help calm a cough, suck on a Lifesavers Pep-O-Mint candy. The volatile oils in peppermint increase saliva production, soothing your throat and suppressing the cough.

- **Lipton Ginger Tea.** To alleviate a cough, drink a cup of strongly brewed Lipton Ginger Tea every two or three hours until the cough subsides. A strong anti-inflammatory, ginger reduces the sore throat pain that might be triggering the cough. (Do not drink ginger tea if you have gallstones. Ginger can increase bile production.)

- **McCormick Black Pepper** and **SueBee Honey.** Place one teaspoon McCormick Black Pepper in a teacup, fill with boiling water, cover with a saucer, and let steep for fifteen minutes. Add two tablespoons SueBee Honey, and drink the peppery tea. The black pepper stimulates circulation and doubles as a decongestant. The mildly antibiotic honey soothes the throat and relieves coughing. (Do not feed honey to infants less than one year of age. Honey often carries a benign strain of *C. botulinum,* and an infant's immune system requires twelve months to develop to fight off disease and infection.)

- **McCormick Thyme Leaves.** To relieve a cough, place a tea infuser filled with two teaspoons McCormick Thyme Leaves in a cup, fill with boiling water, cover with a saucer, and let steep for ten minutes. Sip the tea slowly. The flavonoids in thyme reduce inflammation and relax the tracheal and ileal muscles.

- **Morton Salt** and **Arm & Hammer Baking Soda.** To alleviate a cough, make a saline nose wash to rinse mucus from your nasal passages. Purify eight ounces of water by boiling for three minutes, let cool to room temperature, and dissolve one-quarter teaspoon Morton Salt and one-quarter teaspoon Arm & Hammer Baking Soda in the purified water. Use a bulb syringe or neti pot to rinse the inside of your nose. Postnasal drip frequently causes or worsens coughs, and washing out the mucus that would otherwise drip down your throat relieves the cough.

- **SueBee Honey, Star Olive Oil,** and **ReaLemon.** To make homemade cough syrup, mix one cup SueBee Honey, one-half cup Star Olive Oil, and four tablespoons ReaLemon lemon juice in a saucepan and warm over low heat for five minutes. Stir vigorously for several minutes until the mixture attains the consistency of syrup. To relieve a cough, take one teaspoon of the formula every two hours. Store in an airtight container. (Do not feed honey to infants less than one year of age. Honey often carries a benign strain of *C. botulinum,* and an infant's immune system requires twelve months to develop to fight off disease and infection.)

℞ STRANGE MEDICINE ℞

CAN YOU HACK IT?

- A "productive" cough is the body's way of clearing an irritant—typically mucus or phlegm—from the throat or respiratory system.

- Smoke, fumes, dust, and soot cause a "dry" cough.

- Most coughs clear up on their own within ten days.

- To help ease a cough, drink eight 8-ounce glasses of water every day to moisten mucus membranes.

- Taking a hot shower with plenty of steam or running a humidifier helps liquefy mucus trapped in your airways, making it easier to cough up.

- Never take a cough suppressant to stifle a "productive" cough. Productive coughs purge secretions from the airways.

- Expectorants help thin mucus, making it easier to cough up.

- To relieve a "productive" cough, blow your nose frequently to clear your sinuses and prevent postnasal drip from triggering more coughs.

Doctor's Orders

Cough it up! If your cough lasts longer than two weeks or if you cough up blood, consult a doctor to rule out strep throat or a respiratory disease. If you have chills, chest pains, and a fever higher than 101 degrees Fahrenheit, your cough may be a symptom of pneumonia.

Cuts and Scrapes

- **Bag Balm.** To protect a cut or scrape, keep the scab soft, and speed healing, coat the affected area with Bag Balm, the salve originally developed in Vermont to soothe cows' udders.

- **ChapStick.** If you nick yourself shaving or get a paper cut, stop the bleeding quickly by smearing a dab of ChapStick over the wound. The wax seals the laceration, preventing air from causing the nerve to tingle.

- **Krazy Glue.** To seal a minor cut, simply apply some Krazy Glue along the laceration. The active ingredient in Krazy Glue is ethyl 2-cyanoacrylate, virtually the same active ingredient contained in Band-Aid Brand Liquid Bandage, an instant glue used to seal lacerations.

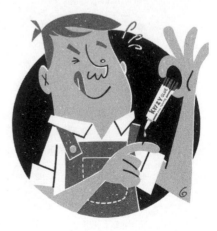

- **Lipton Tea Bags.** Heal a minor laceration by applying a Lipton Tea Bag dampened with cool water to the spot. The tannin in the tea acts like an astringent to stop the bleeding, soothe the skin, and reduce inflammation.

- **Listerine.** To disinfect a cut or scrape, pour original formula Listerine antiseptic mouthwash over the wound. Developed by Dr. Joseph Lawrence in 1857 as a safe and effective antiseptic for use in surgical procedures, Listerine is an astringent and antibacterial.

- **McCormick Black Pepper** or **McCormick Ground (Cayenne) Red Pepper.** To stop a minor cut from bleeding, rinse well with soap and water, sprinkle ground McCormick Black Pepper or McCormick Ground (Cayenne) Red Pepper on the laceration, and cover with a bandage.

- **McCormick Garlic Powder.** To disinfect a cut or scrape, mix one-half teaspoon McCormick Garlic Powder with enough water to make a thick

℞ STRANGE MEDICINE ℞

ALL YOU BLEED IS BLOOD

● To treat a cut or abrasion, stop the bleeding by applying direct pressure with a clean cloth or gauze, disinfect the wound by washing with soap and water to prevent bacterial infection, and then apply a bandage.

● If applying pressure fails to stop the bleeding, elevate the wound above your heart to reduce the blood flow to the area and apply direct pressure.

● If the wound continues bleeding, press the nearest pressure point above the wound for roughly one minute. Pressure points are located inside the wrists, on the inner side of the arms halfway between the elbow and shoulder, and on the inside of the thighs just below the groin.

● If you're unable to wash a wound, lick it with your tongue. A 2008 study published in the *FASEB Journal* found that histatin, a small protein in saliva known to kill bacteria, greatly speeds the healing of wounds. This finding explains why animals lick their wounds and why wounds in the mouth heal much faster than flesh wounds.

● To prevent infection, wash the wound with soap and water twice a day.

● Keeping the wound moist with an antibacterial salve and a bandage speeds up the regeneration of skin cells. Allowing the wound to form a scab actually slows new cell growth.

paste, and apply it to the affected area. Garlic is a natural antibiotic that contains antiseptic compounds.

- **McCormick Ground Cloves.** To protect a cut from infection, sprinkle McCormick Ground Cloves on the laceration. The eugenol in the cloves doubles as an antiseptic and a pain reliever, numbing the wound.

- **McCormick Ground Sage.** In the first century, the ancient Greek physician Dioscorides used sage to stop wounds from bleeding. To do so, simply sprinkle McCormick Ground Sage on the cut.

- **Smirnoff Vodka.** To prevent a laceration or abrasion from getting infected, pour Smirnoff Vodka over the wound. As an antiseptic, the alcohol disinfects the wound.

- **Stayfree Maxi Pads.** To stop a cut or scrape from bleeding, apply direct pressure to the wound with a Stayfree Maxi Pad and raise the wound above heart level.

- **SueBee Honey.** To help heal a minor cut or scrape and prevent infection, coat the laceration or abrasion with SueBee Honey. Honey is hygroscopic, meaning it absorbs moisture from wounds, making the wound an inhospitable environment for bacteria and sealing out contaminants. The honey dries to form a unique bandage.

- **Vaseline Petroleum Jelly.** To expedite healing, rub a few dabs of Vaseline Petroleum Jelly on the cut or scrape. In 1859, Brooklyn chemist Robert Augustus Chesebrough learned from petroleum drilling workers in Titusville, Pennsylvania, that the jelly residue that gunked up oil drilling rods quickened healing when rubbed on a wound.

Doctor's Orders

Cut to the chase! If the bleeding from a cut or scrape doesn't stop after ten minutes, consult a doctor.

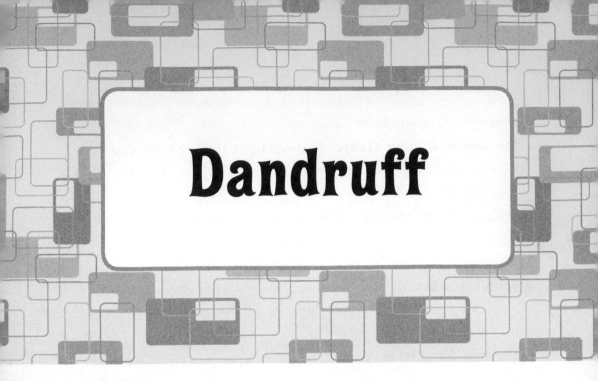

Dandruff

- **Castor Oil.** Using a cotton ball, rub Castor Oil into the scalp, wait ten minutes, then rinse clean. The Castor Oil kills the bacteria on the scalp (that can cause dandruff) and moisturizes the skin, ending dry flakes.

- **Dannon Yogurt.** To remedy dandruff, work Dannon Plain Nonfat Yogurt into your scalp, let sit for thirty minutes, and then rinse thoroughly. The *Lactobacillus acidophilus* bacteria (probiotics) in the yogurt devour the yeast *Pityrosporum* (*Malassezia*) *orbiculare* that feed on sebum oil, causing dandruff.

- **Dickinson's Witch Hazel.** To remove excess oil from your hair, use a cotton ball to apply Dickinson's Witch Hazel to the roots, then comb this natural astringent through your hair.

- **Fruit of the Earth Aloe Vera Gel.** To eliminate dandruff, slather Fruit of the Earth Aloe Vera Gel into your scalp and massage deeply. Let sit for two hours, then rinse clean in the shower (without using any shampoo). No one knows precisely why this works, but studies suggest that aloe vera gel may have antibacterial and antifungal properties.

- **Gerber Carrots, SueBee Honey, Quaker Oats,** and **Now Sweet Almond Oil.** To combat dandruff, mix together five ounces (one small container) Gerber Carrots, two tablespoons SueBee Honey, three tablespoons Quaker Oats, and two teaspoons Now Sweet Almond Oil in a bowl. Massage the mixture into your hair and scalp. Let sit for five minutes, shampoo your hair thoroughly, condition as usual, and rinse with cold water. The carotene in the carrots deeply moisturizes the scalp, and the honey improves the shine of your hair.

- **Heinz Apple Cider Vinegar.** To get rid of dandruff, mix equal parts Heinz Apple Cider Vinegar with water, pour the mixture over your hair, and massage it into the scalp. The acetic acid in the vinegar balances the scalp's pH and simultaneously kills any yeast or bacteria that might also be drying the scalp and causing the flakes.

- **Lipton Green Tea.** Place two Lipton Green Tea bags in one cup of boiling water, cover with a saucer, and let steep for twenty minutes. Squeeze and remove the tea bags, and let the liquid cool to the touch. Massage the tea into your scalp. The antioxidants in the green tea exfoliate the dry skin from your scalp, and tannins in green tea soothe and strengthen the skin.

- **Listerine.** Frequently caused by *Pityrosporum (Malassezia) ovale,* a yeast-like fungus that feeds on the scalp's oils, dandruff can be cured by applying original formula Listerine antiseptic mouthwash to your scalp. After shampooing your hair, rinse with Listerine. The thymol, eucalyptol, menthol, and methyl salicylate in Listerine seem to kill the fungus (and bacteria).

- **McCormick Rosemary Leaves.** To quell dandruff flakes, add two tablespoons McCormick Rosemary Leaves to one cup of boiling water, cover with a saucer, and steep for twenty minutes. Strain and let cool to room temperature. After shampooing, conditioning, and rinsing your hair, use the rosemary tea as a final rinse, massaging it into the scalp. Do not rinse out the rosemary solution. Rosemary impedes your scalp from producing excess sebum, the oil that contributes to dandruff.

- **McCormick Thyme Leaves.** To alleviate dandruff, add three tablespoons McCormick Thyme Leaves to a quart of boiling water, cover the pot, and simmer for twenty minutes. After shampooing, conditioning, and rinsing

℞ STRANGE MEDICINE ℞

SCRATCH THAT

● When the scalp is excessively dry, the glands in the scalp overproduce sebum, which causes the skin to flake and itch.

● Dandruff is not a hair problem, so a dandruff shampoo that treats your hair will not remedy dandruff. If you do use a medicated dandruff shampoo, lather it into your scalp, leave it in for ten minutes (to give the medication a chance to work on your scalp), and rinse clean.

● Shampooing your hair daily with a gentle cleanser controls dandruff. Shampoos cleanse the oil and dead skin cells from your scalp.

● Dandruff appears as tiny white flakes of dead skin that speckle your hair and shoulders, accompanied by an itchy, scaling scalp.

● Dandruff tends to worsen during the fall and winter, when indoor heating dries the skin.

● During the summer, dandruff tends to improve. When exposed to direct ultraviolet light, scaly skin conditions get better.

● Dandruff can also be caused by eczema, psoriasis, sensitivity to hair care products or hair dyes (contact dermatitis), bacteria, or *Pityrosporum* (*Malassezia*) (a yeast-like fungus that feeds on oils in your scalp).

● Men are more prone to dandruff than women, probably because men have larger oil-producing glands on their scalps or possibly due to male hormones.

● A deficiency in zinc, B vitamins, or certain fats might increase your likelihood of dandruff.

● To combat dandruff, cease using hair sprays, styling gels, mousses, and hair waxes. The buildup from these products on your hair and scalp increases oiliness, which triggers itching and flaking.

your hair, use the cooled thyme tea as a final rinse, massaging it into the scalp. Do not rinse it out. The thymol in thyme can kill the fungus and bacteria living in your scalp and likely casuing the dandruff problem.

- **Miracle Whip** and **Saran Wrap.** To remedy a flaky, scaly scalp, rub Miracle Whip into your scalp, wrap your head in a sheet of Saran Wrap (above the eyes, nose, and mouth), and let sit for two hours. Then rinse clean. The oil and vinegar in the Miracle Whip seem to moisturize the dry skin and kill the fungus or bacteria, and simultaneously condition your hair.

- **Purell Instant Hand Sanitizer.** Rub Purell Instant Hand Sanitizer into your scalp, wait five minutes, then rinse clean. The ethyl alcohol in Purell kills the bacteria that may be responsible for your dry scalp.

- **Star Olive Oil** and **Saran Wrap.** To loosen the scaly skin from your scalp before it flakes into dandruff, warm one-half cup Star Olive Oil, wet your hair with water (to prevent it from absorbing any oil), and use a gravy brush to apply the oil to your scalp. Wrap your head in Saran Wrap (above your eyes, nose, and mouth), and let sit for thirty minutes. Then shampoo and rinse thoroughly.

- **Vicks VapoRub** and **Dawn Dishwashing Liquid.** Apply Vicks VapoRub to your hair and scalp, let sit for thirty minutes, and then use Dawn Dishwashing Liquid to shampoo out the balm. The thymol, eucalyptol, and camphor in Vicks VapoRub kill the fungus that can cause dandruff.

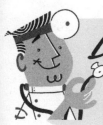

Doctor's Orders

Don't flake out! If your dandruff persists after two months of home remedy treatments, see a dermatologist to rule out a yeast infection of the scalp or hormone imbalances.

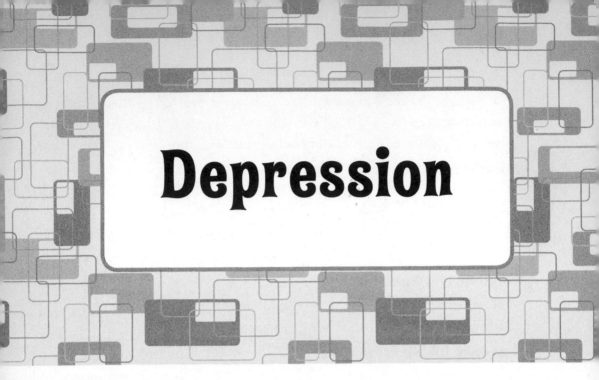

Depression

- **Chicken of the Sea Salmon, Chicken of the Sea Sardines,** or **Chicken of the Sea Tuna.** Eat salmon, sardines, or tuna three or four times a week to add omega-3 fatty acids to your diet. Studies show that people who consume large amounts of fish have one-tenth the rate of depression compared to those who do not eat fish. No one knows how omega-3 oils protect against depression, but doctors do know that the eicosapentaenoic acid (EPA) and docosahexaenoic acid (DHA) in these fish are important to the health of brain cells. Also, one serving of Chicken of the Sea Chunk Light Tuna provides nearly 60 percent of the daily requirement for vitamin B_6, a deficiency of which is linked to depression.

- **Hershey's Special Dark Chocolate Bar.** To lift your mood, eat a Hershey's Special Dark Chocolate Bar. Dark chocolate stimulates the production of endorphins, chemicals in the brain that induce feelings of pleasure. Chocolate also raises levels of the brain chemical serotonin, which acts as an antidepressant. (While eating chocolate may lift depression in the short term, researchers warn that eating it regularly may have a negative effect on health and mood in the long run. Chocolate is also high in saturated fat and calories.)

- **Kellogg's All-Bran, Kellogg's Special K,** or **Total.** To avoid depression, eat one-half cup Kellogg's All-Bran, Kellogg's Special K, or Total cereal every day. Depression is one of the most common symptoms of a folic acid deficiency. Studies find that men who get 234 micrograms of folate for every 1,000 calories they eat are half as likely to become depressed as men who only get 119 micrograms. One-half cup of Kellogg's All-Bran cereal, Kellogg's Special K, or Total contains 400 micrograms of folate, better known as vitamin B_9.

- **McCormick Pure Vanilla Extract.** To lift your mood, saturate a cotton ball with McCormick Pure Vanilla Extract and set it on a saucer. The aroma of vanilla triggers your pituitary gland and hypothalamus to produce endorphins, the neurotransmitters that produce a feeling of well-being. Studies show that the scent of vanilla significantly reduces anxiety.

- **Planters Dry Roasted Cashews.** People with depression have low levels of zinc in their blood, but eating a handful of cashews, which are rich in zinc, provides 50 percent of the recommended daily allowance of zinc.

- **Progresso Lentil Soup.** To help counteract depression, eat one cup Progresso Lentil Soup to increase the amount of vitamin B_9 (also known as folate) in your diet. Depression is one of the most common symptoms of a folic acid deficiency. Studies find that men who get 234 micrograms of folate for every 1,000 calories they eat are half as likely to become depressed as men who only get 119 micrograms. One cup of Progresso Lentil Soup contains 102 micrograms of folate.

- **Quaker Oats.** To lift your mood and keep it even keeled, eat a bowl of Quaker Oats oatmeal for breakfast at least three times a week. Oats contain more than half the recommended daily allowance of fatty acids, folic acid, and zinc. The fiber content keeps your blood sugar balanced.

- **Uncle Ben's Converted Brand Rice.** To lift your mood, eat one cup cooked Uncle Ben's Converted Brand Rice. The carbohydrates in rice can boost the production of serotonin, a neurotransmitter that improves your mood.

℞ STRANGE MEDICINE ℞

DOWN AND OUT

● Depression is a chronic medical illness marked by persistent melancholy and lack of interest, sometimes causing physical symptoms including insomnia, excessive sleeping, irritability, neck or back pain, and loss of appetite.

● Affecting your feelings, thoughts, and behavior, depression can lead to various emotional and physical problems, including suicidal tendencies.

● Usually requiring long-term treatment, depression can be overcome with medication, psychological counseling, or other treatments.

● No one knows exactly what causes depression. Possible triggers include biological changes in the brain, a problem with neurotransmitters in the brain, a hormonal imbalance (caused by thyroid problems, menopause, or another condition), a genetic predisposition toward depression, or traumatic events (like the death of a loved one, financial difficulties, or stress).

● You can resolve depression without taking antidepressant drugs—unless you're suffering from clinical depression, which requires professional care.

● Listening to music dissipates depression. Scientific studies show that listening to Mozart's piano concertos or Vienna waltzes relieves depression.

● Sunlight restores the soul. Spend at least fifteen minutes (ideally thirty minutes) outdoors when the sun is shining. Too little sunlight interrupts the steady production of hormones and brain chemicals.

● To help overcome depression, exercise for one hour a day every day by simply going for a walk in the early morning. Exercise triggers changes in brain chemistry just like an antidepressant drug.

● To prevent and help defeat depression, avoid alcohol and illegal drugs. While alcohol or drugs may seem to temporarily buffer the emotional pain, self-medicating with a depressant (alcohol) or narcotics generally worsens depression, making it more difficult to treat.

Doctor's Orders

Keep your chin up! If you or a loved one feel depressed or have suicidal thoughts, make an appointment to see your doctor immediately. Or speak with a mental health provider, clergy leader, or someone else you trust, or call the National Suicide Prevention Lifeline at 800-273-8255 to talk with a trained counselor.

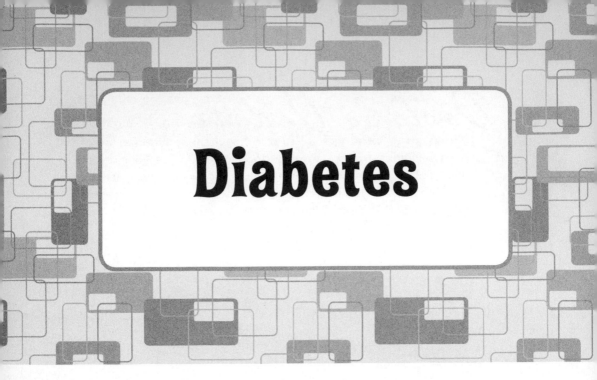

Diabetes

- **Heinz Apple Cider Vinegar.** Taking two tablespoons Heinz Apple Cider Vinegar before a high-carbohydrate meal can counteract the anticipated increase in blood sugar in people with type 2 diabetes, according to a 2004 study conducted at Arizona State University. To make the vinegar palatable, add it to oil to make salad dressing.

- **Hershey's Special Dark Chocolate Bar.** Eating a small square of Hershey's Special Dark Chocolate daily helps lower diabetes risk by increasing insulin sensitivity, according to a 2011 study conducted at Harvard University. (Before you start eating chocolate daily, be aware that chocolate is high in saturated fat and calories.)

- **Jif Peanut Butter.** To lower your risk of type 2 diabetes by 25 percent, eat one-tablespoon Jif Peanut Butter every day, according to a 2002 Nurses' Health Study published in the *Journal of the American Medical Association*. Also, when added to a meal with a high glycemic load, such as a bagel and a glass of juice, peanut butters stabilizes your blood sugar level, preventing it from rising too high too quickly, according to a 2005 study published in the *Journal of the American Dietetic Association*. Getting a

℞ STRANGE MEDICINE ℞

HOW SWEET IT ISN'T

● Diabetes commonly refers to the disease diabetes mellitus, which affects how the body uses blood sugar. In type 1 diabetes, the pancreas produces an insufficient amount of the hormone insulin, inhibiting the body from using and storing sugar. In type 2 diabetes, the pancreas produces sufficient amounts of insulin but the body does not use the insulin properly.

● Ninety to 95 percent of diabetics have type 2 diabetes.

● Common symptoms of diabetes include excessive urination, extreme hunger, increased thirst, and loss of weight and strength.

● Type 1 diabetes usually develops in childhood or adolescence. If the symptoms occur suddenly, accompanied by nausea, vomiting, and difficulty breathing, the victim may go into a diabetic coma unless she receives immediate treatment.

● People with type 1 diabetes require daily insulin injections.

● Type 2 diabetes is preventable and typically strikes overweight people over age forty.

● No one knows what causes diabetes, but obesity, a diet high in saturated fat, inactivity, high blood pressure, low levels of high-density lipoprotein (HDL) or "good" cholesterol, high levels of triglycerides, and age increase the risk of type 2 diabetes.

● Left untreated, diabetes can lead to kidney failure, heart disease, blindness, and limb amputation.

sufficient amount of magnesium in your diet reduces the risk of diabetes, and two tablespoons of Jif Peanut Butter provide 15 percent of the daily value of magnesium.

● **Maxwell House Coffee.** To reduce your risk of developing type 2 diabetes, drink four cups of Maxwell House Coffee every day. A 2011 study at

UCLA showed that women who drink at least four cups of coffee a day are 58 percent less likely to develop diabetes as non-coffee drinkers.

- **McCormick Ground Cinnamon.** To lower your blood sugar and reduce the risk of diabetic complications, sprinkle one-half teaspoon McCormick Ground Cinnamon on your cereal, oatmeal, yogurt, or other foods once a day. A 2003 study published in *Diabetes Care* showed that consuming roughly one-half teaspoon of cinnamon per day leads to dramatic improvements in blood sugar, cholesterol, LDL cholesterol, and triglycerides in people with type 2 diabetes.

- **Planters Dry Roasted Almonds, Planters Dry Roasted Cashews,** or **Planters Dry Roasted Peanuts.** Eating foods high in magnesium—like Planters Dry Roasted Almonds, Planters Dry Roasted Cashews, or Planters Dry Roasted Peanuts—can reduce your risk of getting diabetes. A 2004 study at the Harvard School of Public Health linked low magnesium intake with an increased risk of diabetes. One ounce of almonds provides 80 milligrams of magnesium, one ounce of cashews provides 75 milligrams, and one ounce of dry roasted peanuts provides 50 milligrams.

- **Planters Walnuts.** If you have type 2 diabetes, improve your heart health markers and significantly reduce your fasting insulin level by eating one-half cup Planters Walnuts every day. You can add walnuts to salads, meatloaf, and other recipes, or just eat them plain. Walnuts also lower overall cholesterol, prevent and control high blood pressure, and provide an excellent source of omega-3 fatty acids. (Be aware that one-half cup of walnuts contains 327 calories.)

Doctor's Orders

Sweeten the deal! If you suspect that you or your child may have diabetes, contact your doctor immediately. If you've been diagnosed with diabetes, heed your doctor's counsel to keep your blood sugar levels stabilized.

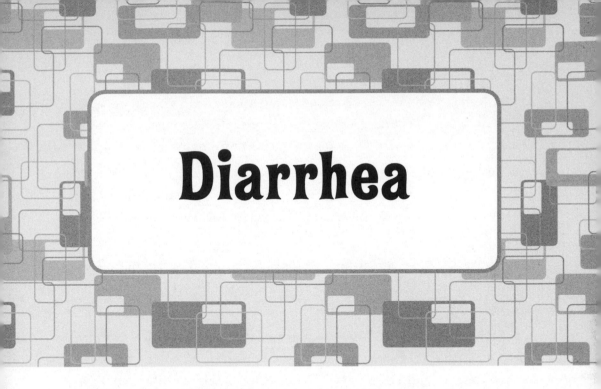

Diarrhea

- **Baker's Angel Flake Coconut.** To bring diarrhea under control, eat two teaspoons Baker's Angel Flake Coconut. A 2010 study published in the *Journal of Ethnopharmacology* showed that coconut extract was just as effective as a leading antidiarrheal medication when tested on rats.

- **CharcoCaps Activated Charcoal.** To relieve diarrhea caused by food poisoning, take four to six 200-milligram CharcoCaps Activated Charcoal capsules every two hours until the symptoms subside. The charcoal absorbs toxins from the digestive track, carrying them out of the body. Charcoal also absorbs nutrients, so be sure to discontinue use after a few days. (Don't confuse activated charcoal with charcoal briquettes. Activated charcoal is a charcoal that has been processed with oxygen to be extremely porous.)

- **Dannon Yogurt.** To ease diarrhea, eat a cup of Dannon Nonfat Yogurt. The beneficial *Lactobacillus acidophilus* (probiotics) in yogurt assist the helpful bacteria in your colon that aid digestion.

- **Gatorade.** To refortify your body with liquid and electrolytes, drink Gatorade to quickly replace essential nutrients and minerals, preventing muscle spasms in your stomach.

- **Heinz Apple Cider Vinegar.** To subdue diarrhea caused by a bacterial infection, drink two tablespoons Heinz Apple Cider Vinegar added to a glass of water. The antibiotic properties of apple cider vinegar combat the bacteria, and the pectin may soothe intestinal spasms.

- **Kellogg's All-Bran.** To clear up diarrhea, eat one cup Kellogg's All-Bran cereal every morning for breakfast. Adding 20 to 35 grams of fiber to your diet daily creates large, soft stools. One cup of Kellogg's All-Bran contains 20 grams of fiber.

- **Knorr Chicken Bouillon.** To replace the liquid, salts, and minerals depleted by diarrhea, dissolve one Knorr Chicken Bouillon cube in a cup of hot water and sip the broth.

- **Lipton Chamomile Tea.** To calm a bout of diarrhea, place two Lipton Chamomile Tea bags in a cup, fill with boiling water, cover with a saucer, and steep for fifteen minutes. Drink a cup of this tea three times a day. Chamomile contains compounds that tame intestinal spasms and reduce inflammation. (Coumarin, an anticoagulant in chamomile, may increase the likelihood of bleeding when taken in combination with the blood thinner Coumadin or other anticoagulant medications.)

- **McCormick Caraway Seed.** Reduce the intensity of intestinal spasms by placing a tea infuser filled with one teaspoon McCormick Caraway Seed in a teacup, pour boiling water into the cup, and cover with a saucer. Steep for fifteen minutes and then drink the tea. The caraway alleviates the discomfort.

- **McCormick Ground Cinnamon** and **McCormick Ground Ginger.** To combat diarrhea caused by food poisoning, mix one teaspoon McCormick Ground Cinnamon and one-half teaspoon McCormick Ground Ginger in a teacup, add boiling water, cover with a saucer, and let steep for fifteen minutes. Strain and then sip the tea. The cinnamon can help kill the responsible bacteria, and the ginger helps quell stomach spasms. (Do not use ginger if you have gallstones. Ginger can increase bile production.)

- **Metamucil.** To add fiber to your diet and absorb excess fluid in your intestines, take one serving of Metamucil (as instructed on the package label) in or with eight ounces of water once a day. Metamucil contains psyllium seed husk, a natural dietary fiber originating from the psyllium plant, which soaks up liquid, bulking up your stool.

- **Minute Maid Orange Juice, ReaLemon,** and **Morton Salt.** To stay well hydrated and replenish electrolytes lost during a bout with diarrhea, mix one cup Minute Maid Orange Juice, three tablespoons ReaLemon lemon juice, one teaspoon Morton Salt, and two cups of water. Drink as needed.

℞ STRANGE MEDICINE ℞

ON THE LOOSE

- With diarrhea, the bowels discharge loose, watery feces with troubling frequency.

- Common causes of diarrhea include viruses, food or water contaminated with bacteria or parasites, medications (most commonly antibiotics), lactose intolerance, fructose, or artificial sweeteners.

- In most cases, diarrhea clears up within a couple of days without any treatment.

- Diarrhea that lasts for weeks can signal a serious disorder, such as inflammatory bowel disease, Crohn's disease, colitis, or irritable bowel syndrome.

- Diarrhea causes the body to lose significant amounts of water and salts. Drink plenty of water and fruit juice (not apple or pear) to prevent dehydration. Fruit juice helps maintain your electrolyte levels and eating soup or chicken bouillon replaces lost sodium and other minerals.

- Diarrhea helps purge harmful bacteria or a parasite from your digestive system.

- The best treatment for a quick recovery from diarrhea is to let it clear up by itself.

- Using an antidiarrheal medication tends to prolong the affliction.

- To help remedy diarrhea, avoid dairy products, fatty foods, high-fiber foods, or highly seasoned foods until the symptoms subside.

- **Mott's Applesauce.** To tame diarrhea, eat Mott's Applesauce. The pectin in the applesauce is a soluble fiber that absorbs fluid in your intestines and helps solidify soft bowel movements. Applesauce also contains malic acid and quercetin, which help inhibit harmful bacteria in your stomach.

- **SueBee Honey.** To cure diarrhea, mix four tablespoons SueBee Honey into a cup of hot water. Let cool and drink. A 1985 study conducted in South Africa and reported in the *British Medical Journal* showed that honey shortens the duration of diarrhea in patients with bacterial gastroenteritis caused by *Salmonella, Shigella,* and *E. coli.* (Do not feed honey to infants less than one year of age. Honey often carries a benign strain of *C. botulinum,* and an infant's immune system requires twelve months to develop to fight off disease and infection.)

- **Uncle Ben's Converted Brand Rice.** To get diarrhea under control, eat small portions of plain, white Uncle Ben's Converted Brand Rice. Rice binds the bowels, creating healthy stools.

- **Wonder Bread.** To help recover from diarrhea, transition slowly to solid foods by starting with some slices of toasted Wonder Bread, which are easy to digest and provide starch.

Doctor's Orders

Put it behind you! If diarrhea lasts more than three days, or if the stools are black or contain green mucus or blood, consult your doctor.

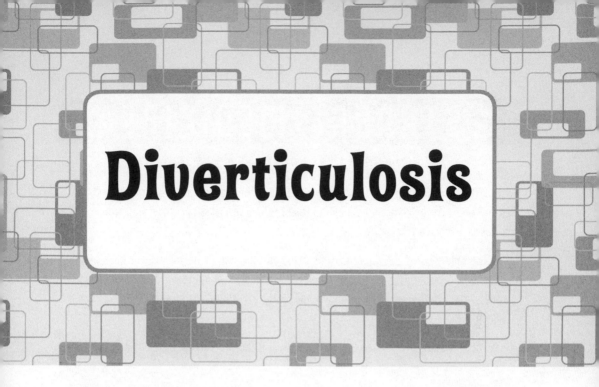

Diverticulosis

- **Dannon Yogurt.** If you're taking antibiotics to fight an infection from diverticulosis, increase the effectiveness of the antibiotics by eating one cup of Dannon Nonfat Yogurt daily (two hours after taking the antibiotics). Yogurt contains beneficial *Lactobacillus acidophilus* bacteria (probiotics) that can replace the "good" bacteria that the antibiotics tend to kill along with the "bad" bacteria.

- **Fiber One.** To help prevent problems from diverticulosis, eat 20 to 35 grams of fiber daily. One cup of Fiber One cereal contains 28 grams of fiber. Adding fiber to your diet lowers the internal pressure in your large intestine and produces soft, regular stools, reducing or eliminating the symptoms of diverticulosis.

- **Heinz Baked Beanz.** To treat and prevent diverticulosis, eat one-half cup Heinz Baked Beanz daily. The high levels of soluble fiber in baked beans (9.5 grams) help keep your stools regular and soft.

- **Kellogg's All-Bran.** One cup of Kellogg's All-Bran contains 20 grams of fiber. To help prevent problems from diverticulosis, eat 20 to

INSIDE INFORMATION

● With diverticulosis, a medical condition commonly affecting the large intestine, small areas of the outer intestinal wall swell to the size of grapes, creating small protuberances called diverticula.

● The only way to cure diverticulosis is to consume more fiber, which, in turn, helps the colon form large, soft stools. Insufficient fiber causes the colon to produce small stools that can be expelled from the body only by producing high internal pressure, which creates diverticula.

● Roughly half of all Americans ages 60 to 80 have diverticulosis, but most never experience any symptoms.

● To help prevent problems from diverticulosis, eat 20 to 35 grams of fiber daily. Adding fiber to your diet lowers the internal pressure in your large intestine, reducing or eliminating the symptoms.

● Drink eight 8-ounce glasses of water a day to help stools pass easily through your system. The straining caused by constipation exacerbates diverticulosis.

● Diverticulosis can advance to diverticulitis, a painful inflammation or infection of the diverticula.

● If you feel the urge to move your bowels, don't suppress it. Delaying bowel movements creates harder stools and can actually cause constipation, worsening your diverticulosis.

● Going for a thirty-minute walk every day helps the digestive system flow smoothly and tones the muscles in your intestines, minimizing straining during bowel movements.

● Contrary to popular belief, eating seeds or nuts does not cause diverticulosis.

35 grams of fiber daily. Adding fiber to your diet lowers the internal pressure in your large intestine, reducing or eliminating the symptoms of diverticulosis.

- **Kretschmer Wheat Germ.** Sprinkle a few tablespoons of Kretschmer Wheat Germ on meals or into a bowl of cereal. Each tablespoon of wheat germ contains 13 grams of fiber, which helps the colon expand when eliminating waste.

- **Metamucil.** If you have difficulty consuming more than 20 grams of fiber daily, take one serving of Metamucil (as instructed on the package label) in or with eight ounces of water once a day. Metamucil contains psyllium seed husk, a natural dietary fiber originating from the psyllium plant, which absorbs liquid, bulking up your stool and allowing it to pass through your system more comfortably.

- **Uncle Ben's Converted Brand Rice.** To soothe the tenderness or cramping, fill a clean sock with Uncle Ben's Converted Brand Rice, tie a knot in the end, and heat in the microwave oven for one to two minutes. Making sure the sock isn't too hot, hold it against the left-hand side of your belly. The rice-filled sock conforms to the shape of your body, allowing the warmth to relieve the pain. The homemade heating pad is also reusable.

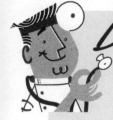

Doctor's Orders

Get the inside story! If you've been diagnosed with diverticulosis, experience recurring symptoms, develop a persistent pain on the left side of your belly, or notice blood in your stool, consult a doctor or gastroenterologist.

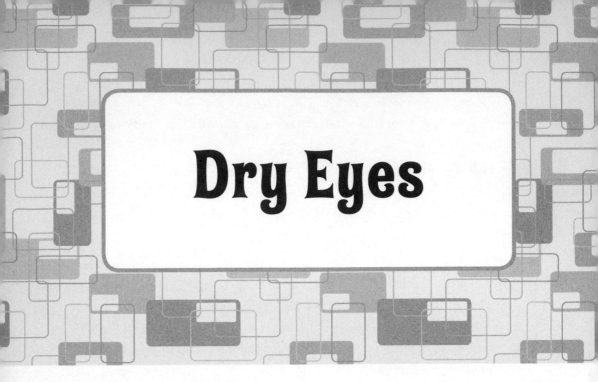

Dry Eyes

- **Betty Crocker Potato Buds.** To soothe dry eyes, mix Betty Crocker Potato Buds with enough water to make a thick paste. Apply the paste to closed eyes (making sure to remove contact lenses or any eye makeup beforehand), cover with a washcloth, and relax for twenty minutes. Rinse clean. Potatoes have astringent properties.

- **Chicken of the Sea Salmon, Chicken of the Sea Sardines,** or **Chicken of the Sea Tuna.** To lower your risk of dry eyes, eat salmon, sardines, or tuna three times a week to add the fatty acids commonly known as omega-3 oils to your diet. A study published in 2005 in the *American Journal of Clinical Nutrition* showed that omega-3 fatty acids help alleviate dry eye symptoms.

- **Dickinson's Witch Hazel** and **Stayfree Maxi Pads.** To soothe dry eyes and reduce puffiness, dampen a Stayfree Maxi Pad with Dickinson's Witch Hazel, lie down, and place the pad on your closed eyelids.

- **Lipton Chamomile Tea.** Place two Lipton Chamomile Tea bags in a cup, fill with boiling water, cover with a saucer, and steep for fifteen minutes. Remove the tea bags and let the liquid cool to the touch. Saturate two cotton balls with the tea, and place them over your eyes for ten minutes.

℞ STRANGE MEDICINE ℞

MORE THAN MEETS THE EYE

● When the eye fails to produce sufficient tears to moisten the eyeball, dry eye results.

● Dry eye causes redness, stinging, burning, itching, excessive tearing, and sensitivity to light.

● To restore moisture to eyes, use natural eyedrops made without preservatives.

● Over-the-counter eyedrops like Visine or Murine eliminate red eyes by constricting the blood vessels without necessarily moistening the dryness effectively.

● Drinking eight 8-ounce glasses of water daily can help keep your eyes moist by keeping your body properly hydrated.

● To get your eyes to produce tears naturally, simply use a knife to carefully cut an onion into slices. When you cut into an onion, the onion produces the chemical irritant syn-Propanethial-S-oxide as a vapor, which, when it comes into contact with your eyes, irritates the lachrymal glands, which respond by producing tears.

● To end dry eyes, eat a banana every day. The roughly 400 milligrams of potassium in a banana relieves dry eye symptoms.

● Blinking once every five seconds lubricates the eyes. Staring intently at a computer or television screen without blinking frequently dries the eyes. Concentrate on blinking once every five seconds until your subconscious mind takes control of the job.

● To prevent dry eye symptoms, avoid air blowing from hair dryers, air conditioners, heaters, or fans toward your eyes.

● On windy days, wear wraparound eyeglasses, and while swimming, wear goggles (to protect your eyes from chemicals in the water that can dry your eyes).

● In winter, run a humidifier in your bedroom or office to add moisture to dry indoor air.

● Smoke can worsen dry eye symptoms. If you smoke, quit. And steer clear of any secondhand smoke.

- **Lipton Tea Bags.** Soothe tired eyes by immersing two Lipton Tea Bags in warm water, squeezing out the excess moisture, and placing them over your closed eyes for twenty minutes. The tannin in the tea reduces the puffiness and revitalizes dry eyes.

- **Sun-Maid Raisins.** To relieve dry eyes, eat a small box of Sun-Maid Raisins every day. People with dry eye frequently have low potassium levels. The 220 milligrams of potassium in a small box of raisins helps relieve dry eye symptoms.

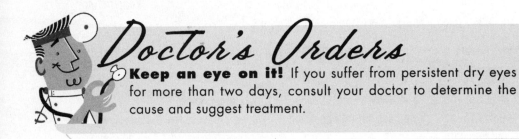

Doctor's Orders

Keep an eye on it! If you suffer from persistent dry eyes for more than two days, consult your doctor to determine the cause and suggest treatment.

Dry Hair and Split Ends

- **Bacardi Rum.** To revitalize dry hair, beat two egg yolks, add one tablespoon Bacardi Rum, and whisk well. Apply to hair, wait thirty minutes, shampoo, and rinse clean.

- **Budweiser.** To give dry hair great body, after shampooing, rinse hair with Budweiser beer, wait five minutes, and then rinse clean with water.

- **Castor Oil.** Treat split ends by rubbing Castor Oil between your palms and then rubbing your palms over the ends of your hair.

- **Cool Whip.** Apply Cool Whip to dry hair, wait thirty minutes, rinse clean, and shampoo. The coconut and palm kernel oils in the dessert topping condition hair, giving you a luxurious shine.

- **Dannon Yogurt.** In a bowl, mix five tablespoons Dannon Plain Yogurt and one egg yolk with a whisk to create a creamy paste. Set aside while you shampoo your hair and dry with a towel. Massage the conditioning mixture into your hair, cover with a plastic shower cap (or wrap your head in Saran Wrap—above the eyes, nose, and mouth), wrap in a warm towel, and wait fifteen minutes. Rinse your hair clean with warm water, followed by a final rinse of cold water. The lecithin in egg yolk helps enrich dry hair, adding volume and body.

- **Downy Fabric Softener.** If you run out of crème rinse, use a drop of Downy Fabric Softener in your final rinse to leave your hair tangle-free, soft, and smelling April fresh.

- **Dr. Teal's Epsom Salt.** Mix three tablespoons of your regular conditioner with three tablespoons Dr. Teal's Epsom Salt, and heat the mixture in a microwave oven. Let cool to the touch, work the warm mixture through your hair, and let sit for twenty minutes. Rinse with warm water. The magnesium sulfate helps revitalize dry hair.

- **Fruit of the Earth Aloe Vera Gel.** To revive dry hair, add one teaspoon Fruit of the Earth Aloe Vera Gel to your shampoo and massage the mixture into your scalp for five minutes when you wash your hair. Rinse thoroughly. Aloe gel heals and moisturizes dry hair.

- **Gerber Pears** and **Knox Gelatin.** Mix a five-ounce container of Gerber Pears with one teaspoon Knox Gelatin powder. After shampooing and rinsing your hair, apply the mixture to hair and massage into the scalp. Wait fifteen minutes, and then shampoo and rinse clean. The pears add texture and volume to hair, and the gelatin strengthens the shafts.

- **Knox Gelatin** and **Heinz Apple Cider Vinegar.** To revitalize dry, fragile, or brittle hair, mix one tablespoon Knox Gelatin powder and one cup of water, and let the mixture set slightly, not completely. Add one tablespoon Heinz Apple Cider Vinegar, and after shampooing and rinsing your hair, work the solution through your hair and let sit for ten minutes. The protein in the gelatin helps fortify and strengthen the hair shafts. Repeat once a week.

- **Kraft Mayo, Heinz Apple Cider Vinegar,** and **ReaLemon.** Mix one tablespoon Kraft Mayo, two tablespoons Heinz Apple Cider Vinegar, and two tablespoons ReaLemon lemon juice. Work into dry hair, wait twenty minutes, and then rinse clean with warm water.

- **Lipton Tea** and **McCormick Rosemary Leaves.** Brew one cup of Lipton Tea, add one tablespoon McCormick Rosemary Leaves, cover with a saucer, and steep for ten minutes. Let cool, pour through your hair, and massage. Rinse clean.

℞ STRANGE MEDICINE ℞

A HAIR-RAISING EXPERIENCE

● Harsh shampoos strip the sebaceous glands in your scalp that produce oil, causing dry, lifeless hair.

● Curly and frizzy hair is excessively porous and tends to be dry.

● Dry hair can result from a diet lacking the nutrients that cause the sebaceous glands to produce oil.

● Excessive blow-drying, sun exposure, swimming, sun or wind exposure, coloring treatments, straightening, or perms can dry out hair.

● Harsh chemicals or intense heat can strip away small sections of your hair's outer layer, and the stripped hair fails to retain moisture.

● Conditioners improve the hair's natural sheen by helping to smooth the hair cuticle.

● Commercial conditioners contain "cationic surfactants," which temporarily coat dry and damaged hair.

● Many people neglect to rinse all traces of conditioner from their hair. Be sure to rinse several times, otherwise the residue of conditioner leaves hair dull and limp.

● A conditioner or crème rinse replaces the oils stripped from the hair by shampooing.

● During the day, the hair follicles produce enough sebum (natural hair oil) to adequately coat the first three inches of hair closest to the scalp. Using a conditioner or crème rinse on the first three inches of hair can over-condition that area. Instead, apply the conditioner or crème rinse on hair three inches from the scalp to the ends, and comb the conditioner through the hair.

● Use the deep conditioning treatments listed in this chapter no more than once a week, otherwise a protein-based deep conditioner meant to strengthen and add body could cause your hair to become dry and brittle, and an oil-based deep conditioner could turn your hair limp and lifeless.

- **Miracle Whip.** Apply Miracle Whip to dry hair, wait thirty minutes, and then rinse several times before shampooing thoroughly. The oils in this miracle treatment revitalize dry hair and give it a great shine.

- **Now Sweet Almond Oil.** Put a few drops of Now Sweet Almond Oil on your fingertips and rub the oil into your hair. Wait twenty minutes, then shampoo and condition.

- **Pam Cooking Spray.** While standing in a shower stall, lightly spray your hair with Pam Cooking Spray and then run your fingers through your hair. The cooking oil conditions your hair and scalp. Shampoo and rinse clean.

- **Star Olive Oil.** Warm one-half cup Star Olive Oil in a microwave oven until slightly warm to the touch. Treat dry hair and split ends by massaging the olive oil into your hair, and then wrapping it in a warm towel for five minutes before shampooing and conditioning.

- **SueBee Honey.** To soften your hair and give it a great shine, mix one-half cup SueBee Honey and one egg. Apply the mixture to dry hair, comb it through, and then wait one hour. Rinse clean.

- **Wesson Canola Oil, Fleishmann's Margarine, SueBee Honey,** and **Aunt Jemima Original Syrup.** To condition damaged hair, mix one tablespoon each of Wesson Canola Oil, Fleishmann's Margarine, SueBee Honey, and Aunt Jemima Original Syrup. Heat briefly in a microwave oven, massage the warm syrupy mixture into your hair, wait fifteen minutes, then shampoo and rinse thoroughly.

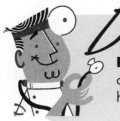

Doctor's Orders

Don't pull your hair out! If you experience persistent dry hair or inexplicable hair loss, consult a doctor to rule out an illness, hormonal imbalance, nutritional deficiency, or stress.

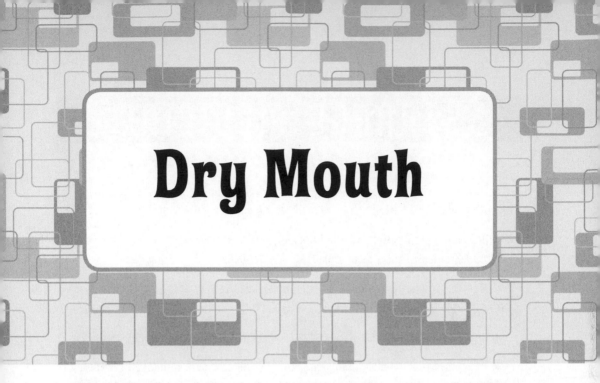

Dry Mouth

- **Arm & Hammer Baking Soda** and **Morton Salt.** Using a mouthwash that contains alcohol dries your mouth further. Instead, dissolve one-quarter teaspoon Arm & Hammer Baking Soda and one-eighth teaspoon Morton Salt in an eight-ounce glass of water, rinse with the homemade mouthwash, and spit out. The baking soda neutralizes acids in your mouth, and the salt kills bacteria.

- **Fruit of the Earth Aloe Vera Gel** and **Q-Tips Cotton Swabs.** To soothe inflamed gums from dry mouth, dip a Q-Tips Cotton Swab in Fruit of the Earth Aloe Vera Gel, and spread the gel on the affected gums. Refrain from eating or drinking for one hour. Aloe gel relieves burning and swollen gum tissue.

- **Heinz Apple Cider Vinegar.** To keep your mouth moist, add one-half teaspoon Heinz Apple Cider Vinegar to an eight-ounce glass of water, and drink eight glasses a day. The water keeps you hydrated and the vinegar stimulates saliva flow.

- **Life Savers Pep-O-Mint.** Sucking on a hard candy triggers saliva production, and the mint in Life Savers Pep-O-Mint stimulates even more saliva.

- **ReaLemon.** To keep your mouth moist, add one-half teaspoon ReaLemon lemon juice to an eight-ounce glass of water, and drink eight glasses a day. The water keeps you hydrated and the lemon juice stimulates saliva flow.

℞ STRANGE MEDICINE ℞

MAKING YOUR MOUTH WATER

- Lack of saliva production causes dry mouth, which, if chronic, allows the acid in your mouth produced by bacteria to decay teeth, erode gums, and cause mouth sores.

- Dry mouth often results from not drinking sufficient amounts of water during the day. Drink at least twelve 8-ounce glasses of water daily.

- Many prescription drugs cause dry mouth as a side effect, most notably anticholinergics, antidepressants, antihistamines, beta-blockers, diuretics, and pain relievers.

- Dry mouth is often the side effect of a disease, a drug, or radiation treatment for cancer.

- To improve your dry mouth symptoms, concentrate on breathing through your nose, rather than your mouth, and use a humidifier to add moisture to your bedroom or office.

- To combat dry mouth, don't rinse your mouth with a mouthwash that contains alcohol, which is a drying agent.

- If you smoke, quit. Smoking or chewing tobacco can increase dry mouth symptoms.

- **Tabasco Pepper Sauce.** Sprinkle a few drops of Tabasco Pepper Sauce on your meals to trigger your salivary glands to generate more saliva.

- **Wrigley's Spearmint Gum.** To spur saliva production and keep your mouth moist, chew a stick of Wrigley's Spearmint Gum. Chewing stimulates the salivary glands.

Doctor's Orders

Open your mouth! If dry mouth lasts for several days, consult your dentist.

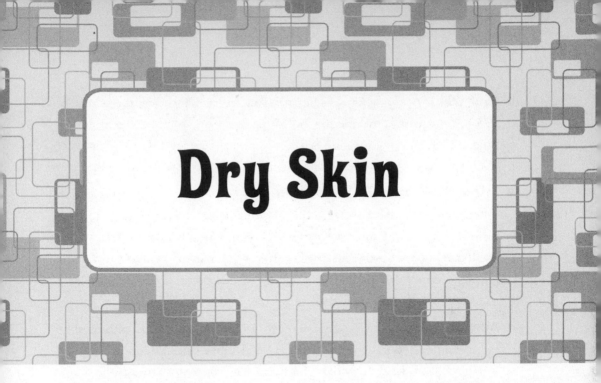

Dry Skin

- **Alberto VO5 Conditioning Hairdressing.** After taking a shower and patting yourself dry, rub a dab of Alberto VO5 Conditioning Hairdressing over your damp skin to seal in moisture.

- **Arm & Hammer Baking Soda.** Give yourself soft, smooth-feeling skin and a relaxing bath by dissolving one-half cup Arm & Hammer Baking Soda in a bathtub filled with warm water.

- **Bag Balm.** To heal and rejuvenate dry skin, apply a thin coat of Bag Balm, the salve developed by Vermont farmers to prevent the udders of cows from chapping, to your damp skin after taking a shower.

- **Castor Oil.** This natural emollient—first used as a skin softener throughout Mesopotamia and ancient Egypt—doubles as a moisturizer. Rub a few drops into your skin to seal in moisture.

- **Chicken of the Sea Salmon, Chicken of the Sea Sardines,** or **Chicken of the Sea Tuna.** To keep your skin healthy, eat salmon, sardines, or tuna at least twice a week. All these fish add the essential fatty acids commonly known as omega-3 oils to your diet, helping the body regenerate skin.

- **Cool Whip.** Applying Cool Whip as a skin cream moisturizes the skin. The coconut and palm kernel oils in Cool Whip revive and soothe the skin. For an invigorating and moisturizing facial, cover your face with Cool Whip, wait twenty minutes, and then wash clean with warm water followed by cold water.

- **Crisco All-Vegetable Shortening.** Cover your face with a washcloth dampened with warm water and soak your hands in warm water for five minutes. Seal in the moisture by coating your damp hands and face with a small dab of Crisco All-Vegetable Shortening. Or, after taking a shower and patting yourself dry, moisturize your damp body by rubbing in a few dabs of Crisco All-Vegetable Shortening.

- **Dannon Yogurt.** Before taking a shower, cover your entire body with Dannon Plain Yogurt (add an optional teaspoon Star Olive Oil, if desired), wait ten minutes, then rinse clean with warm water. The yogurt moisturizes the skin.

- **Dove.** Rather than using harsh soaps that strip too much natural oil from your skin, switch to Dove, a superfatted soap made with one-quarter pure moisturizing cream and mild cleansers. Dove leaves skin feeling clean, soft, and smooth—unlike ordinary soaps whose drying ingredients rob skin of its natural moisture.

- **Dr. Teal's Epsom Salt.** To relieve dry skin, fill the bathtub with warm water and add two cups Dr. Teal's Epsom Salt. Soak for twenty minutes, giving the magnesium in the Epsom Salt plenty of time to moisturize your skin.

- **Dynasty Sesame Seed Oil.** For a natural moisturizer, use Dynasty Sesame Seed Oil, an emollient extracted from sesame seeds that blocks roughly 30 percent of UV rays and is a common ingredient in sunscreen lotions.

- **Fleischmann's Margarine.** To moisturize and soften dry skin, massage softened Fleischmann's Margarine over your entire body, let it penetrate the skin, then shower clean in warm water. The vegetable oils in the margarine soften skin.

- **Fruit of the Earth Aloe Vera Gel.** To moisturize dry skin, rub soothing Fruit of the Earth Aloe Vera Gel into your face and body.

- **Grapeola Grape Seed Oil.** This all-natural oil extracted from grape seeds makes an excellent moisturizer because it is a nonallergenic emollient and the least greasy oil there is.

- **Hain Safflower Oil.** For a natural moisturizer, rub a few drops of Hain Safflower Oil into your skin.

- **Heinz Apple Cider Vinegar.** Adding one cup Heinz Apple Cider Vinegar—which contains iron, phosphorous, potassium, magnesium, and sodium—to bathwater softens skin and helps restore its natural acid balance. Soak for roughly twenty minutes.

- **Johnson's Baby Oil.** To relieve extremely dry skin, after your shower or bath, apply a few drops of Johnson's Baby Oil while your skin is still moist. The mineral oil lasts longer than a moisturizer and prevents moisture from evaporating from the surface of your skin.

- **Loriva Extra Sunflower Oil.** A few drops of sunflower oil, extracted from sunflower seeds, makes an excellent moisturizer, leaving skin soft and smooth.

- **Lubriderm.** To relieve dry, flaky skin, apply Lubriderm two times during the day. The moisturizer lubricates the skin and seals in moisture.

- **McCormick Pure Vanilla Extract** and **Crisco All-Vegetable Shortening.** Mix one-half tablespoon McCormick Pure Vanilla Extract and one tablespoon Crisco All-Vegetable Shortening, and massage the mixture into your hands. The vanilla provides aromatherapy, and the shortening moisturizes the skin.

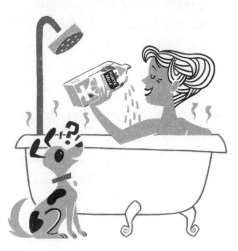

- **Minute Maid Orange Juice.** Add one cup Minute Maid Orange Juice to warm bathwater, and soak for twenty minutes to rejuvenate dull skin.

- **Miracle Whip.** Applying Miracle Whip as a skin cream moisturizes and rejuvenates dry skin. You can also give yourself a facial by applying Miracle Whip as a face mask. Leave it on for twenty minutes, and then wash off with warm water, followed by cold water. Miracle Whip cleanses the skin and tightens the pores. Or exfoliate dead skin by rubbing a dab of Miracle Whip into your feet, knees, elbows, or face. Let sit for a few minutes, then massage with your fingertips.

- **Nestlé Carnation Nonfat Dry Milk.** Add a handful of Nestlé Carnation Nonfat Dry Milk powder to warm running bathwater for a luxurious milk bath worthy of Cleopatra. The lactic acid in the milk exfoliates the skin, and the proteins in the milk leave the skin feeling silky smooth.

- **Now Sweet Almond Oil.** For a fragrant moisturizer, use Now Sweet Almond Oil, an emollient that rejuvenates the skin.

- **Noxzema.** Noxzema, the skin cream originally invented in 1914 by pharmacist Dr. George Bunting in the prescription room of his Baltimore drugstore as a sunburn remedy, moisturizes dry skin. The camphor, menthol, and eucalyptus oil also provide soothing aromatherapy.

- **Quaker Oats** and **L'eggs Sheer Energy Panty Hose.** To relieve dry skin, grind one cup uncooked Quaker Oats in a blender, pour a few tablespoons of the fine powder into the foot cut from a clean, used pair of L'eggs Sheer Energy Panty Hose, and tie a knot in the open end. Fill a bathtub with lukewarm water, pour the remaining powdered oats into the tub, and, while soaking for fifteen minutes, saturate the panty hose sachet with water, and gently rub it over the affected area.

- **Quaker Oats, SueBee Honey,** and **ReaLemon.** In a blender, grind two cups Quaker Oats into a fine powder. In a bowl, mix the powdered Quaker Oats with enough SueBee Honey and ReaLemon lemon juice to make a thick paste. Apply the sticky substance to your body, let sit for ten minutes, and then rinse with warm water. The citric acid in the lemon juice disinfects the pores, and the honey is hygroscopic, moisturizing the skin.

- **ReaLemon** and **Johnson's Baby Oil.** Mix one tablespoon ReaLemon lemon juice and one-half cup Johnson's Baby Oil, and add the mixture to your bathwater to soften skin and infuse the air with soothing aromatherapy.

- **Star Olive Oil.** Warm one-half cup Star Olive Oil in a microwave oven until slightly warm to the touch and massage this restorative emollient into

℞ STRANGE MEDICINE ℞

SAVING YOUR OWN SKIN

- Dry skin typically results from exposure to hot or cold weather with low humidity levels, living in an environment with central heating or cooling, excessive bathing, or using harsh soaps and shampoos.

- Immediately after bathing, pat yourself with a towel without drying yourself completely and apply moisturizer to your damp skin. The moisturizer helps trap water in the surface cells, keeping your skin moist and healthy.

- After applying a moisturizer that contains humectants, gently mist your face with a trigger-spray bottle filled with water. Mist your face three times a day or as frequently as possible. The humectants in the moisturizer retain water.

- A simple bar of soap with a pH value between 11 and 14 can be used to cleanse skin. If you have dry skin, use a superfatted soap with moisturizer added. If you have sensitive skin, use a fragrance-free mild soap without any unnecessary ingredients.

- Drinking a minimum of eight 8-ounce glasses of water a day moisturizes the skin from the inside out.

- To keep your skin moist and healthy, limit your showers and baths to less than fifteen minutes, and use warm (not hot) water. Long hot showers remove the natural oils from your skin.

- To prevent dry skin, use a humidifier in your bedroom or office to moisten hot, dry indoor air.

dry skin. The monounsaturated fat in the oil hydrates the skin without leaving a greasy film.

- **SueBee Honey** and **Heinz White Vinegar.** Add one-quarter cup SueBee Honey and one-quarter cup Heinz White Vinegar to your bathwater to leave your skin feeling baby smooth.

- **Uncle Ben's Instant Brown Rice** and **L'eggs Sheer Energy Panty Hose.** Cut off one foot from a pair of clean, used L'eggs Sheer Energy Panty Hose, fill the foot with Uncle Ben's Instant Brown Rice, tie a knot in the open end, and rub the sachet all over your skin while you take a bath. Brown rice doubles as a moisturizing exfoliant.

- **Vaseline Petroleum Jelly.** After getting out of the shower or bathtub, apply a thin coat of Vaseline Petroleum Jelly as a safe, effective moisturizer that thwarts dry skin.

- **Wesson Canola Oil.** A few drops of this fragrant emollient, rubbed into your body, moisturizes the skin.

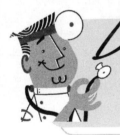

Doctor's Orders

Left high and dry? If you experience dry skin or itching for more than a few weeks, consult a dermatologist to diagnose the cause of the rash.

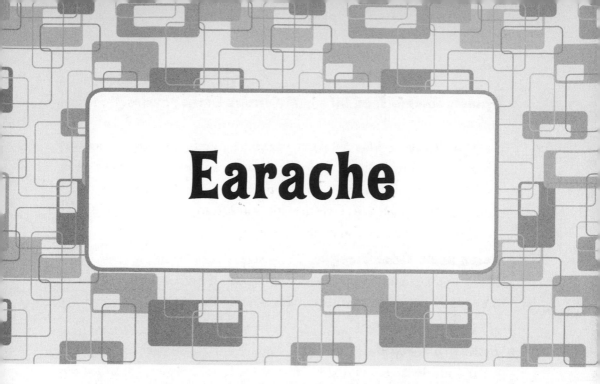

Earache

- **Campbell's Chicken Noodle Soup** and **Tabasco Pepper Sauce.** Add one teaspoon Tabasco Pepper Sauce to a bowl of Campbell's Chicken Noodle Soup, mix well, and eat. The hot soup and the capsaicin in the Tabasco Pepper Sauce spurs mucus production, which can drain your Eustachian tubes, relieving the pressure causing the ear pain.

- **Conair Hair Dryer.** Set a Conair Hair Dryer on warm, hold it roughly twelve inches from your head, and blow warm air into your ear. The warmth stimulates circulation to the ear and helps relieve the pressure responsible for the pain.

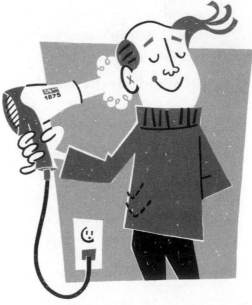

- **Dynasty Sesame Seed Oil** and **McCormick Garlic Powder.** To relieve an earache, add one-quarter teaspoon McCormick Garlic Powder to one teaspoon Dynasty Sesame Seed Oil, warm the mixture to body temperature (98 degrees Fahrenheit) in a microwave oven, and using a dropper, place four drops in the ear canal. Let sit for ten minutes, and then tilt your head to drain out the oil. Rinse clean with water from a bulb syringe. Garlic doubles as an antibiotic and antibacterial.

- **Heinz Apple Cider Vinegar.** To assuage earache pain, mix equal parts Heinz Apple Cider Vinegar and warm water, and use a dropper to put four drops of the solution in the ear canal. Let sit for ten minutes and then drain. Do this four times a day.

- **Hydrogen Peroxide.** To soothe an earache, use a dropper to fill the ear canal with Hydrogen Peroxide every three to four hours. Let sit for five minutes and then drain. The hydrogen peroxide kills bacteria, helps reduce inflammation, and numbs the pain.

- **Johnson's Baby Oil.** To reduce the discomfort of an earache, warm some Johnson's Baby Oil to 98 degrees Fahrenheit (by holding the bottle under running hot water for a few minutes), and then use a dropper to fill the ear canal with the warm oil. Let sit for a few minutes, and then use a bulb syringe filled with warm water to gently flush the oil from your ear, draining it onto a hand towel.

- **McCormick Garlic Powder.** To combat an earache and give your immune system a boost, use McCormick Garlic Powder in your cooking, or once a day eat a slice of lightly buttered bread sprinkled with one-half teaspoon garlic powder. As a natural antibiotic, garlic helps fight bacteria and viruses.

- **Morton Salt.** To alleviate an earache, dissolve one teaspoon Morton Salt in an eight-ounce glass of warm water, and gargle with the salty solution. The warmth from the liquid helps increase blood flow to the Eustachian tubes, providing relief.

BELIEVING YOUR EARS

- Children get frequent ear infections because the developing Eustachian tubes run horizontally from the nasal cavity to the middle ear, allowing bacteria to enter. In adults, Eustachian tubes run vertically, preventing bacteria from infiltrating.

- Earaches can be caused by an infection of the outer ear, an infection of the middle ear behind the eardrum, a cold, allergies, a sore throat, or tooth pain.

- Flying in an airplane while suffering from ear problems can result in excruciating pain. Taking an over-the-counter decongestant an hour before the flight can relieve congestion in the Eustachian tubes, preventing pain during changes in air pressure.

- A bacterial or viral infection of the middle ear causes inflammation and fluid build up of in the small chamber behind the eardrum that contains three tiny bones—the *malleus* (hammer), *incus* (anvil), and *stapes* (stirrup).

- Inflammation and fluid buildup in the middle ear can be excruciatingly painful.

- Most ear infections clear up on their own within a week to ten days.

- Elevating your head at night when you sleep can help prevent postnasal drip from clogging your Eustachian tubes.

- The mere act of swallowing, yawning, or drinking a glass of water opens the Eustachian tubes, allowing them to drain.

- Doctors tend to prescribe antibiotics to treat an ear infection in children under two years of age or in anyone with moderate to severe pain.

- **Smirnoff Vodka.** To kill the bacteria that might be causing the earache, use a dropper to put four drops of Smirnoff Vodka in the sore ear. Let sit for ten minutes and drain.

- **Star Olive Oil.** To relieve an earache, warm one teaspoon Star Olive Oil to body temperature (98 degrees Fahrenheit) in a microwave oven, and using a dropper, place four drops in the ear canal. Let sit for ten minutes, and then tilt your head to drain out the oil onto a hand towel. Rinse clean with water from a bulb syringe.

- **Trident.** To stymie a middle-ear infection, chew two pieces of Trident sugarless gum for five minutes five times a day. The mere act of chewing opens the Eustachian tubes. The sweetener xylitol—an organic sugar substitute extracted from corn husks, birch, and various berries—impedes the growth of *Streptococcus pneumoniae*, the bacteria responsible for middle-ear infections. A 1996 study in Finland showed that children who chewed two pieces of sugarless gum sweetened with xylitol for five minutes five times a day for two months had 25 percent fewer ear infections.

- **Uncle Ben's Converted Brand Rice.** Fill a clean sock with Uncle Ben's Converted Brand Rice, tie a knot in the end, and heat in the microwave oven for one to two minutes. Making sure the sock isn't too hot, hold it against the painful ear. The rice-filled sock conforms to the shape of the ear, allowing the warmth to soothe the pain. The homemade heating pad is also reusable.

Doctor's Orders

Play it by ear! If you suffer from a severely painful earache, experience discharge from the ear, or have a fever above 100 degrees Fahrenheit, consult your doctor immediately.

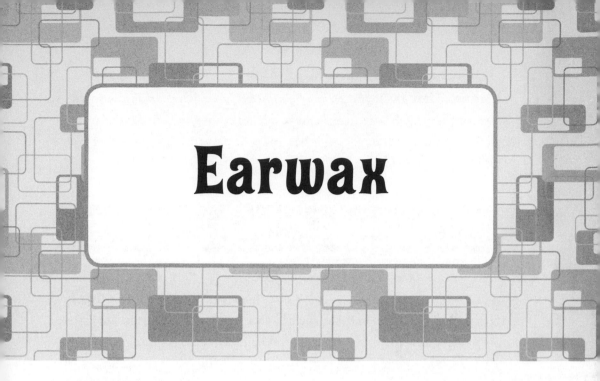

Earwax

- **Conair Hair Dryer.** After washing wax from your ears with any of the tips in this section, set a Conair Hair Dryer on the coolest setting and hold it roughly twelve inches from your ear to air-dry each ear.

- **Hydrogen Peroxide.** To soften earwax buildup, lie down with your head tilted to one side, and using a dropper, fill the ear canal with Hydrogen Peroxide. Let sit for three minutes, allowing the liquid to bubble away at the wax, and then let the hydrogen peroxide flow out onto a hand towel. Use a bulb syringe to gently fill the ear canal with warm water, let sit, and then drain onto the hand towel, cleaning away the softened wax. Repeat for the other ear. The hydrogen peroxide softens the wax.

- **Johnson's Baby Oil.** Soften the wax in your ears by tilting your head to one side and placing a few drops of warm Johnson's Baby Oil in the ear canal with a dropper. (You can warm the oil by holding the bottle under running hot water for a few minutes.) Let sit for fifteen minutes, and then use a bulb syringe filled with warm water to gently flush the oil from your ear, draining onto a hand towel. The warm mineral oil melts the wax and carries it out of the ear.

● **Kleenex Tissues.** If you wear a hearing aid, use a Kleenex Tissue to wipe it clean every night when you remove it before going to bed. The tissue collects the wax residue from the hearing aid, preventing excess wax from building up in your ear.

℞ STRANGE MEDICINE ℞

THE WHOLE BALL OF WAX

● Produced by glands in the ear canal, earwax (medically known as cerumen) lubricates the skin, helps ward off bacteria and other microorganisms, and traps dust and dirt.

● Some people produce excess earwax, which can clog the ear canal, limit hearing, and cause itching, pain, ringing in the ear, or equilibrium problems.

● When earwax hardens, forming a plug next to the eardrum, a doctor is needed to remove the wax.

● Having a doctor remove earwax may seem excessive, but attempting to remove hardened earwax can easily damage the ear canal or eardrum.

● Never stick a cotton swab in your ear to clean wax from the ear canal. A cotton swab pushes the wax further into the ear canal, where the wax hardens. A cotton swab inserted into your ear can also puncture your eardrum.

● Never insert a bobby pin, paper clip, or pencil tip into your ear. Doing so risks tearing your eardrum.

● Never use "ear candling" to remove earwax. This misguided method involves placing a long hollow candle into the ear, lighting the protruding end, and letting the flame burn for roughly fifteen minutes with the intent of creating negative pressure to get the earwax to stick to the candle. Ear candling has caused burns, ear canal obstructions, and perforations of the eardrum. A 1996 study by Spokane Ear, Nose and Throat Clinic showed that a burning candle does not produce any negative pressure in the ear, and that the only deposit removed from the ear is candle wax.

- **Star Olive Oil.** To loosen excess earwax, lean your head to one side and, using a dropper, put a few drops of warm Star Olive Oil in your ear. Let sit for fifteen minutes. Drain and rinse clean. Repeat for the other ear. Give yourself this treatment four times a day. The olive oil softens and gradually loosens the wax, which eventually migrates out of your ear on its own.

- **Vaseline Petroleum Jelly.** To prevent hardened wax buildup from forming in your ear, apply a light coat of Vaseline Petroleum Jelly inside the opening of each ear canal. The lubricant keeps earwax moist and stops it from drying out and building up into a crust.

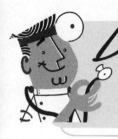

Doctor's Orders

Come clean! If none of these home remedies work to remove excess wax from your ear, see your doctor for an ear lavage to wash the impacted wax from your ear with a stream of water.

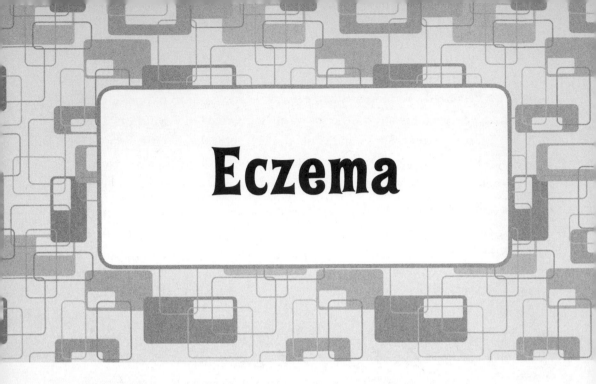

Eczema

- **Band-Aid Bandages.** To stop yourself from unconsciously scratching an eczema–affected area within easy reach, cover the spot with a small Band-Aid Bandage to remind yourself to cease scratching the patch.

- **Chicken of the Sea Salmon, Chicken of the Sea Sardines,** or **Chicken of the Sea Tuna.** To reduce eczema, eat salmon, sardines, or tuna three times a week. All these fish add the essential fatty acids commonly known as omega-3 oils to your diet, reducing inflammation and helping the body regenerate skin.

- **Cortaid.** To stop the itching, apply a thin coat of Cortaid. This hydrocortisone cream is an anti-inflammatory preparation that treats the symptoms, not the cause. Use the cream only until the rash subsides. (Be aware that daily use of a hydrocortisone cream for more than three weeks can thin and damage the skin.)

- **Crisco All-Vegetable Shortening.** To seal in moisture and protect the eczema from irritants, apply a thin coat of Crisco All-Vegetable Shortening to the affected skin after bathing.

- **Dannon Yogurt.** If you suffer from eczema, eat a cup of Dannon Plain Nonfat Yogurt every day. The beneficial *Lactobacillus acidophilus* (probiotics) in yogurt help maintain a healthy balance of bacteria in your digestive system, which, studies show, reduces eczema.

- **Dove** and **Johnson's Baby Shampoo.** To help avoid drying the skin further and prevent eczema from flaring up, use Dove Sensitive Skin Unscented (a hypoallergenic, fragrance-free moisturizing soap) and Johnson's Baby Shampoo (a mild shampoo) in the bath or shower.

- **Fruit of the Earth Aloe Vera Gel.** To heal eczema outbreaks, slather Fruit of the Earth Aloe Vera Gel on the affected area several times a day. Aloe vera gel abounds with anti-inflammatory and healing compounds.

- **Johnson's Baby Oil.** After taking a shower or bath, apply a few drops of Johnson's Baby Oil to your damp skin. Mineral oil lasts longer than ordinary moisturizers do and prevents water from evaporating from the surface of your skin.

- **Krazy Glue.** To repair a painful crack in your skin, hold the skin together, apply Krazy Glue over the crack, and let dry. Krazy Glue contains nearly the identical ingredients as Band-Aid Brand Liquid Bandage, an instant glue used to seal lacerations.

- **Lipton Green Tea.** To soothe eczema, brew a strong cup of Lipton Green Tea, let cool, and lay a washcloth dampened with the tea over the affected area for ten minutes. The tannins in green tea soothe and strengthen the epidermis and reduce inflammation.

- **McCormick Ground Turmeric.** To fight eczema, take one tablespoon McCormick Ground Turmeric daily by simply sprinkling it on your food or using the spice in recipes for rice, casseroles, soups, and stews. Curcumin, an antioxidant in turmeric, doubles as an anti-inflammatory and also stimulates the immune system. (Turmeric may increase the likelihood of bleeding when taken in combination with the blood thinner Coumadin or other anticoagulant medications.)

- **Miracle Whip.** To remedy flaky, scaly skin and soothe eczema, rub Miracle Whip into the affected area and let sit for fifteen minutes. The oil and vinegar in the Miracle Whip seem to moisturize and rejuvenate the dry skin and relieve the itch of eczema. To exfoliate dead skin, rub a dab of Miracle Whip into the affected area, let sit for a few minutes, and then massage with your fingertips. You can also give yourself a facial by applying Miracle Whip as a face mask.

SCRATCHING THE SURFACE

● An itchy inflammation of the skin, eczema is a chronic condition that periodically flares and subsides, generally appearing on the hands, feet, arms, and behind the knees.

● No one knows exactly what causes eczema, but doctors suspect that a genetic tendency for sensitive skin combined with a malfunction in the body's immune system may be responsible.

● To relieve eczema, keep your skin away from water as much as possible. Water washes away the oils that keep your skin moist. Avoid washing your hands, doing the dishes, or taking long baths or showers. Limit your baths and showers to less than ten minutes and use lukewarm water.

● The most common form of eczema—atopic eczema—causes red, itchy skin and sometimes fluid-filled blisters.

● Contact dermatitis, another type of eczema, results from contact with an irritant like cosmetics, detergent, or soap.

● Scratching an eczema rash can increase the itch and cause additional inflammation. Breaking the skin invites bacteria that commonly live on the skin—most notably *Staphylococcus aureus*—to infect the broken skin. To prevent yourself from scratching, cover the itchy area, trim your nails, and wear gloves to bed at night.

● Cutting your fingernails short helps prevent damage to the skin should you inadvertently scratch yourself.

● To help reduce itching and soothe inflammation, run a humidifier in your bedroom or office to put moisture in the air. Hot, dry indoor air can worsen itching and flaking.

● To prevent eczema from flaring up, bathe less frequently and when doing so, limit your showers or baths to less than ten minutes and use warm (not hot) water. Immediately after bathing, pat yourself with a towel without drying yourself completely and apply moisturizer to your damp skin. The moisturizer helps trap water in the surface cells, keeping your skin moist and healthy.

Leave it on for twenty minutes, and then wash off with warm water, followed by cold water. Miracle Whip cleanses the skin and tightens the pores.

- **Nestlé Carnation Condensed Milk.** To relieve the itch from eczema, saturate a washcloth with Nestlé Carnation Condensed Milk, and lay the cloth over the affected area for fifteen minutes. Repeat when necessary.

- **Noxzema.** When a customer told Dr. George Bunting, "Your sunburn cream sure knocked my eczema," Bunting changed the name of Dr. Bunting's Sunburn Remedy to Noxzema—a clever combination of the misspelled word *knocks* and the last two syllables of the word *eczema*. While still used primarily as a sunburn cream and moisturizer, Noxzema soothes eczema. Simply apply a thin coat to the affected area.

- **Pam Cooking Spray.** After bathing, seal in moisture by spraying your skin with a light coat of Pam Cooking Spray. The vegetable oil moisturizes dry skin. (Do not go out in the sun with your unprotected skin coated with vegetable oil; otherwise you risk sunburn.)

- **Planters Walnuts.** To reduce inflammation caused by eczema, eat Planters Walnuts. One ounce of walnuts contains 2.6 grams of omega-3 fatty acids, which decrease inflammation and strengthen the immune system.

- **Quaker Oats.** To relieve eczema, grind one cup uncooked Quaker Oats in a blender, and add the oats to your bathwater. Oats soothe itchy skin.

- **Vaseline Petroleum Jelly.** After bathing, apply a thin coat of Vaseline Petroleum Jelly to your skin as a moisturizer. The petroleum jelly seals in moisture and protects the skin from irritants.

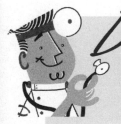

Doctor's Orders

Have a thick skin? If your eczema spreads, constantly recurs, shows signs of infection, or prevents you from sleeping at night, contact your doctor to rule out a food allergy or obtain a prescription for a medicated ointment.

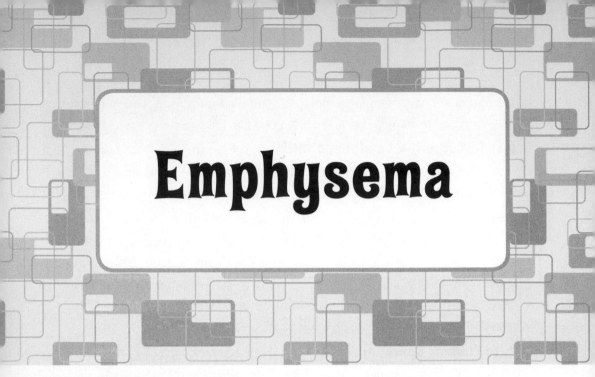

Emphysema

- **Chicken of the Sea Salmon, Chicken of the Sea Sardines,** or **Chicken of the Sea Tuna.** To decrease lung inflammation and ease breathing, try eating salmon, sardines, or tuna four times a week. All these fish add the fatty acids commonly known as omega-3 oils to your diet, reducing inflammation and pain, strengthening the immune system, and increasing resistance to stress. A 1994 study at the University of Minnesota found that current or former smokers who ate four servings of fish every week had one-third the risk of getting emphysema compared with smokers who ate little fish.

- **Kretschmer Wheat Germ.** To help treat the symptoms and side effects of emphysema, sprinkle a few tablespoons of Kretschmer Wheat Germ on your morning bowl of oatmeal. The vitamin E, B vitamins, magnesium, potassium, iron, and zinc in wheat germ boost the immune system.

- **McCormick Garlic Powder.** To alleviate the symptoms of emphysema and give your immune system a boost, use McCormick Garlic Powder in your cooking, or once a day eat a slice of lightly buttered bread sprinkled with one-half teaspoon garlic powder. Aside from being a natural antibiotic, garlic contains alliin, a chemical that liquefies mucus.

☙ STRANGE MEDICINE ☙

BREATHE A SIGH OF RELIEF

● Smoking cigarettes causes emphysema, an irreversible lung disease that causes mild to severe shortness of breath. The oxidants in cigarette smoke damage the alveoli, the tiny air sacs in the lungs that transport oxygen from the air into the blood and pump out carbon dioxide.

● Corticosteroids, the drugs used to treat emphysema, cause side effects that include diabetes and osteoporosis.

● A respiratory infection in a person with emphysema can quickly snowball into a fatal case of pneumonia.

● Unless you quit smoking, no home remedy will help relieve emphysema. For ways to quit smoking, see page 343.

● Cigarette smoke and other airborne irritants exacerbate emphysema. Steer clear of smoke-filled rooms, air fresheners, aerosol sprays, or any environment tainted with fumes.

● A high-quality HEPA air filter can remove irritants from the air in your home, bedroom, and office.

● To avoid catching respiratory infections that can worsen emphysema, get an annual flu shot and a pneumonia vaccination. Stay away from people with a cold or flu. And during cold and flu season, wash your hands frequently and keep a small bottle of hand sanitizer nearby to use whenever necessary.

● Exercising regularly can significantly increase your lung capacity. Walk thirty minutes every day, or lift small two-pound weights to exercise the muscles in your neck, shoulders, and chest.

● To protect yourself from complications from emphysema, wear a soft scarf over your mouth and nose before going outside in cold weather. Breathing cold air can cause the bronchial tract to spasm. Breathing through the scarf warms the air before it enters your lungs, preventing this problem.

- **Planters Dry Roasted Almonds, Planters Dry Roasted Cashews,** or **Planters Dry Roasted Peanuts.** Eating foods high in magnesium—like Planters Dry Roasted Almonds, Planters Dry Roasted Cashews, or Planters Dry Roasted Peanuts—helps keep healthy lungs functioning properly. One ounce of almonds provides 80 milligrams of magnesium, one ounce of cashews provides 75 milligrams, and one ounce of dry roasted peanuts provides 50 milligrams.

- **Planters Sunflower Kernels** or **Planters Dry Roasted Almonds.** To help protect your body from some of the damaging effects of smoking, eat one-quarter cup Planters Sunflower Kernels or Planters Dry Roasted Almonds every day. Sunflower seeds and almonds are packed with vitamin E, which can help protect your body from some of the damaging effects of smoking and enhance the immune response. One-quarter cup of sunflower seed kernels provides 22.68 milligrams of vitamin E, or 143 percent of the recommended daily allowance. One-quarter cup of almonds provides 15 milligrams of vitamin E, or 100 percent of the recommended daily allowance.

- **ReaLemon.** To relieve the symptoms of emphysema, take one teaspoon ReaLemon lemon juice several times a day before or between meals.

Doctor's Orders

As I live and breathe! Emphysema is a serious disease requiring professional medical attention.

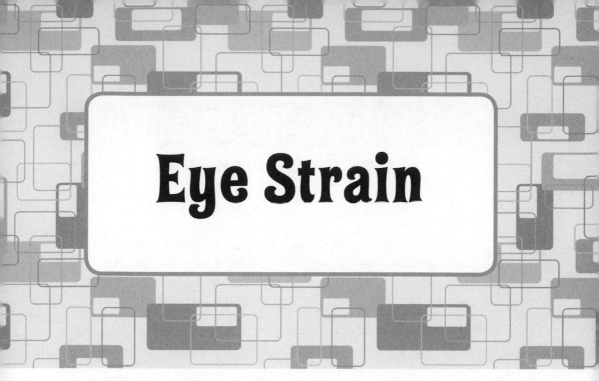

Eye Strain

- **Birds Eye Frozen Peas** and **Bounty Paper Towels.** To reduce the swelling of puffy eyes, ease the pain, and constrict the blood vessels to prevent discoloration, cover a bag of Birds Eye Frozen Peas with a sheet of Bounty Paper Towels, and place the bag over your puffy eyes for ten minutes. The frozen peas act like small ice cubes, soothing and reducing the inflammation, and the bag of peas conforms to the shape of your face. The paper towel creates a layer of insulation to prevent frostbite. Refreeze the bag of peas for future ice-pack use. Be sure to label the bag for ice-pack use only. If you want to eat the peas, cook them after they thaw the first time, never after refreezing.

- **Fruit of the Earth Aloe Vera Gel** and **Dynasty Sesame Seed Oil.** Mix two tablespoons Fruit of the Earth Aloe Vera Gel and one tablespoon Dynasty Sesame Seed Oil with a whisk. Apply to the area around your eye with the fingertip of your middle finger in a gentle circular motion. The sesame seed oil reduces puffiness, and the aloe vera gel moisturizes the skin.

- **Gerber Bananas.** To reduce circles under your eyes, spread the contents of a five-ounce container of Gerber Bananas over your clean, dry face, wait ten minutes, and then rinse clean with cool water. The bananas leave your

A SIGHT FOR SORE EYES

● The best way to relieve eye strain is to simply close your weary eyes and give them a brief rest.

● To prevent eye strain caused by staring at a computer or television screen for hours at a time, every twenty minutes stare at a faraway object for thirty seconds to let your eyes readjust. Doing so exercises the muscles that focus your eyes and gives them a reprieve.

● Wear sunglasses in bright sunlight. Otherwise, squinting will inevitably bring on a case of eye ache.

● Drinking eight 8-ounce glasses of water daily can help keep your eyes moist by keeping your body properly hydrated.

● Blinking once every five seconds lubricates the eyes and relaxes the eye muscles. Staring intently at a computer or television screen without blinking frequently dries the eyes. Concentrate on blinking once every five seconds until your subconscious mind takes control of the job.

● To soothe your tired eyes quickly and efficiently, rub your hands together briskly and place the heel of your palms against your closed eyes for ten seconds. The warmth from your hands relaxes the eye muscles.

● For another simple way to relieve eye strain, dampen a washcloth with cool water, fold it in half, and place it over your eyes for five minutes.

● To make working at the computer less straining on your eyes, increase the brightness or contrast of your display to increase the clarity. Also, increase the zoom in whatever program you're using to enlarge your view of the type.

● Make sure you have sufficient light when reading a book, newspaper, or magazine to avoid straining your eyes.

skin feeling soft, and the potassium content helps eliminate circles under your eyes.

- **Lipton Tea Bags.** Dampen two Lipton Tea Bags with warm water, lie down, and cover your eyes with the tea bags for five to ten minutes. The tannin from the tea relieves eye strain.

- **Preparation H.** Reduce puffy bags under your eyes by carefully rubbing Preparation H into the skin around the eyes. The hemorrhoid ointment acts as a vasoconstrictor and relieves swelling. (Just be careful not to get it in your eyes.)

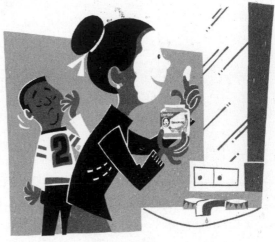

- **Quaker Oats.** Soothe puffy eyes by mixing up one-half cup Quaker Oats according to the directions on the canister, chill in the refrigerator, then apply to your closed eyes. Wait ten minutes, then wash clean.

- **Uncle Ben's Converted Brand Rice.** Fill a clean sock with uncooked Uncle Ben's Converted Brand Rice, tie a knot in the end, and heat the sock in a microwave oven for sixty seconds. Let cool to the touch, and then place the warm sock over your closed eyes for ten minutes to relieve any soreness. The homemade heating pad conforms to the shape of your face and is reusable.

Doctor's Orders

Don't bat an eye! If you experience pain in your eye or sensitivity to light, consult a doctor immediately.

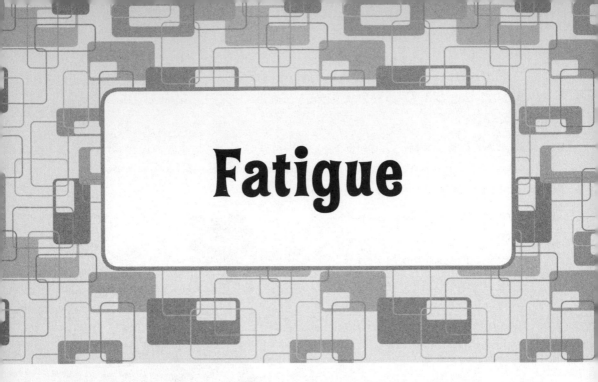

Fatigue

- **Angostura Aromatic Bitters** and **Canada Dry Club Soda.** To revitalize your being, add several dashes of Angostura Aromatic Bitters to an eight-ounce glass of Canada Dry Club Soda, and drink the elixir. The tincture of the gentian root stimulates digestion, possibly reversing fatigue due to a nutritional deficiency. In any case, the bitter tonic is sure to reinvigorate your senses.

- **Grandma's Robust Molasses.** The most common cause of fatigue is an iron deficiency. Eating one tablespoon Grandma's Robust Molasses, which provides 3.5 milligrams of iron (approximately 43 percent of the recommended daily allowance), can help rejuvenate you. Dissolve a tablespoon of the blackstrap molasses in a cup of hot water, add it to a cup of tea, or spread it on a cracker.

- **Heinz Apple Cider Vinegar.** To reenergize yourself, drink two tablespoons Heinz Apple Cider Vinegar added to a glass of water. The amino acids in apple cider vinegar counteract the fatigue-causing lactic acid built up in your body from stress and exercise, and the potassium and enzymes in the vinegar relieve lethargy.

- **Heinz Baked Beanz.** To keep your energy levels humming along smoothly, eat one-half cup Heinz Baked Beanz. Baked beans slow the release of blood sugar into your bloodstream, giving your body and brain a steady source of fuel, keeping you energized.

- **Kellogg's All-Bran.** To give yourself more energy, eat one cup Kellogg's All-Bran cereal every day. One cup of Kellogg's All-Bran contains 70 percent of the daily value of phosphorous, a mineral that the body uses to metabolize carbohydrates, fat, and protein, converting them into energy.

- **Kellogg's Rice Krispies.** To help boost your energy levels, start your day with a bowl of Kellogg's Rice Krispies. One serving contains 25 percent of the daily recommended allowance of thiamine, which helps the body break down carbohydrates and release energy.

- **Kretschmer Wheat Germ** and **Dannon Yogurt.** Mix three tablespoons Kretschmer Wheat Germ into a cup of Dannon Nonfat Yogurt for breakfast or lunch. The thiamine in the wheat germ helps the body break down carbohydrates and release energy. Three tablespoons of wheat germ contain 33 percent of the recommended daily allowance of thiamine.

- **Lipton Black Tea.** To reduce fatigue and enhance alertness, drink a cup of Lipton Black Tea rather than a cup of coffee. Black tea contains both caffeine and the amino acid L-theanine, and studies show that the combination fights fatigue. L-theanine increases the body's production of the neurotransmitters dopamine, serotonin, and gamma-aminobutyric acid, reversing the effects of mental fatigue.

- **McCormick Pure Peppermint Extract** and **Kleenex Tissues.** Put two or three drops McCormick Pure Peppermint Extract on a Kleenex Tissue, hold it under your nose, and breathe deeply. The aroma of peppermint stimulates the brain.

- **McCormick Rosemary Leaves** and **L'eggs Sheer Energy Panty Hose.** To boost your alertness and ability to concentrate, place one teaspoon McCormick Rosemary Leaves in the foot cut from a pair of clean, used

℞ STRANGE MEDICINE ℞

NO REST FOR THE WEARY

- Fatigue typically stems from poor nutrition or lack of sleep.

- Not drinking enough water every day causes dehydration, which, in turn, causes fatigue. Water helps the body transport nutrients, enables cells to perform at optimum levels, and helps oxygenate the blood. To boost your energy, drink eight to ten 8-ounce glasses of water a day.

- Skipping breakfast can result in fatigue. A bowl of cereal with milk provides complex carbohydrates and protein. Other sources of carbohydrates are wheat toast and muffins. A cup of low-fat yogurt or scrambled egg whites supply protein. Avoid sugary cereals or doughnuts, which create a jolt of insulin and a drop in blood sugar, producing the lethargy you are trying to overcome.

- Exercise gives you energy and improves your mood. Walking briskly for twenty to thirty minutes three to five times a week invigorates you, reduces stress, and helps you sleep better at night.

- Taking a multivitamin daily can help prevent a vitamin deficiency from zapping your strength and energy.

- Minimize your alcohol consumption. As a depressant, alcohol slows your central nervous system and decreases your blood sugar level.

- To prevent fatigue, sleep eight hours a night. Go to bed and wake up at the same time every day, even on weekends.

- Limit the amount of caffeinated beverages you drink. Yes, coffee and caffeinated soda give you a short burst of energy, but the subsequent crash tends to make you even more lethargic.

- Taking a mid-afternoon "power nap" for fifteen to thirty minutes can rejuvenate and refresh your mind. Napping longer than thirty minutes puts your body into deep sleep, which is difficult to wake from and will likely make you groggy.

L'eggs Sheer Energy Panty Hose, tie a knot in the open end, and sniff the sachet throughout the day. Studies show that the scent of rosemary prompts the brain to increase its production of beta waves.

- **Mott's Applesauce.** To raise your energy, eat one cup Mott's Applesauce every day. The malic acid in applesauce helps the mitochondria, the microscopic organelles in every cell in your body, produce adenosine triphosphate (ATP) more efficiently, giving your cells more energy.

- **Sun-Maid Raisins.** To give yourself a quick energy boost, snack on a small box of Sun-Maid Raisins. The carbohydrates and protein in raisins kick you back into high gear.

- **Wrigley's Spearmint Gum.** To reinvigorate yourself, chew a stick of Wrigley's Spearmint Gum. The minty flavor and scent reawaken your senses, and the act of chewing gives you a burst of energy.

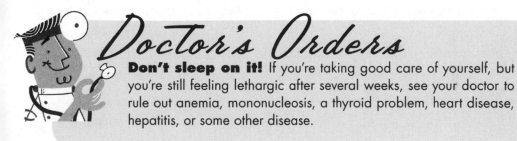

Doctor's Orders

Don't sleep on it! If you're taking good care of yourself, but you're still feeling lethargic after several weeks, see your doctor to rule out anemia, mononucleosis, a thyroid problem, heart disease, hepatitis, or some other disease.

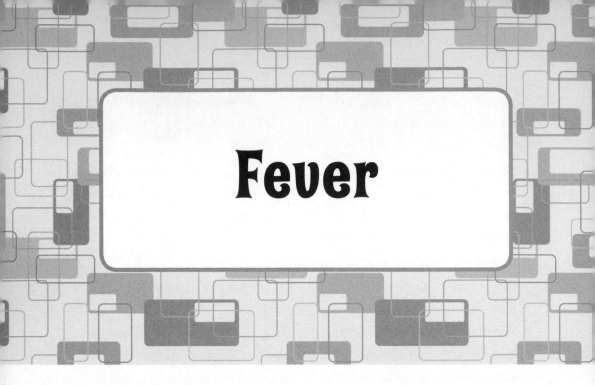

Fever

- **Campbell's Chicken Noodle Soup** and **Tabasco Pepper Sauce.** When you regain your appetite, add one teaspoon Tabasco Pepper Sauce to a bowl of Campbell's Chicken Noodle Soup, mix well, and eat. The hot soup and the capsaicin in the Tabasco Pepper Sauce promote sweating, which reduces the body's temperature. Chicken soup is also known as "Jewish penicillin."

- **Colman's Mustard Powder.** To ease a fever, dissolve two teaspoons Colman's Mustard Powder in a quart of warm water in a basin large enough to hold your feet. Soak your feet in the mustard footbath for fifteen minutes. The warmth of the mustard draws blood to the feet, significantly improving circulation.

- **Gatorade.** To prevent yourself from becoming dehydrated from a fever, drink plenty of Gatorade. The sports drink quickly replaces fluid, electrolytes, and important minerals.

- **Heinz White Vinegar** and **Bounty Paper Towels.** To help break a fever, fold a sheet of Bounty Paper Towels like a washcloth, saturate it with Heinz White Vinegar, and apply it to your forehead as a compress until the sheet of paper towel heats up. The vinegar increases evaporation from the skin, which cools the blood as it circulates close to the skin.

℞ STRANGE MEDICINE ℞

THE HEAT IS ON

● A fever typically signals that your body is fighting off a bacterial or viral infection. To combat the intruders, your white blood cells release chemicals to raise your body temperature, turning your body into an inhospitable habitat for the infection.

● A fever typically subsides within a few days.

● To take your temperature accurately, wait fifteen minutes after eating, drinking, or taking a bath before placing the thermometer in your mouth. Place the bulb tip of the thermometer under your tongue, hold the thermometer in place with your lips (not your teeth), and breathe through your nose (to prevent the room temperature from altering the reading). Wait three to five minutes, and then read the thermometer.

● To reduce your temperature, apply a washcloth dampened with hot (yes, hot) water to your forehead. The hot water actually lowers your body temperature. (If your fever rises above 103 degrees Fahrenheit, apply cool compresses.)

● To help reduce a fever, give yourself a sponge bath with cool water, concentrating on the areas that produce the most heat—your armpits and groin. The evaporating water cools the body.

● Taking a bath in lukewarm (not cold) water helps lower your body temperature.

● When you have a fever, your body perspires so that the subsequent evaporation helps cool you down. Drinking eight to twelve 8-ounce glasses of water a day helps prevent dehydration and enables the body to continue perspiring to help you cope with the fever.

● To hasten your recovery, get plenty of rest to allow your body to concentrate its energy on fighting off the infection.

● If you get the chills, wrap yourself in a blanket. Your body shivers to raise its internal temperature. The quivering muscles generate heat to produce more fever to fight the infection.

● To avoid getting fevers, simply wash your hands frequently to reduce your exposure to infectious diseases.

- **Jell-O Vanilla Pudding.** When you begin to regain your appetite, eat Jell-O Vanilla Pudding to help revive your strength. It's easy to eat and goes down smoothly.

- **Lipton Ginger Tea.** To induce the sweating that helps break a fever, drink a cup of Lipton Ginger Tea. Some of the anti-inflammatory compounds in ginger also act like aspirin. (Do not drink ginger tea if you have gallstones. Ginger can increase bile production.)

- **McCormick Ground (Cayenne) Red Pepper.** To help break a fever, sprinkle McCormick Ground (Cayenne) Red Pepper on your food. The capsaicin in the pepper fosters sweating and promotes rapid blood circulation.

- **Popsicle.** If you feel too nauseous to drink water or juice to rehydrate yourself, suck on your favorite flavor Popsicle.

- **ReaLemon, McCormick Cream of Tartar,** and **SueBee Honey.** Mix three tablespoons ReaLemon lemon juice and one teaspoon McCormick Cream of Tartar in a sixteen-ounce glass of water. Sweeten to taste with SueBee Honey and sip the concoction slowly. This German folklore remedy helps reduce a fever. (Do not feed honey to infants less than one year of age. Honey often carries a benign strain of *C. botulinum*, and an infant's immune system requires twelve months to develop to fight off disease and infection.)

- **Wonder Bread.** When you regain your appetite, eat some slices of toasted Wonder Bread, which are easy to digest and reenergize your body with carbohydrates.

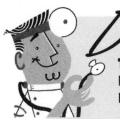

Doctor's Orders

Too hot to handle! If your temperature reaches 103 degrees Fahrenheit or more, or if your temperature exceeds 101 degrees Fahrenheit for more than three days, call a doctor immediately.

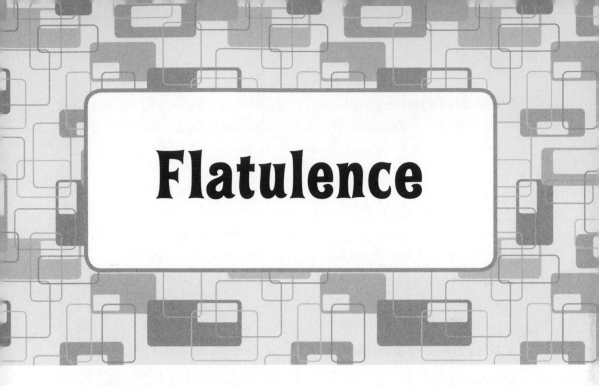

Flatulence

- **Angostura Aromatic Bitters.** To prevent flatulence, add several dashes of Angostura Aromatic Bitters to a glass of water, and drink the concoction after meals. The tincture of the gentian root stimulates digestion.

- **Arm & Hammer Baking Soda** and **ReaLemon.** To neutralize the stomach acid causing gas, dissolve one-half teaspoon Arm & Hammer Baking Soda in four ounces of warm water, add a few drops of ReaLemon lemon juice, and drink the solution. The alkaline baking soda neutralizes stomach acid and the lemon juice dispels some of the gas generated by the baking soda. (Do not use this remedy if you're on a sodium-restricted diet. Read the directions on the side of the box of baking soda before administering.)

- **CharcoCaps Activated Charcoal.** To prevent or eliminate excessive gas, take one to two 200- to 500-milligram CharcoCaps Activated Charcoal capsules. The charcoal absorbs toxins, gases, and other irritants in the digestive track, carrying them out of the body. Charcoal also absorbs nutrients, so be sure to discontinue use after a few days. (Don't confuse activated charcoal with charcoal briquettes. Activated charcoal is a charcoal that has been processed with oxygen to be extremely porous and absorb odors or other substances.)

- **Dannon Yogurt.** Eating a cup of Dannon Nonfat Yogurt a few times a week can help reduce flatulence. The *Lactobacillus acidophilus* (probiotics) in yogurt break down milk sugars, relieving gas problems created by dairy products. Yogurt also helps maintain a healthy balance of beneficial bacteria in your digestive system. Also, taking antibiotics can give you gas because they kill the beneficial bacteria in the intestines, allowing other bacteria and microorganisms to propagate and generate toxins that cause gas. Eating a cup of yogurt daily restores the bacterial balance and clears up the flatulence.

- **Hennessy Cognac.** To reduce flatulence after a meal, take one teaspoon Hennessy Cognac. A sip or two of brandy to relieve gas has been a folklore remedy touted for centuries.

- **Lifesavers Pep-O-Mint.** To minimize flatulence, suck on a Lifesavers Pep-O-Mint candy upon finishing each meal. Peppermint helps reduce gas and improve digestion.

- **Lipton Ginger Tea.** To prevent or alleviate flatulence, drink a cup of strongly brewed Lipton Ginger Tea after each meal. Ginger stimulates digestion and relaxes the muscles in the digestive tract, enabling food to pass more quickly through the intestines. (Do not drink ginger tea if you have gallstones. Ginger can increase bile production.)

- **Lipton Peppermint Tea.** To quiet flatulence, place a Lipton Peppermint Tea bag in a cup of boiling water, cover with a saucer, steep for ten minutes, and sip slowly after each meal. The peppermint soothes digestion and clears up the gas.

- **McCormick Basil Leaves.** To prevent beans and other starchy foods from giving you gas, sprinkle McCormick Basil Leaves over the dish. As a carminative herb, basil prevents the formation of gas in the gastrointestinal tract, enabling you to evade the problem.

- **McCormick Fennel Seed.** To relieve flatulence, chew five to ten McCormick Fennel Seeds thoroughly after eating a meal and then swallow the seeds. Or make fennel tea by placing a tea infuser filled with one tablespoon crushed McCormick Fennel Seed in a teacup, adding boiling water, covering with a saucer, and steeping for ten minutes. The volatile oil in the fennel aids the digestive process, dispersing gas from the intestinal tract. In India, fennel seeds are served after meals like after–dinner mints.

℞ STRANGE MEDICINE ℞

GONE WITH THE WIND

● Flatulence results when bacteria in your large intestine ferment carbohydrates that your small intestine did not digest, producing gas that your body subsequently expels through the rectum.

● Healthy, high-fiber foods, which keep your digestive tract running smoothly and regulate blood sugar and cholesterol levels, also lead to the formation of gas.

● The average person expels gas six to twenty-one times a day.

● Flatulence problems often stem from lactose intolerance.

● To reduce flatulence, avoid highly flatulogenic foods such as apricots, asparagus, bananas, beans, broccoli, Brussels sprouts, cabbage, cauliflower, onions, prunes, and radishes.

● Beans cause gas because humans do not produce the enzyme alpha-galactosidase, which breaks down the difficult-to-digest sugars in beans. The bacteria in the colon ferment these sugars, producing gases including hydrogen, carbon dioxide, methane, and hydrogen sulfide.

● Before cooking beans, soak them in water for twelve hours and then drain off the water to significantly remove the amount of carbohydrates that produce gas.

● If you feel bloated from a build-up of gas in your intestines, go for a short walk to stimulate gas dispersal.

● Other causes of excess gas include antibiotics, artificial sweeteners, constipation, laxatives, or swallowed air.

- **McCormick Ground Turmeric.** Boil one teaspoon McCormick Ground Turmeric in one cup of water, strain, and drink immediately. Those who practice Ayurvedic medicine, the traditional medicine of India, insist that turmeric quickly relieves gas. (Turmeric may increase the likelihood of bleeding when taken in combination with the blood thinner Coumadin or other anticoagulant medications.)

- **Pepto-Bismol.** Taking one teaspoon Pepto-Bismol does not bring excessive flatulence under control, but it does significantly reduce the odor.

Doctor's Orders

Spill the beans! If you suffer from excessive flatulence, consult your doctor to rule out diverticulitis, ulcerative colitis, Crohn's disease, or another inflammatory bowel disease.

Flu

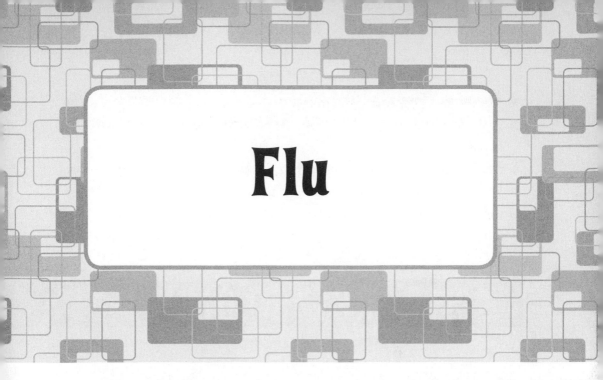

- **Campbell's Chicken Noodle Soup.** To soothe flu symptoms, eat a bowl of Campbell's Chicken Noodle Soup. Scientific studies verify that chicken soup, nicknamed "Jewish penicillin," stops specific white blood cells called neutrophils from causing the inflammation that triggers the body to produce large amounts of mucus.

- **Colman's Mustard Powder.** To relieve congestion, dissolve two teaspoons Colman's Mustard Powder in a quart of warm water in a basin large enough to hold your feet. Soak your feet in the mustard footbath for fifteen minutes. The warmth of the mustard draws blood to the feet, improving circulation and alleviating congestion.

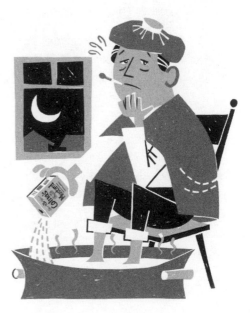

- **Cream of Wheat.** As you recover from the flu and regain your appetite, start with soft, bland foods like Cream of Wheat, which is soothing and easy to digest.

- **Dr. Bronner's Eucalyptus Castile Soap.** To relieve a stuffy nose, use Dr. Bronner's Eucalyptus Castile Soap in the shower or bath. The penetrating scent of eucalyptus clears congestion and opens nasal passages.

⚗ STRANGE MEDICINE ⚗

WHAT'S THE CATCH?

- The flu, more accurately called influenza, is a viral infection in the respiratory system that attacks the nose, throat, and lungs. (A stomach flu isn't caused by the influenza virus at all. Known medically as gastroenteritis, the stomach flu is caused by a variety of different viruses, resulting in diarrhea and vomiting.)

- If you have all the symptoms of a cold plus a temperature of 102 degrees Fahrenheit or more, muscle aches, headache, and extreme fatigue, you most likely have the flu.

- A runny nose, sore throat, and sneezing are common symptoms of a cold. A fever, headache, hacking cough, muscle aches, and extreme fatigue rarely accompany a cold, but are symptoms of the flu. Unlike colds, the flu is rarely associated with sneezing.

- The flu tends to strike suddenly. A cold usually develops gradually.

- When you have the flu, your immune system produces toxins to destroy the virus, and your body expels water to flush out the toxins. To replenish the lost liquid and help your body flush out the flu, drink at least twelve 8-ounce glasses of water a day. Drinking water also helps thin mucus, making it easier to expel.

- The flu is a viral infection, meaning antibiotics cannot kill it.

- While suffering from the flu, avoid dairy products, which increase mucus production and worsen nasal congestion.

- **French's Mustard.** Spread French's Mustard on your chest and cover with a washcloth dampened with warm water. Let sit for fifteen minutes and wash clean. The penetrating warmth from the mustard plaster thins the mucus in your chest.

- **Gold's Horseradish** and **Nabisco Original Premium Saltine Crackers.** To break through congestion, eat one teaspoon Gold's Horseradish

- Keeping a humidifier running in your bedroom for the duration of the flu helps moisten mucous membranes so you can expel mucus easily.

- Getting plenty of bed rest allows your body to focus the bulk of its energy on fighting the infection.

- The single best way to avoid getting the flu? Get a yearly flu shot in the fall, several weeks before the start of flu season. The vaccine takes roughly two weeks to build up your immunity. If you still get the flu, the vaccine lessens the severity of the disease.

- The flu is transmitted when an infected person spews droplets in the air by coughing, sneezing, blowing his nose carelessly, or talking. Others get the influenza virus by inhaling the droplets or touching a contaminated object or surface and then touching their eyes, nose, or mouth.

- Washing your hands frequently and thoroughly with soap and water for at least fifteen seconds (or using an alcohol-based hand sanitizer) helps you avoid getting and spreading the flu.

- Every time you catch a flu, your body produces antibodies to fight that particular strain of the influenza virus. Those antibodies may prevent infection from influenza viruses similar to what you had before or lessen the severity of the malady.

- Typically, the common cold lasts longer than the flu.

spread on a Nabisco Original Premium Saltine Cracker. Horseradish is a scientifically proven decongestant.

- **Lipton Chamomile Tea.** To clear congestion from your nose and sinuses, fill a large bowl with boiling water and add three Lipton Chamomile Tea bags. Wearing a towel over your head to form a tent over the bowl, hold your face close to the steaming tea for ten minutes. Keep a box of tissues nearby to blow your nose repeatedly.

- **Lipton Ginger Tea.** To alleviate flu symptoms, drink a cup of strongly brewed Lipton Ginger Tea every two or three hours until you beat the flu. Ginger relieves nasal congestion, helps eliminate the chills and muscle aches (by improving circulation), and reduces sore throat pain. (Do not drink ginger tea if you have gallstones. Ginger can increase bile production.)

- **McCormick Garlic Powder.** To strengthen your immune system and reduce nasal and sinus congestion, add one teaspoon McCormick Garlic Powder when making Campbell's Chicken Noodle Soup (see page 189). The garlic liquefies mucus.

- **McCormick Oregano Leaves.** To clear congestion, place a tea infuser filled with one or two tablespoons McCormick Oregano Leaves in a teacup, add boiling water, cover with a saucer, steep for ten minutes, and drink the medicinal tea. Oregano contains compounds that help loosen phlegm, making it easier to cough up.

- **Morton Salt.** To relieve a sore throat accompanying the flu, dissolve one teaspoon Morton Salt in an eight-ounce glass of warm water, and gargle with the solution. Salt water soothes the pain and washes out secretions.

- **Mott's Applesauce.** You'll most likely loose your appetite during the worst stage of the flu, but when you're feeling hungry again, Mott's Applesauce makes an excellent starting point. The bland food is substantial yet easy on your recovering system.

- **ReaLemon.** To ward off a sore throat caused by the flu, mix one teaspoon ReaLemon lemon juice in an eight-ounce glass of warm water, and gargle with the lemon solution. The combination of acids in the lemon juice works as an antiseptic.

- **Tabasco Pepper Sauce.** To soothe sore throat pain, mix ten drops Tabasco Pepper Sauce in a glass of water, and gargle with the spicy solution. The capsicum in the Tabasco Pepper Sauce numbs the throat.

- **Tabasco Pepper Sauce** and **Campbell's Tomato Juice.** To help clear sinuses and raise your body temperature to fight off the influenza virus, add ten to twenty drops Tabasco Pepper Sauce to a glass of Campbell's Tomato Juice, and drink this mixture several times a day. The hot sauce doubles as a decongestant.

- **Tootsie Roll Pops.** To soothe a sore throat, suck on a Tootsie Roll Pop. Sucking on candy moistens your throat and the sugar provides necessary glucose.

- **Uncle Ben's Converted Brand Rice.** When you get your appetite back, start by eating bland, starchy foods, like Uncle Ben's Converted Brand Rice.

- **Vaseline Petroleum Jelly.** To prevent your nostrils from getting sore from blowing your nose too often, lubricate them with a thin coat of Vaseline Petroleum Jelly.

- **Vicks VapoRub.** To keep your respiratory passages moist and open, rub a thick coat of Vicks VapoRub on your chest and neck. The penetrating smell of menthol and eucalyptus oil help clear congestion and fight infection.

- **Wonder Bread.** When you regain your appetite, transition slowly to solid foods by starting with some slices of toasted Wonder Bread, which are easy to digest and provide starch.

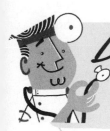

Doctor's Orders

Shake it off! If the flu lasts for more than five days, you experience difficulty breathing or pains in your chest, or you start coughing up yellow or green phlegm, consult a doctor.

Food Poisoning

- **Canada Dry Ginger Ale.** Drinking Canada Dry Ginger Ale—flat—helps settle your stomach. The ginger seems to relax the muscles in the stomach. Contrary to popular belief, Canada Dry Ginger Ale does indeed contain genuine ginger, included in the list of ingredients as "natural flavors." (Do not drink ginger ale if you have gallstones. Ginger can increase bile production.)

- **CharcoCaps Activated Charcoal.** To relieve diarrhea caused by food poisoning, take four to six 200-milligram CharcoCaps Activated Charcoal capsules every two hours until the symptoms subside. The charcoal absorbs toxins from the digestive track, carrying them out of the body. Charcoal also absorbs nutrients, so be sure to discontinue use after a few days. (Don't confuse activated charcoal with charcoal briquettes. Activated charcoal is a charcoal that has been processed with oxygen to be extremely porous and absorb odors or other substances.)

- **Coca-Cola.** Drinking flat Coca-Cola helps settle your queasy stomach. Pharmacies sell cola syrup that can be taken in small doses to relieve nausea. The concentrated sugars are believed to relax the gastrointestinal tract. Letting the bubbles out of the soda prevents the carbonation from further upsetting your stomach.

- **Gatorade.** To avoid dehydration and refortify your body with liquid and electrolytes after a bout of diarrhea and vomiting, drink Gatorade to quickly replace essential nutrients and minerals. The sports drink helps prevent muscle spasms in your stomach.

- **Knorr Chicken Bouillon.** To replace the liquid, salts, and minerals depleted by diarrhea and vomiting, dissolve one Knorr Chicken Bouillon cube in a cup of hot water and sip the soothing broth.

- **McCormick Ground Cinnamon** and **McCormick Ground Ginger.** To combat nausea, vomiting, and diarrhea caused by food poisoning, mix one teaspoon McCormick Ground Cinnamon and one-half teaspoon McCormick Ground Ginger in a teacup, add boiling water, cover with a saucer, and steep for fifteen minutes. Strain and then sip the tea. The cinnamon can help annihilate the responsible bacteria, and the ginger suppresses stomach spasms. (Do not use ginger if you have gallstones. Ginger can increase bile production.)

- **Mott's Apple Juice, SueBee Honey,** and **Morton Salt.** To stay well hydrated and replenish electrolytes lost during a bout of food poisoning, mix one cup Mott's Apple Juice, three tablespoons SueBee Honey, one teaspoon Morton Salt, and two cups of water. Drink the solution throughout the day or as needed. The apple juice provides potassium, the honey supplies glucose, and the salt furnishes sodium.

- **Mott's Applesauce.** Once the diarrhea and vomiting have subsided, eat Mott's Applesauce. The pectin in the applesauce is a soluble fiber that absorbs fluid in your intestines and helps solidify soft bowel movements. Applesauce also contains malic acid and quercetin, which help inhibit harmful bacteria in your stomach.

- **Nabisco Original Premium Saltine Crackers.** When you feel up to eating something, eat a few Nabisco Original Premium Saltine Crackers.

℞ STRANGE MEDICINE ℞

WHAT'S YOUR POISON?

● Food poisoning is caused by eating food contaminated with infectious bacteria, viruses, or parasites.

● Food poisoning typically causes nausea, cramping, vomiting, or diarrhea—generally within hours of eating contaminated food (but sometimes up to two weeks later).

● Food poisoning usually resolves itself without medical treatment within forty-eight hours. However, a severe case may require hospitalization.

● To ease discomfort after the onset of food poisoning, let your stomach settle by not eating or drinking for a few hours.

● To prevent dehydration, the most common complication posed by food poisoning, drink between eight and sixteen 8-ounce glasses of water, fruit juice, or a sports drink daily to replace the fluid lost from vomiting and diarrhea.

● Drinking fruit juice helps maintain your electrolyte levels and eating chicken bouillon replaces lost sodium.

● Diarrhea and vomiting help purge harmful bacteria or an unwelcome parasite from your digestive system.

● To speed your recovery, avoid dairy products, caffeine, alcohol, nicotine, fatty foods, or highly seasoned foods—until your stomach has returned to normal.

● Between bouts of vomiting and diarrhea, get plenty of sleep and rest. Sleep and idleness help your body regain energy and focus attention on fighting the infection.

● If you suspect a specific restaurant, grocery store, butcher, or canned good as the source of your food poisoning, file a report with your local health department to help prevent other customers from getting sick and to stop a potential outbreak.

High in carbohydrates, the crackers help settle your stomach and help you regain your strength.

- **Popsicle.** If you feel too nauseous to drink water or juice to rehydrate yourself, suck on your favorite flavor Popsicle.

- **7-Up.** To help rehydrate yourself and settle your stomach, drink flat 7-Up.

- **SueBee Honey.** To cure diarrhea, mix four tablespoons SueBee Honey into a cup of hot water. Let cool and drink. A 1985 study conducted in South Africa and reported in the *British Medical Journal* showed that honey shortens the duration of diarrhea in patients with bacterial gastroenteritis caused by *Salmonella, Shigella,* and *E. coli.* (Do not feed honey to infants less than one year of age. Honey often carries a benign strain of *C. botulinum,* and an infant's immune system requires twelve months to develop to fight off disease and infection.)

- **Uncle Ben's Converted Brand Rice.** Once the vomiting and diarrhea have subsided, eat small portions of plain, white Uncle Ben's Converted Brand Rice. Rice binds the bowels, creating healthy stools.

- **Wonder Bread.** To help yourself recover from the diarrhea and vomiting, transition slowly to solid foods by starting with some slices of toasted Wonder Bread, which are easy to digest and provide starch.

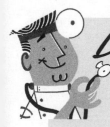

Doctor's Orders

What's eating you? If you experience severe diarrhea for more than three days, frequent vomiting that prevents you from keeping liquids down, severe abdominal cramping, or digested blood in your vomit (looks like black coffee grounds) or bowel movements (black stools), seek medical attention.

Foot and Heel Pain

- **Birds Eye Frozen Peas** and **Bounty Paper Towels.** To relieve heel pain, cover a bag of Birds Eye Frozen Peas with a sheet of Bounty Paper Towels, and place the bag on the sore heel for twenty minutes three times a day. The frozen peas act like small ice cubes, soothing and numbing the pain, and the bag of peas conforms to the shape of your heel. The paper towel creates a layer of insulation to prevent frostbite. Refreeze the bag of peas for future ice-pack use. Be sure to label the bag for ice-pack use only. If you want to eat the peas, cook them after they thaw the first time, never after refreezing.

- **Campbell's Soup.** To give your sore foot a rejuvenating massage, roll your foot over a Campbell's Soup can placed on its side.

- **Dr. Teal's Epsom Salt** and **Lubriderm.** To ease foot pain, dissolve two tablespoons Dr. Teal's Epsom Salt in a basin filled with warm water, and soak your feet in the solution for fifteen minutes. Rinse with clean water, pat your feet dry with a towel, and rub in a dab of Lubriderm, massaging your feet.

- **Johnson's Baby Oil.** Give yourself a soothing foot massage with a few drops of Johnson's Baby Oil to lubricate the skin. Or have a partner rub your feet for you.

- **Lipton Peppermint Tea.** Place four Lipton Peppermint Tea bags in two cups of boiling water, cover with a saucer, and let steep for ten minutes. Pour the tea in a basin filled with one gallon of warm water, and soak your feet in the aromatic solution for ten minutes. The warmth of the water and the essential oils in the peppermint help resuscitate your feet.

- **McCormick Ground (Cayenne) Red Pepper.** To keep your feet warm on a winter's day, sprinkle McCormick Ground (Cayenne) Red Pepper in your socks and shoes before putting them on and going out in the cold. The hot pepper brings blood to the surface of the skin, relieving cold feet.

- **McCormick Thyme Leaves.** To relieve foot pain, add two tablespoons McCormick Thyme Leaves to a quart of boiling water, cover the pot, and simmer for twenty minutes. Let cool until comfortable to the touch, and soak your feet in the solution in a basin for twenty minutes. A study published in the January 2010 issue of *Journal of Lipid Research* reported that the antioxidant carvacrol in thyme suppresses inflammation by inhibiting the COX-2 enzyme in cells by nearly 75 percent.

- **Star Olive Oil** and **Heinz White Vinegar.** To relieve foot pain and stimulate circulation, mix equal parts Star Olive Oil and Heinz White Vinegar, and massage your feet with the mixture.

- **Stayfree Maxi Pads.** To make a temporary shoe insert to relieve pain caused by flat feet or fallen arches, place your foot on top of a flattened Stayfree Maxi Pad, trace around your foot with a marker, and use a pair of scissors to carefully cut off the excess pad. Pull off the adhesive strip and place the pad inside your shoe to cushion your foot.

- **Tabasco Pepper Sauce** and **Crisco All-Vegetable Shortening.** To relieve the burning pain of sore feet, mix one-quarter teaspoon Tabasco Pepper Sauce with two tablespoons Crisco All-Vegetable Shortening, and apply the spicy homemade ointment to the affected areas up to five times a day. The capsaicin in the Tabasco Pepper Sauce helps numb the pain. (Do not apply this salve on open sores and avoid contact with eyes and nose.)

☥ STRANGE MEDICINE ☥

LANDING ON BOTH FEET

● To rejuvenate sore feet, take off your shoes, sit in a chair with your feet elevated, wiggle your toes, rotate each foot in a circle, and relax for twenty minutes. Doing so stimulates the circulation in your toes and reduces swelling.

● To relieve foot and heel pain quickly and effectively, soak your feet in cold water for five minutes, then soak them in hot water for five minutes, and repeat the process. The hot water opens the blood vessels, stimulating circulation, and the cold water constricts them—essentially massaging your tired, achy feet from within.

● For a surefire way to reduce foot aches, stop wearing high heels. They may look fashionable, but high heel shoes force the calf muscles to contract, which gradually causes your feet to ache. Instead, wear sensible flat shoes or running shoes.

● To prevent achy feet, buy your shoes in the afternoon, when your feet are most swollen, and consider insoles, which add protective cushioning. Be sure you buy a pair of shoes with plenty of room in the toe area. From the tip of the shoe, your longest toe should have space measuring the width of your thumb.

● Stretching your calf muscles helps soothe your feet and heels. To do so, stand three feet from a blank wall, place your palms on the wall at head level, step forward with one foot, and lean toward the wall, bending your elbows. You'll feel your calf muscle stretching. Then repeat with the other leg.

● To relieve a foot ache, have a friend or partner massage your feet, or roll your feet over a rolling pin.

● **Vicks VapoRub.** To alleviate a foot ache, rub Vicks VapoRub into your foot. The camphor and menthol in the balm reduce pain and inflammation by stimulating blood flow to the foot.

● **Wilson Tennis Balls.** Insert three Wilson Tennis Balls into a sock, tie a knot in the open end of the sock, place the sock on the floor, and roll your bare feet over it. The tennis balls massage the soles of your feet.

- **Ziploc Storage Bags.** If your shoes are too tight, fill two Ziploc Storage Bags halfway with water, seal the bags shut securely (so the water doesn't leak out), and insert one water-filled bag snuggly inside each shoe. Place the shoes in the freezer overnight. When water freezes to ice, it expands, stretching the shoes. (If you have difficulty removing the frozen bags of ice from the shoes, simply let the ice melt.)

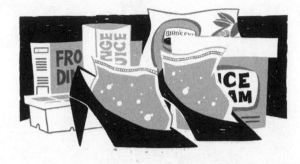

Doctor's Orders

Dead on your feet? If you experience difficulty walking when you wake up, the pain in your feet regularly increases throughout the day, or you can no longer wear shoes without pain, see your doctor.

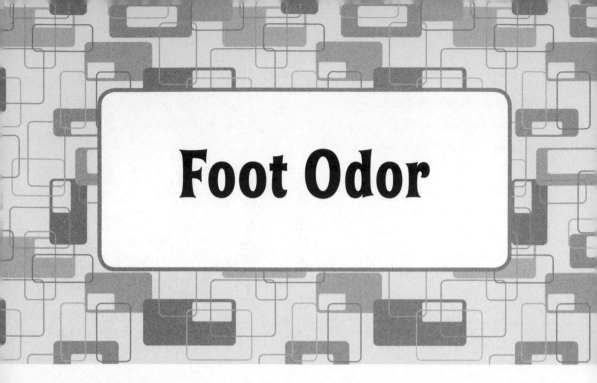

Foot Odor

- **Arm & Hammer Baking Soda.** To minimize the perspiration on which odor-causing bacteria thrive, dust your feet with Arm & Hammer Baking Soda before putting on your socks and shoes. The baking soda absorbs moisture and simultaneously neutralizes odors.

- **Arm & Hammer Baking Soda.** To kill the odor-causing bacteria on your feet, dissolve one tablespoon Arm & Hammer Baking Soda in one quart of water in a basin. Soak your feet in the solution for fifteen minutes twice a week. The sodium bicarbonate increases the acidity of the skin's surface, reducing the number of bacteria.

- **Clearasil.** To kill the bacteria that cause foot odor, apply Clearasil to your clean, dry feet. The benzoyl peroxide in Clearasil combats the bacteria.

- **Conair Hair Dryer.** After washing your feet and toweling them dry, blow-dry your feet with a Conair Hair Dryer set on low. Drying your feet eliminates the moisture that provides a breeding ground for bacteria.

- **Dial Soap.** To rid your feet of the bacteria that cause foot odor, wash your feet daily in warm water using Dial Antibacterial Soap, which contains Triclosan, an antibacterial agent. Dry your feet thoroughly.

- **Dr. Teal's Epsom Salt.** Mix two cups Dr. Teal's Epsom Salt in one gallon of warm water in a basin, and soak your feet in the solution for fifteen minutes two times a day. The Epsom Salt minimizes perspiration and may kill bacteria.

- **Heinz White Vinegar.** To deodorize smelly feet, add one cup Heinz White Vinegar to a basin of warm water, and soak your feet in the solution for twenty minutes a day for two weeks. The acetic acid in the vinegar kills the offending bacteria. (Do not soak your feet in vinegar if you have open sores on your feet.)

- **Jell-O.** To prevent your feet from perspiring, mix up a box of Jell-O according to the directions on the box, and soak your feet in the gelatin solution. Like an antiperspirant, the gel fills and obstructs the sweat glands.

- **Johnson's Baby Powder.** To keep the insides of your shoes dry and smelling sweet, sprinkle them with Johnson's Baby Powder. The talc absorbs moisture.

- **Kingsford's Corn Starch.** For another good foot powder to absorb perspiration from your feet, dust your feet and powder the insides of your shoes with Kingsford's Corn Starch. The cornstarch helps keep your feet dry, denying bacteria a moist breeding ground.

- **Lipton Black Tea.** Steep four Lipton Black Tea bags in one quart of boiling water for ten minutes. Let cool to room temperature (or add cool water to the tea). Soak your feet in the tea for thirty minutes, dry your feet thoroughly, and apply Arm & Hammer Baking Soda (opposite) or Kingsford's Corn Starch (above). Do this twice a day for two weeks. The tannin in the tea kills the odor-causing bacteria and dries the skin.

- **Listerine.** To eliminate the bacteria that cause foot odor, saturate a cotton ball with original formula Listerine antiseptic mouthwash and apply to your feet and between your toes. The thymol in Listerine kills the odor-causing bacteria. (Do not apply Listerine to your feet if you have broken skin or open sores.)

- **McCormick Ground Sage.** To minimize foot odor, sprinkle McCormick Ground Sage in your shoes. Sage neutralizes odors.

☙ STRANGE MEDICINE ☙

CREATING A BIG STINK

● Oddly, the same bacteria responsible for ripening Limburger cheese into the smelliest cheese consume the fat molecules in human perspiration and excrete foul-smelling isovaleric acid.

● Eliminating the bacteria that feast on human perspiration gets rid of foot odor.

● To keep your feet dry when combating foot odor, change your socks at least once a day (or as often as necessary) and never wear the same pair of shoes two days in a row. After wearing a pair of shoes for one day, let them air dry for twenty-four hours in a well-lit, well-ventilated area. Exposure to sunlight can kill the offending microbes. If the shoes have removable insoles, remove them to dry as well.

● Wool socks wick moisture away from the skin. Cotton socks hold moisture against the skin.

● Wearing sandals, flip-flops, or open-toe shoes allow your feet to breathe, rather than confining them in a closed environment that fosters bacterial growth.

● The sweat glands in your feet produce up to eight fluid ounces of perspiration daily.

● The sweat glands, including the ones in your feet, secrete the extracts from oils— and the accompanying smell—from cumin, curry, garlic, onion, and fish for hours after you eat them.

● An orthotic shoe insert that provides arch support may reduce the amount of perspiration your feet produce by simply allowing your foot muscles to work less.

● **Neosporin.** To kill the bacteria causing the foot odor, before going to bed, rub a thin coat of Neosporin into your feet and toenails, put on a pair of socks, and go to sleep. The antibiotic ointment eradicates the bacteria by morning. If your feet smell the following evening, repeat the process for a second night.

- **ReaLemon.** To deodorize smelly feet, add three tablespoons ReaLemon lemon juice to a basin of warm water, and soak your feet in the solution for twenty minutes a day for two weeks. The acidic lemon juice doubles as an antiseptic, killing the offending bacteria. (Do not soak your feet in lemon juice if you have open sores on your feet.)

- **Secret Antiperspirant.** Gliding a stick of Secret Antiperspirant between your toes and on your feet stops perspiration, controlling the subsequent odor. (Applying an antiperspirant to feet plagued by athlete's foot will sting.)

- **Smirnoff Vodka.** To kill the odor-producing bacteria thriving on your feet, use a cotton ball to apply Smirnoff Vodka to your feet and between your toes. The alcohol in the vodka eliminates the microbes.

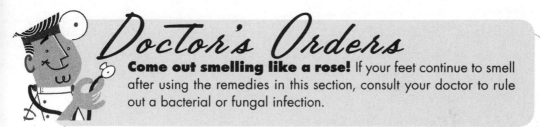

Doctor's Orders

Come out smelling like a rose! If your feet continue to smell after using the remedies in this section, consult your doctor to rule out a bacterial or fungal infection.

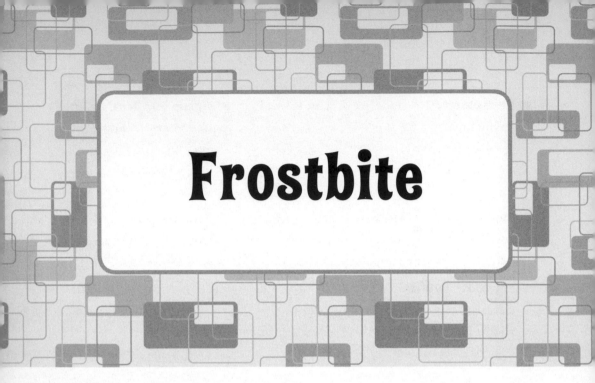

Frostbite

- **Colman's Mustard Powder.** To help prevent frostbite, sprinkle Colman's Mustard Powder in socks and shoes before putting them on and going out in the cold. The mustard powder brings blood to the surface of the skin, relieving cold feet.

- **Fruit of the Earth Aloe Vera Gel.** To speed the healing of frostbite after being treated by a doctor, slather Fruit of the Earth Aloe Vera Gel on the affected area four times a day—until the damaged skin heals. Aloe vera gel relieves the pain, fosters healing, and prevents infection. Frostbite blisters contain the tissue-damaging chemical thromboxane, and aloe vera gel helps inhibit thromboxane production. (Be sure to secure your doctor's blessing before adding aloe vera gel to your frostbite treatment.)

- **Knorr Chicken Bouillon.** To raise the temperature of your body core and improve circulation to your extremities, dissolve a cube of Knorr Chicken Bouillon in a cup of hot water and drink the warm, nonalcoholic, non-caffeinated beverage.

- **McCormick Ground (Cayenne) Red Pepper.** To help prevent frostbite, eat one-quarter teaspoon McCormick Ground (Cayenne) Red Pepper,

℞ STRANGE MEDICINE ℞

FREEZING YOUR TAIL OFF

● Exposure to temperatures of −4 to −10 degrees Fahrenheit (or a higher temperature exacerbated by high winds) for more than six hours typically produces frostbite. Getting wet or touching metal can expedite frostbite.

● With frostbite, the fluid in the cells freeze and the resulting ice crystals kill the cells. The blood clots, discontinuing circulation to the affected area, and the skin turns white and becomes numb.

● The parts of the human body most susceptible to frostbite are the fingers, toes, earlobes, chin, and tip of the nose.

● Frostbite occurs when the body constricts circulation to your extremities in an attempt to preserve its core temperature.

● To prevent frostbite, dress in layers so that air trapped between the layers provides insulation and wear a hat to avoid losing half your body heat through your head. Wool socks keep your feet warm by wicking away any moisture.

● Before going out in the cold, remove all metal jewelry, which conducts cold.

● Frostbite begins with a feeling of coldness in the skin that progresses to stinging, burning, throbbing, and ultimately numbness. Frostbitten skin is white and feels firm.

● If you can't get inside immediately, warm your fingers and hands with your own body heat by placing them in your armpits or between your thighs.

● Never let a frostbitten body part defrost and then refreeze. The part refreezes with larger water crystals, causing greater tissue damage.

sprinkled on food. The capsaicin in cayenne pepper helps your blood circulate to your extremities, keeping them warm.

● **Planters Sunflower Kernels** or **Planters Dry Roasted Almonds.** To help heal frostbite, eat one-quarter cup Planters Sunflower Kernels or Planters

Dry Roasted Almonds every day until the skin recovers. Sunflower seeds and almonds are packed with vitamin E, which helps repair damaged skin. One-quarter cup of sunflower seed kernels provides 22.68 milligrams of vitamin E, or 143 percent of the recommended daily allowance. One-quarter cup of almonds provides 15 milligrams of vitamin E, or 100 percent of the recommended daily allowance.

- **Tabasco Pepper Sauce** and **Star Olive Oil.** To help protect your feet from frostbite, mix ten drops Tabasco Pepper Sauce in one-quarter cup Star Olive Oil, and rub the mixture into your feet before putting on your socks and boots to go out into the cold. The capsaicin in this folk remedy, commonly used in developing countries, improves the circulation of blood to the capillaries in the skin. (Do not apply the mixture to broken skin or athlete's foot.)

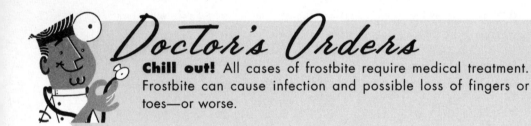

Doctor's Orders

Chill out! All cases of frostbite require medical treatment. Frostbite can cause infection and possible loss of fingers or toes—or worse.

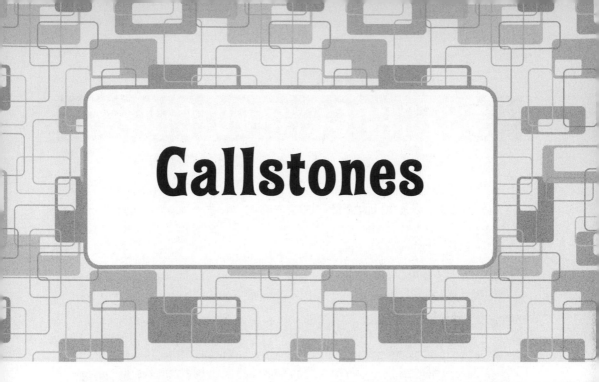

Gallstones

- **Chicken of the Sea Salmon, Chicken of the Sea Sardines,** or **Chicken of the Sea Tuna.** To prevent gallstones, eat salmon, sardines, or tuna three times a week to add the fatty acids commonly known as omega-3 oils to your diet. Omega-3 fatty acids improve the solubility of bile, preventing the growth of stones.

- **Kellogg's All-Bran.** One cup of Kellogg's All-Bran contains 20 grams of fiber. To help prevent problems from gallstones, eat 20 to 35 grams of fiber daily. Eighty percent of all gallstones are composed of cholesterol, but adding fiber to your diet helps remove excess cholesterol from the body. A daily minimum of five servings of fruits and vegetables, three servings of whole-grain foods, and one serving of beans adds sufficient fiber to your body to lower cholesterol.

- **McCormick Ground Turmeric.** To prevent the formation of gallstones, eat plenty of Indian curries spiced with McCormick Ground Turmeric. Turmeric contains curcumin, which increases the solubility of bile stored in the gallbladder. (If you are already suffering from gallstones, avoid turmeric.

℞ STRANGE MEDICINE ℞

LEAVE NO STONE UNTURNED

- The gallbladder stores bile, a digestive liquid produced by the liver. When this bile becomes too thick in the gallbladder, hard stones can form—anywhere from the size of a grain of sand to the size of a golf ball. If the stones get stuck in the ducts leading to the small intestine, intense pain results.

- Some people develop one gallstone at a time. Others develop many gallstones at the same time.

- Stuck gallstones sometimes pass through the duct or return to the gallbladder.

- Doctors treat painful gallstones by either removing the gallbladder (allowing bile to flow directly from your liver into your small intestine) or, in rare instances, by prescribing medication to dissolve the gallstones.

- Roughly one million Americans are diagnosed with gallstones every year.

- No one knows for certain what causes the formation of gallstones, but doctors believe gallstones may result from more cholesterol in the liver than the bile can dissolve, excess bilirubin in the bile, and the failure of your gallbladder to empty correctly.

- Approximately 500,000 Americans have their gallbladders removed every year to eliminate problems with gallstones.

- To prevent a lack of proper hydration from making bile more concentrated and more apt to produce gallstones, drink one ounce of water daily for every two pounds you weigh. In other words, if you weigh 160 pounds, drink eighty ounces (or ten 8-ounce glasses) of water daily.

Also, turmeric may increase the likelihood of bleeding when taken in combination with the blood thinner Coumadin or other anticoagulant medications.)

- **Minute Maid Orange Juice.** If you're a woman, help prevent gallstones by drinking an eight-ounce glass of Minute Maid Orange Juice daily.

According to one study, women with higher levels of vitamin C were 39 percent less likely to get gallstones than women with lower levels. Vitamin C lowers bile cholesterol levels. An 8-ounce glass of Minute Maid Orange Juice contains 71 milligrams of vitamin C, which is 120 percent the recommended daily allowance.

● **Star Olive Oil** and **ReaLemon.** To flush small gallstones from your system on your own, mix one-quarter cup Star Olive Oil and one-quarter cup ReaLemon lemon juice. One hour before you go to bed, drink the solution. Afterwards, take the herbal laxative cascara sagrada according to the directions on the label. Lie on your right side for thirty minutes, and then go to bed. If you see tiny green stones in your stool the following morning, the treatment worked. Repeat the treatment for two or three more days. (Do not perform this treatment without first obtaining your doctor's approval.)

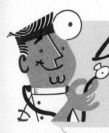

Doctor's Orders

Don't sink like a stone! If you experience severe pain in your abdomen lasting anywhere from several minutes to several hours, see a doctor immediately.

Genital Herpes

- **Conair Hair Dryer.** To relieve genital sores and speed healing, use a Conair Hair Dryer set on low or cool to blow the genital area dry after a bath or shower. The air from the dryer helps soothe and dry the sores.

- **Dannon Yogurt.** To reduce your susceptibility to a herpes outbreak, eat two cups of Dannon Nonfat Yogurt daily. Yogurt contains high amounts of lysine, an amino acid that inhibits the herpes virus from using other amino acids to construct the protein sheath that surrounds it, reducing and preventing herpes outbreaks. The beneficial *Lactobacillus acidophilus* bacteria (probiotics) in the yogurt are also believed to impede herpes.

- **Dial Soap.** During a herpes outbreak, keep the affected area clean by washing gently with Dial Antibacterial Soap and water. Triclosan, the antibacterial ingredient in the soap, prevents a secondary bacterial infection. Pat the area dry with a second towel solely for your genitals, and wash the towel after each use.

- **Heinz Baked Beanz.** To decrease the frequency of herpes outbreaks, eat one cup Heinz Baked Beanz every day. High in the amino acid lysine, baked beans inhibit the herpes virus from using other amino acids to construct the protein sheath that surrounds it, reducing and preventing herpes outbreaks. One cup of baked beans contains 986 milligrams of lysine.

● **Kingsford's Corn Starch.** To absorb moisture, keep the affected area dry, and promote healing, use a cotton ball to powder the open sores with Kingsford's Corn Starch. The cornstarch absorbs any excess moisture and reduces itching. (Refrain from double-dipping the cotton ball and contaminating the unused cornstarch.)

℞ STRANGE MEDICINE ℞

TOO CLOSE FOR COMFORT

● Genital herpes is a sexually transmitted, incurable virus that can erupt repeatedly with itchy, burning blisters and sores in the genital area for seven to ten days.

● The herpes simplex virus type 2 causes most cases of genital herpes.

● Roughly 25 percent of adults in the United States have genital herpes, but approximately 90 percent of them have no idea they have genital herpes.

● The first outbreak of genital herpes is frequently the most severe, followed by an average of four to five outbreaks a year.

● The antiviral drugs famciclovir, acyclovir, and valacyclovir, available by prescription through a medical doctor, help speed healing, reduce the severity, and suppress outbreaks of genital herpes.

● At the first sign of an outbreak, drink plenty of water (at least eight 8-ounce glasses a day) to flush toxins from your body and help prevent the outbreak from occurring.

● Never use a cortisone cream on genital sores. Cortisone suppresses the immune system, which may fuel the virus.

● To speed the healing of genital sores, wear loose-fitting cotton underwear, which allows the skin to breathe.

● A person infected with the herpes virus can pass the disease on to a partner through sexual contact.

- **Kretschmer Wheat Germ.** To prevent a herpes outbreak, add three teaspoons Kretschmer Wheat Germ to a cup of yogurt or bowl of oatmeal every day. Kretschmer Wheat Germ contains high amounts of the amino acid lysine, which helps discourage herpes outbreaks.

Doctor's Orders

Put it to bed! If you get small, fluid-filled blisters and burning, red, itchy sores on your genitals, consult a doctor for diagnosis and treatment. A herpes infection in a pregnant woman can infect the newborn baby and requires medical treatment.

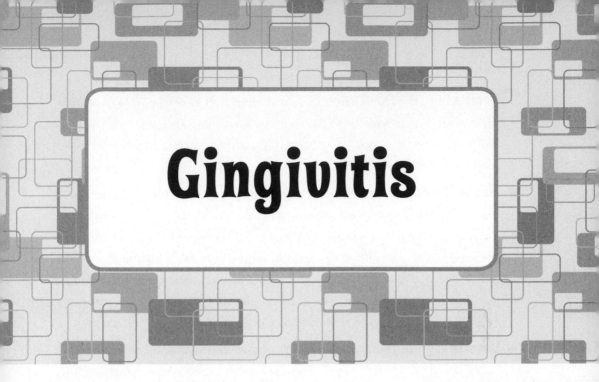

Gingivitis

- **Arm & Hammer Baking Soda.** Dampen your toothbrush bristles with water, dip them in an open box of Arm & Hammer Baking Soda, brush your teeth and along the gumline, and spit out. The mildly abrasive baking soda simultaneously cleans your teeth, kills bacteria that cause gingivitis, neutralizes the acids emitted by bacteria, and deodorizes your breath.

- **Fruit of the Earth Aloe Vera Gel.** If your gums continue bleeding after a faithful regimen of brushing and flossing, mix one tablespoon Fruit of the Earth Aloe Vera Gel with four ounces of warm water, rinse your mouth with the solution for thirty seconds, and spit out. The aloe vera gel soothes the gums.

- **Hydrogen Peroxide.** To augment your brushing and flossing, mix equal parts hydrogen peroxide and water, and rinse your mouth with the solution. The hydrogen peroxide kills the bacteria that excrete the chemicals that stimulate the proliferation of plaque.

- **Kellogg's All-Bran, Kellogg's Special K, or Total.** To heal damaged gums, eat one-half cup Kellogg's All-Bran, Kellogg's Special K, or Total cereal every day. Folate, better known as vitamin B$_9$, helps repair and replenish gum cells that have been damaged by gingivitis. One-half cup of Kellogg's All-Bran, Kellogg's Special K, or Total contains 100 percent of the daily value of folate.

- **Lipton Black Tea** or **Lipton Green Tea.** To prevent plaque from adhering to your teeth, drink one or two cups of Lipton Black Tea or Lipton Green Tea daily or use it as a mouthwash. The polyphenols in black and green teas are antioxidant compounds that inhibit plaque buildup, which leads to gum disease. A 2009 study at Kyushu University in Fukuoka, Japan, published in the *Journal of Periodontology,* found that men who drank a cup of green tea every day showed less risk and incidence of periodontal (gum) disease.

- **Listerine.** To ward off plaque buildup, rinse your mouth for thirty seconds two times daily with Listerine antiseptic mouthwash. A study reported in the *Journal of Clinical Periodontology* in 1993 showed that Listerine prevents plaque from developing, reducing the incidence of gingivitis.

- **McCormick Cardamom Seed.** To reduce inflamed gums, chew on a few McCormick Cardamom Seeds. The abundance of the antiseptic cineole in cardamom seeds helps minimize the bacteria in your mouth.

- **Morton Salt, Arm & Hammer Baking Soda,** and **Hydrogen Peroxide.** To kill the germs in your mouth that cause gingivitis, pour four ounces Morton Salt and four ounces Arm & Hammer Baking Soda into a clean, empty one-gallon jug, fill the rest of the jug with warm water, cap the bottle securely, and shake vigorously. Let sit for five minutes until a thin layer of undissolved solids rests on the bottom of the jug, indicating a concentrated solution. If there is no thin layer, add more salt and baking soda to the solution until one appears. Immediately before using the solution, add two teaspoons Hydrogen Peroxide to the jug. Fill a Waterpik with the solution, irrigate your gums with it, and do not swallow. Add one cup of water to the jug after each use. The solution in the jug is good for ten irrigations. The combination of salt, baking soda, and hydrogen peroxide dehydrates, kills, and washes away much of the bacteria that cause gum disease.

℞ STRANGE MEDICINE ℞

GETTING THE BRUSH-OFF

● Red, puffy gums that bleed when you brush or floss your teeth are the first signs of gingivitis, also known as gum disease.

● The buildup of bacterial plaque on your teeth below the gumline causes gingivitis.

● Plaque is a clear, sticky film of bacteria that adheres to your teeth. Left on your teeth, plaque hardens into mineral deposits called tartar.

● The simplest way to prevent gingivitis is to brush your teeth properly after meals and floss your teeth once a day.

● To remove plaque from your gumline before it hardens into tartar and causes gingivitis, brush your gumline with a toothbrush positioned at a 45-degree angle to your teeth.

● Studies show that brushing your teeth with an electric toothbrush removes more plaque than brushing manually with a regular toothbrush.

● Apples contain compounds that inhibit the enzymes secreted by the bacteria in your mouth. So eating an apple a day really can keep the dentist away.

● A thorough professional teeth cleaning combined with a consistent regimen of good daily oral hygiene can clear up gingivitis within a few days or weeks.

● **Ocean Spray Cranberry Juice.** Drinking cranberry juice, according to a 1998 study at Tel Aviv University School of Dental Medicine in Israel, prevents plaque-forming bacteria from adhering to teeth, thwarting gingivitis and gum disease.

● **Visa.** To remove the bacteria and toxins festering on your tongue, use a clean, expired Visa credit card to scrape your tongue from back to front ten to fifteen times.

- **Wrigley's Big Red Cinnamon Gum.** To prevent plaque buildup, chew a stick of Wrigley's Big Red Cinnamon Gum for twenty minutes. A 2011 study at the University of Illinois at Chicago showed that the cinnamic aldehyde in the gum reduces the amount of oral bacteria in your saliva by 50 percent and kills 40 percent of the types linked to bad breath.

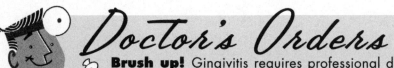

Doctor's Orders

Brush up! Gingivitis requires professional dental attention. If your gums bleed during brushing and flossing, they are red and swollen, or you have persistent bad breath, see your dentist. Otherwise, untreated gingivitis leads to periodontitis and the subsequent loss of teeth.

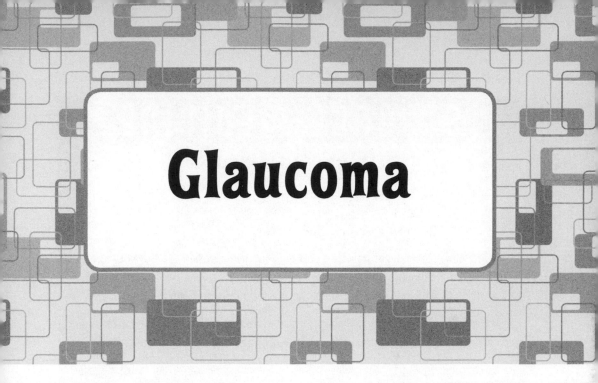

Glaucoma

- **Chicken of the Sea Salmon, Chicken of the Sea Sardines,** or **Chicken of the Sea Tuna.** Eating salmon, sardines, or tuna three times a week adds the fatty acids commonly known as omega-3 oils to your diet, which reduce inflammation and pain, strengthen the immune system, and increase resistance to stress. If your eye's drainage system is clogged due to inflammation, omega-3 fatty acids in fish oil can help decrease the inflammation, open the clog, and release excess pressure.

- **Jif Peanut Butter.** Magnesium can relax the blood vessel walls and improve blood flow to the eye. While eating a wide range of legumes, nuts, whole grains, and vegetables will help you meet your daily dietary need for magnesium, you can quickly replace magnesium in your body by eating Jif Peanut Butter (straight from the jar or in a sandwich). Four tablespoons of peanut butter contain 100 milligrams of magnesium (or 25 percent of the daily value).

- **Lewis Labs Brewer's Yeast.** To lower pressure inside your eyeballs, mix one or two tablespoons Lewis Labs Brewer's Yeast into your food, juice, or water once a day. Brewer's yeast contains chromium, a nutrient that facilitates the ability of the eye muscles to focus. Studies show a distinct correlation

℞ STRANGE MEDICINE ℞

A BLANK LOOK

● With glaucoma, a fluid called aqueous humor steadily builds up in the eyeballs, creating intense pressure that gradually damages nerves inside the eye, causing a slow loss of peripheral vision, giving you tunnel vision.

● Ordinarily, the eye naturally produces aqueous humor inside the front of the eye, and the fluid normally drains out where the iris and cornea meet. When the drainage system stops working properly, the aqueous humor builds up inside the eye.

● Glaucoma, nicknamed the "silent thief of sight," is the second leading cause of blindness, damaging vision gradually without any other noticeable symptoms.

● Glaucoma cannot be completely cured, and damage to your vision caused by the condition is irreversible, but proper treatment can prevent vision loss in people with glaucoma detected in its early stages, and can slow or prevent further vision loss in people with later-stage glaucoma.

● To prevent irreversible damage to your vision from glaucoma, have your eyes examined every three to five years after age 40 and annually after age 60. A thorough eye exam can help detect glaucoma in its early stages when it can be treated to slow or prevent further damage.

● Doctors treat glaucoma by prescribing medicated eyedrops, oral medications, or surgery to help the aqueous fluid flow out from the eye, and/or reduce the production of the fluid, reducing the pressure inside the eye.

● To prevent glaucoma, protect your eyes from injury by wearing proper eye protection when participating in activities where you risk being hit in the eye, such as playing sports involving a small ball or working with power tools.

between low chromium levels and an increased risk of glaucoma. The chromium in brewer's yeast provides the daily value of 120 micrograms of chromium. (Consult your doctor before supplementing your diet with brewer's yeast. Too much chromium can result in iron-deficiency anemia. If you have diabetes, chromium may lower your blood sugar level and reduce your need for insulin.)

- **Planters Dry Roasted Almonds, Planters Dry Roasted Cashews, or Planters Dry Roasted Peanuts.** Eating foods high in magnesium—like Planters Dry Roasted Almonds, Planters Dry Roasted Cashews, or Planters Dry Roasted Peanuts—can relax the blood vessel walls and improve blood flow to the eye. One ounce of almonds provides 80 milligrams of magnesium, one ounce of cashews provides 75 milligrams, and one ounce of dry roasted peanuts provides 50 milligrams.

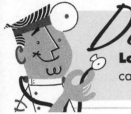

Doctor's Orders

Look out! If you suspect you have glaucoma, get under a doctor's care. Otherwise, glaucoma can lead to blindness.

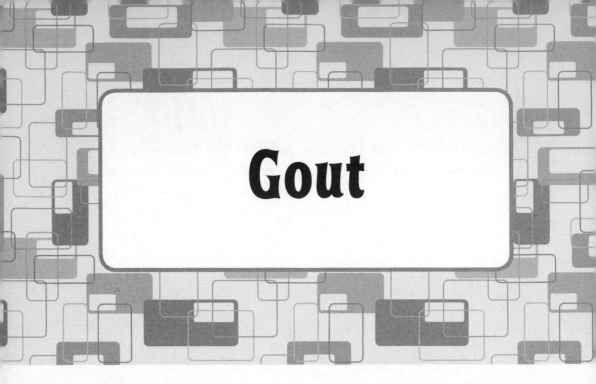

Gout

- **Advil.** To relieve the pain of a gout attack, take Advil according to the directions on the label. Ibuprofen, the active ingredient in Advil, helps reduce the inflammation around the affected joint responsible for the pain. Do not take aspirin (which can impede the body from excreting uric acid) or Tylenol (acetaminophen provides insufficient aid against inflammation).

- **Birds Eye Frozen Peas** and **Bounty Paper Towels.** To relieve gout pain, cover a bag of Birds Eye Frozen Peas with a sheet of Bounty Paper Towels, and place the bag on the painful joint for twenty minutes three times a day. The frozen peas act like small ice cubes, soothing and numbing the pain, and the bag of peas conforms to the shape of your body. The paper towel creates a layer of insulation to prevent frostbite. Refreeze the bag of peas for future ice-pack use. Be sure to label the bag for ice-pack use only. If you want to eat the peas, cook them after they thaw the first time, never after refreezing.

- **Heinz Apple Cider Vinegar.** To prevent gout attacks, take one table-spoon Heinz Apple Cider Vinegar every morning. For severe cases, take a second tablespoon in the evening.

℞ STRANGE MEDICINE ℞

CRYSTAL CLEAR

● Gout is a form of arthritis.

● During a gout attack, abnormally high levels of uric acid in the body cause some of the liquid uric acid to form sharp, painful crystals in the fluid that cushions the joints, causing intense pain, swelling, redness, and heat.

● No one knows why some people develop excessively high levels of uric acid, although scientists suspect genetics, diet, and obesity. They've also linked thiazide diuretics, prescribed for high blood pressure, to the disease.

● Half of all gout attacks affect the big toe.

● One gout attack increases the likelihood of further gout attacks.

● If left untreated, a gout attack can last for days.

● If you're diagnosed with high levels of uric acid, drink one gallon of distilled water (or water filtered by reverse osmosis) daily to dilute the uric acid and flush the crystals from your system.

● Eating anywhere between one-half cup to one pound of cherries a day helps prevent a gout attack. The anthocyanosides in cherries lower uric acid levels.

● A study conducted at the University of British Columbia and published in 2008 in *BMJ* (formerly called the *British Medical Journal*) revealed that men who drank two or more sugar-sweetened sodas each day had an 85 percent increased risk of gout compared to men who drank one soda or less each month.

● To lessen the frequency of gout attacks, avoid eating foods rich in purine, a compound that the body converts into uric acid. Foods high in purine include anchovies, herring, kidney, liver, mackerel, mussels, mushrooms, sardines, and sweetbreads.

● To control gout, cease drinking alcoholic beverages of any kind. All alcoholic beverages—beer, wine, and liquor—contain ethyl alcohol, which the body converts to uric acid.

- **Lakewood Black Cherry Juice.** To lower your uric acid levels (which trigger gout attacks), drink one or two cups of Lakewood Black Cherry Juice every day. A study conducted in 2002 at the University of California, Davis, showed that eating cherries provoked a significant decrease in plasma urate, found in uric acid.

- **Maxwell House Coffee.** If you're a male looking for an extreme way to lower your risk of gout, drink six or more cups of Maxwell House Coffee every day. A University of British Columbia study in 2007 revealed that men who drank six of more cups of coffee daily had a 59 percent lower risk of developing gout than men who did not drink any coffee. Men who drank four or five cups of coffee a day had a 40 percent lower risk than non-coffee drinkers. Components in coffee lower uric acid levels in the blood.

- **McCormick Thyme Leaves.** To relieve gout pain, place one teaspoon McCormick Thyme Leaves in a cup, fill with boiling water, cover with a saucer, and let steep for ten minutes. Strain out the leaves and drink the tea. A 2010 study in Japan revealed that carvacrol, a compound in thyme, prevents the body from producing prostaglandins, which cause inflammation.

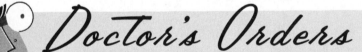

Doctor's Orders

Ouch! If you experience intense pain in a joint, consult a doctor to be tested for a high level of uric acid. A doctor can also administer colchicine, a drug that dissolves uric acid crystals.

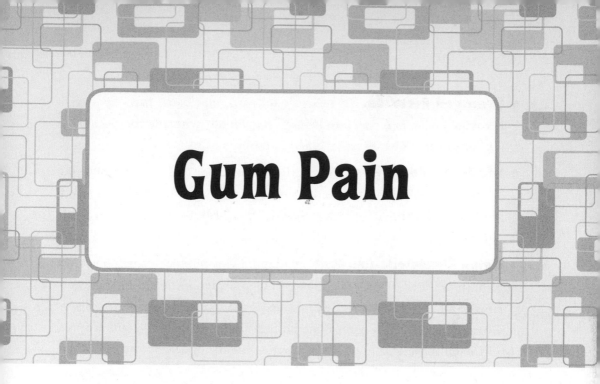

Gum Pain

- **Arm & Hammer Baking Soda.** To soothe gum pain until you can get to a dentist, mix one tablespoon Arm & Hammer Baking Soda with enough water to make a thick paste, and use your index finger to dab a light coat of the mixture on your tender gums. The sodium bicarbonate kills bacteria and neutralizes their acidic secretions. Do not swallow the baking soda.

- **Birds Eye Frozen Peas** and **Bounty Paper Towels.** To assuage gum pain, wrap a bag of Birds Eye Frozen Peas with a sheet of Bounty Paper Towels, and apply the bag to your cheek near the spot where your gums are causing you pain. The frozen peas act like small ice cubes, reducing inflammation and numbing the pain, and the bag of peas conforms to the shape of your face. The paper towel creates a layer of insulation to prevent frostbite. Refreeze the bag of peas for future ice-pack use. Be sure to label the bag for ice-pack use only. If you want to eat the peas, cook them after they thaw the first time, never after refreezing.

- **Fruit of the Earth Aloe Vera Gel.** To soothe irritated gums, use a soft-bristled toothbrush to rub Fruit of the Earth Aloe Vera Gel on your gums. The aloe vera gel relieves the irritation, heals damaged tissue, and stimulates blood circulation.

- **Hydrogen Peroxide.** To relieve gum pain, mix equal parts hydrogen peroxide and warm water and rinse your mouth with the solution. The hydrogen peroxide kills bacteria and numbs the pain.

- **Life Savers Pep-O-Mint.** To relieve sore gums due to dry mouth, suck on a Life Savers Pep-O-Mint candy. Sucking on a hard candy triggers saliva production, and the mint in Life Savers Pep-O-Mint stimulates even more saliva output.

- **Lipton Chamomile Tea.** Place two Lipton Chamomile Tea bags in a cup of boiling water, cover with a saucer, steep for ten minutes, let cool, and rinse your mouth with the entire cup of tea. Repeat this routine daily. Chamomile tea lessens gum pain and helps fight gingivitis. (Coumarin, an anticoagulant in chamomile, may increase the likelihood of bleeding when

☥ STRANGE MEDICINE ☥

GUMMING UP THE WORKS

- Minor gum irritation means you need to do a better job brushing and flossing your teeth.

- Never apply aspirin directly to your gum in the hopes of relieving pain. The salicylic acid in the aspirin burns the gum tissue.

- Gum pain is not the first sign of periodontal (gum) disease. The pain may likely signal that gingivitis (inflammation of the gums) has advanced to periodontitis (inflammation of the tissue around the teeth, causing gums to recede and teeth to loosen).

- If you smoke or chew tobacco, quit immediately. Smoking weakens the gums, and chewing tobacco irritates the gums and causes gum cancer.

- Sores on the gums, including abscesses and canker sores, can cause gum pain.

- The hormonal changes of pregnancy can increase sensitivity of the gums, causing soreness, pain, and bleeding.

taken in combination with the blood thinner Coumadin or other anticoagulant medications.)

- **Lipton Tea Bags.** To soothe bleeding or swollen gums, dampen a Lipton
Tea Bag with warm water, and press it against the affected area. The tannin
in the tea is an astringent that reduces inflammation and stops bleeding.

- **McCormick Thyme Leaves.** To strengthen your gums, place one teaspoon
McCormick Thyme Leaves in a cup, fill with boiling water, cover with a
saucer, and let steep for fifteen minutes. Strain out the leaves and let the tea
cool to room temperature. Rinse your mouth with the tea two or three
times a day. The thymol in thyme kills bacteria, reduces inflammation, and
numbs pain.

- **Morton Salt.** To soothe gum pain and reduce inflammation, dissolve one
teaspoon Morton Salt in an eight-ounce glass of warm water, and swish the
salt water around in your mouth for one minute.

- **Orajel.** To numb a gum infection or a burn, cut, or ulceration on the gum,
apply a dab of Orajel to the affected area. The benzocaine in the ointment
anesthetizes the spot, instantly blocking the pain.

- **Planters Sunflower Kernels.** To strengthen gum tissues, slowly chew a
teaspoon of Planters Sunflower Kernels every day. The minerals in sunflower seeds help keep gums healthy.

- **Popsicle.** If dry mouth is causing gum irritation, suck on your favorite
flavor Popsicle to spur the salivary glands into action, and press it against the
affected area to help soothe the pain.

Doctor's Orders

Don't just flap your gums! If you experience gum pain, see
a dentist to rule out the possibility of periodontal (gum) disease—
even if the pain subsides.

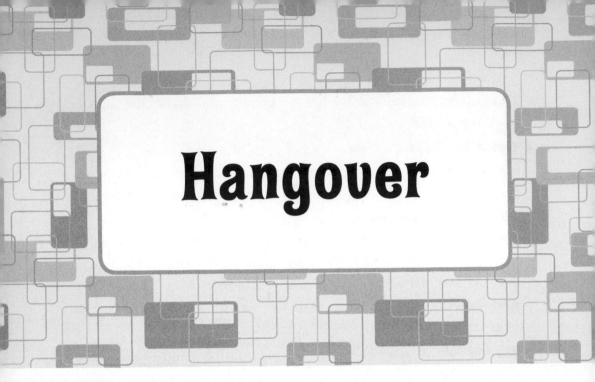

Hangover

- **Aunt Jemima Original Syrup.** To help relieve a hangover, eat two table-spoons Aunt Jemima Original Syrup. The fructose in the corn syrup raises blood sugar depleted by alcohol.

- **Birds Eye Frozen Peas** and **Bounty Paper Towels.** To relieve a headache caused by a hangover, wrap a bag of Birds Eye Frozen Peas with a sheet of Bounty Paper Towels, and hold it against your head. The frozen peas act like small ice cubes, shrinking the swollen blood vessels that cause the throbbing, and the bag of peas conforms to the shape of your head. The paper towel creates a layer of insulation to prevent frostbite. Refreeze the bag of peas for future ice-pack use. Be sure to label the bag for ice-pack use only. If you want to eat the peas, cook them after they thaw the first time, never after refreezing.

- **Campbell's Chicken Noodle Soup** or **Knorr Chicken Bouillon.** To relieve a hangover, once the nausea subsides, have a warm bowl of Campbell's Chicken Noodle Soup or a cup of Knorr Chicken Bouillon to replace the salt and potassium that alcohol depletes from the body.

- **Gatorade.** To restore your equilibrium from a hangover, drink Gatorade to rehydrate your cells and replace the electrolytes, minerals, and nutrients drained from your body by the alcohol.

- **Life Savers Pep-O-Mint.** To help calm the stomach upset accompanying a hangover, suck on a Lifesavers Pep-O-Mint candy. The volatile oils in peppermint help counteract nausea.

- **Lipton Ginger Tea** and **SueBee Honey.** To alleviate hangover pain, place a Lipton Ginger Tea bag in a cup of boiling water, cover with a saucer, and steep for ten minutes. Sweeten with two teaspoons SueBee Honey, and then drink the tea. The ginger eases nausea, and the honey helps your body burn off any alcohol remaining in your system. (Do not drink ginger tea if you have gallstones. Ginger can increase bile production.)

- **Maxwell House Coffee.** To alleviate the pain of a hangover, drink one or two cups of Maxwell House Coffee. As a vasoconstrictor, coffee reduces

STRANGE MEDICINE

DRUNK AS A SKUNK

- Hangover symptoms typically start eight to sixteen hours after drinking to intoxication and generally include headache, nausea, red eyes, dizziness, vomiting, fatigue, sensitivity to light, and difficulty concentrating.

- The vomiting that accompanies a hangover helps purge the body of toxins.

- Alcohol dehydrates and depletes the body of minerals, dilates the blood vessels in the head, and makes the blood excessively acidic.

- To avert a severe hangover after drinking excessively, drink several glasses of water. Alcohol dehydrates the body, and water replenishes the lost liquid and helps flush the alcohol from your system.

- Eating something before imbibing beer, wine, or liquor slows the body's ability to absorb alcohol, tempering the effects of inebriation and helping to prevent a hangover.

- Do not take a pain reliever that contains acetaminophen (such as Tylenol) to combat the headache accompanying a hangover. Mixing acetaminophen with the alcohol remaining in your system can harm your liver.

the width of the swollen blood vessels in your head. (Be aware that coffee is a diuretic that may dehydrate your body further.)

- **Minute Maid Orange Juice, Minute Maid Grapefruit Juice,** or **Campbell's Tomato Juice.** To help relieve a hangover, drink a tall glass of orange, grapefruit, or tomato juice. The fruit sugar, or fructose, in these juices helps the body metabolize alcohol more rapidly, removing the toxins from your system.

- **ReaLime** and **Domino Sugar.** When you wake up in the morning with a hangover, mix two teaspoons ReaLime lime juice, one-quarter teaspoon Domino Sugar, and one cup of water, and drink the solution slowly. The lime is believed to revitalize the liver, the sugar raises blood sugar depleted by alcohol, and the water rehydrates your body.

- **SueBee Honey** and **Nabisco Original Premium Saltine Crackers.** Once the nausea from a hangover subsides, eat some SueBee Honey spread on Nabisco Original Premium Saltine Crackers to help replace the fructose in your body and flush the remaining alcohol from your system.

- **Tabasco Pepper Sauce** and **Campbell's Tomato Juice.** To cure a hangover, mix one-quarter teaspoon Tabasco Pepper Sauce in an eight-ounce glass of Campbell's Tomato Juice, and drink the tonic. The capsaicin in the Tabasco Pepper Sauce helps inhibit the body from producing substance P, which causes inflammation and pain, and the tomato juice replenishes your electrolytes.

- **Wonder Bread.** To help regain your strength and balance in the wake of a hangover, eat a few slices of toasted Wonder Bread. The carbohydrates quickly provide your body with energy, raise the blood sugar depleted by alcohol, and soothe an upset stomach.

Doctor's Orders

It's high time! If you can't remember what happened while you were drunk, or if you get hangovers on a regular basis, you may have a drinking problem. Contact a doctor to discuss possible treatments.

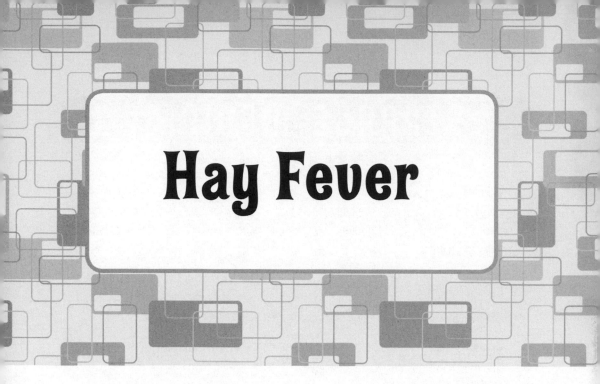

Hay Fever

- **Heinz Apple Cider Vinegar.** Mix two tablespoons Heinz Apple Cider Vinegar in two cups of water, and either sip the mixture throughout the day or drink the entire concoction in one sitting. For more severe cases of hay fever, drink the solution up to three times a day. If you consume the mixture at the onset of hay fever symptoms, the symptoms should dissipate within three hours. If taken after experiencing the symptoms for a day or more, the mixture should quell the symptoms within twenty-four hours. Continue taking the mixture until the symptoms vanish.

- **Lipton Tea Bags.** To soothe itchy eyes caused by hay fever, dampen two Lipton Tea Bags with warm water, lie down, and cover your closed eyes with the tea bags for five to ten minutes. The tannin in the tea relieves the itch and revitalizes irritated eyes.

- **Maxwell House Coffee.** Drinking a cup of Maxwell House Coffee can alleviate some symptoms of hay fever, according to researchers at Wonkwang University in South Korea. Turns out that coffee is a natural antihistamine that prohibits the mast cells from overproducing histamine, which leads to hay fever symptoms. The caffeine in coffee also increases the effectiveness of pain relievers by 40 percent when treating a sinus headache, according

STRANGE MEDICINE

HIT THE HAY

● Hay fever, clinically known as allergic rhinitis, is triggered when a person with the allergy breathes in pollen. The body reacts by releasing chemicals, including histamine, which cause symptoms such as itching, swelling, mucus production, itchy sinuses and eyes, and teary eyes.

● Taking vitamin C can alleviate hay fever symptoms. Several U.S. studies suggest that taking 500 milligrams of vitamin C daily and increasing the dosage to 2,000 milligrams over a six-week period can reduce histamine levels by 40 percent.

● To avoid hay fever triggers, limit your time outdoors, wear a face mask while doing yard work or sitting outside, and keep your doors and windows closed when the pollen count is high.

● To avoid pollen, use air conditioning in your house and car and be sure to use an allergy-grade filter in the ventilation system. In the car, use a car air ionizer to generate negative ions to reduce airborne pollen.

● Run a high-efficiency particulate air (HEPA) filter in your bedroom to remove pollen from the air.

● Use a dehumidifier to reduce indoor humidity. Allergens thrive in humid conditions.

● During hay fever season, refrain from hanging laundry outside to dry, where pollen can stick to sheets, towels, and clothes.

● Avoid outdoor activities in the early morning when pollen counts are highest.

● On dry, windy days stay indoors to avoid gusts of airborne allergens.

● Avoid mowing the lawn or raking leaves, which stirs up pollen.

● Bathe your pets on a weekly basis, if possible, to rinse off any pollen they may be tracking through your home, and keep your pets out of your bedroom.

to the National Headache Foundation. When treating hay fever with coffee, be sure to drink plenty of water. Caffeinated beverages are diuretics, which can lead to dehydration, increasing nasal congestion. Consult your doctor before treating hay fever with coffee.

- **McCormick Garlic Powder.** To alleviate the symptoms of hay fever and give your immune system a boost, use McCormick Garlic Powder in your cooking, or once a day eat a slice of lightly buttered bread sprinkled with one-half teaspoon garlic powder. Aside from being a natural antibiotic, garlic contains alliin, a chemical that mucus liquefies, clearing the sinuses.

- **McCormick Ground Turmeric.** For relief from hay fever within fifteen minutes, stir one teaspoon McCormick Ground Turmeric into an eight-ounce glass of water and drink it. The bioflavonoids in turmeric are antioxidants that suppress histamine production. (Turmeric may increase the likelihood of bleeding when taken in combination with the blood thinner Coumadin or other anticoagulant medications.)

- **Morton Salt** and **Arm & Hammer Baking Soda.** To make a saline nose wash to rinse allergens, irritants, and mucus from your nasal passages, purify eight ounces of water by boiling for three minutes, let cool to room temperature, and dissolve one-quarter teaspoon Morton Salt and one-quarter teaspoon Arm & Hammer Baking Soda in the purified water.

- **Vaseline Petroleum Jelly.** To prevent your nostrils from becoming irritated during a bout of hay fever, apply a small dab of Vaseline Petroleum Jelly inside your nose at the beginning of each day.

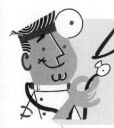

Doctor's Orders

Make hay! If hay fever is making your life unbearable, consult a doctor who can prescribe appropriate allergy medications or advise other treatments.

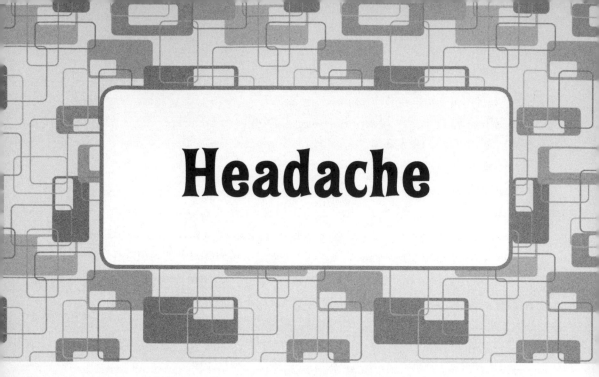

Headache

- **Birds Eye Frozen Peas** and **Bounty Paper Towels.** To soothe a headache, cover a bag of Birds Eye Frozen Peas with a sheet of Bounty Paper Towels, and apply to your forehead or the back of your neck for fifteen minutes. The frozen peas act like small ice cubes, constricting the blood vessels so they stop pressing against the nerves, and the bag of peas conforms to the shape of your head or neck. The paper towel creates a layer of insulation to prevent frostbite. Refreeze the bag of peas for future ice-pack use. Be sure to label the bag for ice-pack use only. If you want to eat the peas, cook them after they thaw the first time, never after refreezing.

- **Colman's Mustard Powder.** To soothe a headache, dissolve two teaspoons Colman's Mustard Powder in a quart of warm water in a basin large enough to hold your feet. Soak your feet in the mustard footbath for fifteen minutes. The warmth of the water and the mustard draws blood to the feet, easing the pressure on the blood vessels in your head.

- **Jif Peanut Butter.** A large number of clinical studies have shown that magnesium can prevent headaches by relaxing arteries and muscles in the body. While eating a wide range of legumes, nuts, whole grains, and vegetables will help you meet your daily dietary need for magnesium, you can quickly replace magnesium in your body by eating Jif Peanut Butter (straight from the jar or in a sandwich). Four tablespoons of peanut butter contain 100 milligrams of magnesium (or 25 percent of the daily value).

- **Lipton Chamomile Tea.** To relieve a headache, slowly sip a cup of Lipton Chamomile Tea, steeped for ten minutes. Chamomile acts like a sedative to calm your nerves. (Coumarin, an anticoagulant in chamomile, may increase the likelihood of bleeding when taken in combination with the blood thinner Coumadin or other anticoagulant medications.)

- **Lipton Ginger Tea.** To alleviate headache pain, place a Lipton Ginger Tea bag in a cup of boiling water, cover with a saucer, steep for ten minutes, and then drink the tea. Ginger inhibits prostaglandin production, thus reducing inflammation in blood vessels in the brain. (Do not drink ginger tea if you have gallstones. Ginger can increase bile production.)

- **Maxwell House Coffee.** Drinking a cup of Maxwell House Coffee can relieve a headache. The caffeine, an ingredient in many pain relievers, doubles as a vasoconstrictor, narrowing the blood vessels.

- **McCormick Pure Peppermint Extract** and **Kleenex Tissues.** Put two or three drops McCormick Pure Peppermint Extract on a Kleenex Tissue, hold it under your nose, and breathe deeply. The aroma of peppermint stimulates the brain and then relaxes the nerves responsible for the headache pain.

- **McCormick Rosemary Leaves.** Place a tea infuser filled with one teaspoon McCormick Rosemary Leaves in a teacup, add boiling water, cover with a saucer, and steep for ten minutes. Drink the tea (unless you're pregnant) to prevent the headache from getting worse.

- **Planters Dry Roasted Almonds, Planters Dry Roasted Cashews,** or **Planters Dry Roasted Peanuts.** Eating foods high in magnesium—like Planters Dry Roasted Almonds, Planters Dry Roasted Cashews, or Planters Dry Roasted Peanuts—can reduce headache pain by relaxing arteries and muscles in the body. A large number of clinical studies have shown that magnesium can prevent headaches. One ounce of almonds provides 80 milligrams of magnesium, one ounce of cashews provides 75 milligrams, and one ounce of dry roasted peanuts provides 50 milligrams.

☥ STRANGE MEDICINE ☥

KEEPING A COOL HEAD

● To avoid headaches, eat a healthy breakfast, and have lunch and dinner at about the same time every day. Otherwise, going without food causes a drop in blood sugar, which can trigger a headache.

● Getting eight hours of continuous sleep at night prevents headaches. For the best results, go to bed and wake up at the same times every day, even on weekends.

● To prevent frequent headaches, avoid taking over-the-counter headache medications more than twice a week. Doing so can actually cause a rebound effect, increasing the severity and frequency of your headaches.

● Get thirty minutes of exercise—walking, bicycling, or swimming—at least three days a week. Exercise relieves the stress that may be responsible for your headaches.

● Grinding your teeth or clenching your jaw while you sleep can cause headache pain. If you do either of these things, have your dentist fit you with a mouthguard.

● Massaging the muscle beneath the web of flesh between the thumb and index finger helps relieve headache pain.

● Reducing stress, a common trigger of headaches, prevents headaches. By meditating, doing yoga, relaxing, listening to music, or taking a hot bath, you can reduce stress and minimize headaches.

● To reduce the frequency of headaches, minimize or eliminate the amount of caffeine you consume. While caffeine can lessen existing headache pain, moderate consumption of caffeine often causes headaches. A 1984 study at the University of Sydney in Australia, published in the *International Journal of Epidemiology*, demonstrated that consuming 240 milligrams of caffeine (the equivalent of approximately two 8-ounce cups of coffee) per day significantly increased the risk of headaches.

● If wearing a helmet, tight hat, headband, or goggles gives you a headache, simply remove the headgear to relieve the continuous pressure on your forehead or scalp.

- **Uncle Ben's Converted Brand Rice.** Fill a clean sock with Uncle Ben's Converted Brand Rice, tie a knot in the end, and heat in a microwave oven for one minute. Place the homemade heating pad over your forehead for ten minutes to relieve the headache pain. If the heating pad is too hot, place a paper towel between your skin and the sock. The rice-filled sock can be reheated often and stored in the pantry closet for future use.

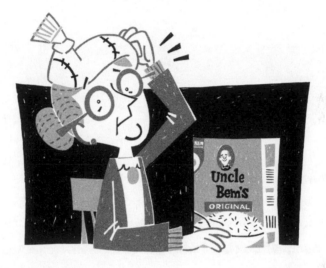

- **Vicks VapoRub.** To soothe headache pain, rub a dab of Vicks VapoRub on your temples and forehead. The scent of the menthol stimulates and then relaxes the nerves causing the pain.

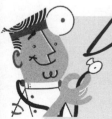

Doctor's Orders

Heads up! If you get three or more headaches a week, or if you get a sudden, severe headache accompanied by blurry vision, consult a doctor.

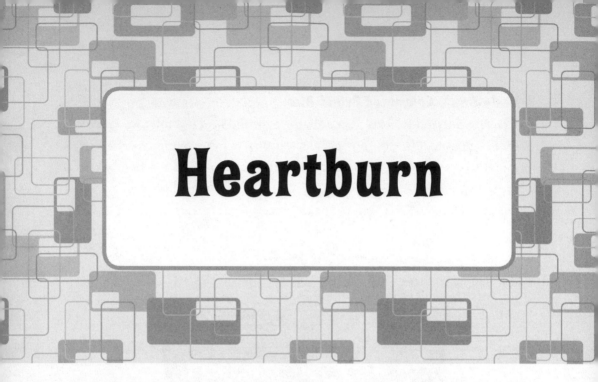

Heartburn

- **Angostura Aromatic Bitters.** To prevent heartburn, add several dashes of Angostura Aromatic Bitters to a glass of water, and drink the concoction before dining. The tincture of the gentian root stimulates digestion.

- **Arm & Hammer Baking Soda** and **ReaLemon.** To neutralize the stomach acid causing heartburn, dissolve one-half teaspoon Arm & Hammer Baking Soda in four-ounces of warm water, add a few drops of ReaLemon lemon juice, and drink the solution. The alkaline baking soda neutralizes stomach acid and the lemon juice dispels some of the gas generated by the baking soda. (Do not use this remedy if you're on a sodium-restricted diet. Read the directions on the side of the box of baking soda before administering.)

- **CharcoCaps Activated Charcoal.** To alleviate heartburn, take one to two 200- to 500-milligram CharcoCaps Activated Charcoal capsules. The charcoal soaks up the excess acid in your throat and stomach, carrying it out of the body. Charcoal also absorbs nutrients, so be sure to discontinue use after a few days. (Don't confuse activated charcoal with charcoal briquettes. Activated charcoal is a charcoal that has been processed with oxygen to be extremely porous and absorb odors or other substances.)

- **French's Mustard.** To prevent heartburn, take one teaspoon French's Mustard before your meal or add it to the dish you're about to eat. The vinegar in the mustard stimulates saliva production and reduces the acidity in your stomach.

- **Fruit of the Earth Aloe Vera Gel.** To relieve the symptoms of heartburn, drink one cup Fruit of the Earth Aloe Vera Gel. Fruit of the Earth Aloe Vera Gel is 100 percent pure aloe gel and edible. The aloe vera gel helps protect and heal the inner lining of the esophagus.

- **Heinz Apple Cider Vinegar.** To soothe heartburn caused by too much food stuck in your belly, mix one teaspoon Heinz Apple Cider Vinegar in four ounces of water, and sip the concoction during or after your meal. Too little stomach acid causes as many cases of heartburn as too much stomach acid. Without an adequate supply of stomach acid, improperly digested food remains in the stomach, causing the lower esophageal sphincter (the valve at the base of the esophagus) to relax, allowing partially digested food (and stomach acid) to travel back up the esophagus. Apple cider vinegar aids in the overall digestive process by stimulating the stomach to secrete more hydrochloric acid.

- **Lakewood Papaya Juice.** To relieve heartburn, drink a glass of Lakewood Papaya Juice. The enzyme papain helps diminish heartburn. Dr. George Herschell, writing in the *British Medical Journal* dated April 3, 1886, reported: "This drug papain is extremely valuable in this form of indigestion."

- **Lakewood Pure Carrot Juice.** To tame the stomach acid causing heartburn, drink a glass of Lakewood Pure Carrot Juice. The alkaline vegetable juice helps subdue the intensity of the stomach acid.

- **Lipton Chamomile Tea.** To relieve heartburn, drink a cup of Lipton Chamomile Tea, steeped for ten minutes, three times a day for two to three weeks. Chamomile, an officially approved heartburn treatment in Germany, eases spasms and acts like a sedative to calm your nerves. (Coumarin, an anticoagulant in chamomile, may increase the likelihood of bleeding when taken in combination with the blood thinner Coumadin or other anticoagulant medications.)

℞ STRANGE MEDICINE ℞

WHERE'S THE FIRE?

● Heartburn, medically called gastroesophageal reflux, occurs when a weakened lower esophageal sphincter (the valve at the bottom of the esophagus) lets stomach acid flow up into the esophagus. The acid burns the inner lining of the tube, causing pain.

● Antacids subdue the harshness of stomach acid, but in order for your digestive system to work properly, the stomach needs adequate hydrochloric acid to break down proteins into amino acids that your body can use. In fact, having too little hydrochloric acid also causes the symptoms of heartburn.

● A simple cure for heartburn: Immediately upon feeling the initial tinge of heartburn, drink a glass of water to flush the stomach acid back down into the stomach.

● To avoid getting heartburn, eat five or six small meals a day (rather than two or three big meals); avoid high-fat foods; do not eat for three or four hours before bedtime; eliminate coffee, tea, and chocolate from your diet; drink fewer carbonated beverages; avoid spicy foods; stop smoking; and cut down on the amount of citrus fruits and tomatoes you eat.

● While you might be tempted to drink milk to cool your throat, milk stimulates the stomach to produce more acid.

● To discourage heartburn at night, sleep with your head elevated four to six inches by placing bricks or blocks under the legs of the bed, letting gravity prevent the stomach acids from traveling up into your esophagus.

● Taking a twenty-minute walk after eating a big meal prevents heartburn for the simple reason that walking aids digestion.

● Wearing clothes with a generous waistband or switching from a belt to suspenders can alleviate heartburn.

- **Lipton Ginger Tea.** To alleviate heartburn pain, place a Lipton Ginger Tea bag in a cup of boiling water, cover with a saucer, steep for ten minutes, and then drink the tea. Do this two or three times a day. Ginger helps relax the muscles lining the inner walls of the esophagus, discouraging them from carrying the stomach acid upward. (Do not drink ginger tea if you have gallstones. Ginger can increase bile production.)

- **McCormick Fennel Seed.** To ease heartburn, place a tea infuser filled with one tablespoon McCormick Fennel Seed in a teacup, add boiling water, cover with a saucer, steep for ten minutes, and drink the tea. Herbalists claim that the volatile oil in the fennel soothes heartburn.

- **McCormick Ground Cardamom.** To relieve heartburn, add one teaspoon McCormick Ground Cardamom to eight ounces of water, boil for ten minutes, strain, and drink the hot tea. Those who practice Ayurvedic medicine claim that tea made from cardamom soothes heartburn.

- **Wesson Canola Oil.** To soothe heartburn, take one tablespoon Wesson Canola Oil, ideally on an empty stomach. The vegetable oil coats the lining of the esophagus with a protective layer, reducing inflammation.

- **Wrigley's Juicy Fruit Gum.** To temporarily relieve heartburn, chew a stick of Wrigley's Juicy Fruit Gum. Chewing gum stimulates the salivary glands to double the production of saliva, which neutralizes acid and pushes the digestive juices back down into the stomach. (Avoid gums flavored with peppermint or spearmint, which relax the lower esophageal sphincter, exacerbating the problem.)

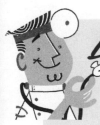

Doctor's Orders

Take heart! If heartburn is accompanied by chest pain or other symptoms, see a doctor immediately to rule out a heart attack. If your heartburn doesn't clear up after one week of using home remedies, see a doctor to make sure you don't have a more serious medical problem.

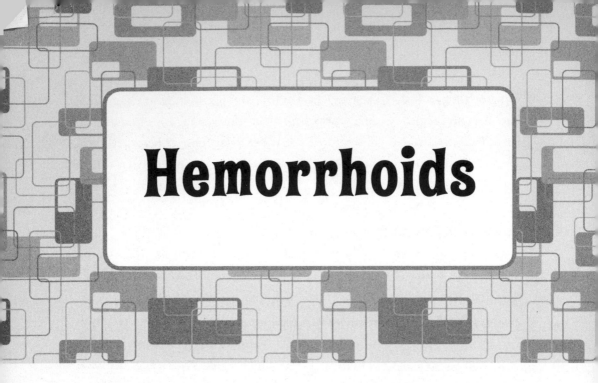

Hemorrhoids

- **Betty Crocker Potato Buds.** To soothe hemorrhoids, mix one-half cup Betty Crocker Potato Buds and one-half cup of hot water into a thick paste, let cool to room temperature, and, lying face down, apply the mashed potatoes to the affected area. Let sit for ten minutes. Potatoes have antibacterial and astringent properties.

- **Birds Eye Frozen Peas** and **Bounty Paper Towels.** To shrink a hemorrhoid and relieve the pain, wrap a bag of Birds Eye Frozen Peas with a sheet of Bounty Paper Towels, hold it between the cheeks of your buttocks, gently pressed against the anus. The frozen peas act like small ice cubes, shrinking the swollen blood vessels and numbing the pain. The bag of peas also conforms to the shape of your body. The paper towel creates a layer of insulation to prevent frostbite. Refreeze the bag of peas for future ice-pack use, making sure to label the bag for ice-pack use only. If you want to eat the peas, cook them after they thaw the first time, never after refreezing.

- **Conair Hair Dryer.** To avoid scratching hemorrhoids after bathing, gently pat the surrounding area dry with a towel and then finish the job by aiming the nozzle of a Conair Hair Dryer set on cool to dry the tender spot.

- **Crisco All-Vegetable Shortening.** To relieve itching and soothe hemorrhoids, apply a dab of Crisco All-Vegetable Shortening. The soybean oil and cottonseed oil moisturize the area.

- **Desitin.** To baby the pain and itch of hemorrhoids, apply a dab of Desitin, the diaper rash remedy, to the affected area. The zinc oxide helps relieve hemorrhoid itch.

- **Dickinson's Witch Hazel** and **Stayfree Maxi Pads.** To help shrink and soothe external hemorrhoids, chill a bottle of Dickinson's Witch Hazel in the refrigerator, saturate a Stayfree Maxi Pad with the cold witch hazel, and hold it against the hemorrhoid until the cold dissipates. Repeat if desired. The cold provides relief, and as a vasoconstrictor, the witch hazel shrinks inflamed blood vessels. Witch hazel is a main ingredient in Tucks medicated pads.

- **Dr. Teal's Epsom Salt.** To relieve hemorrhoid pain rapidly, fill a bathtub with four or five inches of warm water, add a handful of Dr. Teal's Epsom Salt, and take a "sitz bath," soaking your anal area in the solution for ten minutes. Repeat this several times a day. The warm water prompts increased blood flow, which shrinks the inflamed veins, as does the Epsom Salt.

- **Fruit of the Earth Aloe Vera Gel.** To soothe hemorrhoid pain, apply a dab of Fruit of the Earth Aloe Vera Gel to the affected area. The aloe lubricates the anus, preventing further irritation, and helps the tissue heal.

- **Grandma's Robust Molasses.** To cure hemorrhoids, take one teaspoon Grandma's Robust Molasses twice a day. Within a few weeks, the hemorrhoids will diminish significantly and possibly disappear. Grandma's Robust Molasses contains calcium, cooper, iron, manganese, and potassium—minerals that help strengthen veins.

- **Heinz Apple Cider Vinegar.** To relieve a throbbing hemorrhoid, saturate a cotton ball with Heinz Apple Cider Vinegar and hold it against the hemorrhoid for ten minutes. The astringent and anti-inflammatory properties of apple cider vinegar reduce swelling and relieve pain.

BRINGING UP THE REAR

- Hemorrhoids are a group of swollen veins protruding like small balloons from the inside of the anal canal. Hemorrhoids tend to burn, itch, and occasionally bleed.

- The quickest way to relieve hemorrhoid discomfort is to sit in a bathtub filled with four or five inches of warm water for ten minutes several times a day. The warm water prompts increased blood flow, which shrinks the inflamed veins.

- The easiest way to subdue hemorrhoids and prevent them from recurring is to add sufficient fiber to your diet (see Kellogg's All-Bran tip on the opposite page) and drink plenty of water to soften your stools.

- The American Society of Colon and Rectal Surgeons reports that more than half of adult Americans develop hemorrhoids, typically after age thirty.

- Chronic constipation, chronic diarrhea, pregnancy, and childbirth can all cause or exacerbate hemorrhoids.

- Doctors remove hemorrhoids with rubber-band ligation (cutting off circulation to the hemorrhoid, causing it to dry up and fall off), coagulation (laser, infrared light, or heat), or surgery.

- Gently push a protruding hemorrhoid back into the anal canal. Otherwise, the protuberance may clot.

- Walking briskly for twenty to thirty minutes a day aids digestion, keeping your bowels flowing smoothly with far less stress and strain.

- When you feel the urge to defecate, comply with it. Otherwise, trying to suppress your bowel movement can make your stool dry and harder to pass.

- Never strain or hold your breath to force a bowel movement. Doing so puts excessive pressure on the veins in your anal canal.

- **Huggies Baby Wipes.** To avoid irritating hemorrhoids after a bowel movement, clean yourself gently using pre-moistened Huggies Natural Care Baby Wipes. These convenient, hypoallergenic, fragrance-free, alcohol-free wipes also contain soothing aloe and vitamin E.

- **Kellogg's All-Bran.** To prevent hemorrhoids, eat one cup Kellogg's All-Bran cereal every morning for breakfast. Adding 20 to 35 grams of fiber to your diet daily creates large, soft stools that are easy to pass without the straining that damages anal veins. One cup of Kellogg's All-Bran contains 20 grams of fiber. (Be sure to drink plenty of fluids to stay well hydrated to avoid constipation.)

- **Kingsford's Corn Starch.** To absorb moisture and keep the anal area dry, use a cotton ball to powder a protruding hemorrhoid with Kingsford's Corn Starch. The cornstarch absorbs any moisture, protecting the anal area from irritation and infection.

- **Lipton Tea Bags.** To soothe an external hemorrhoid, apply a Lipton Tea Bag dampened with warm water. The tannin anesthetizes the pain, reduces swelling, and stops any bleeding.

- **Metamucil.** For another way to add fiber to your diet and prevent hemorrhoids, take one serving of Metamucil (as instructed on the package label) in or with eight ounces of water once a day. Metamucil contain psyllium seed husk, a natural dietary fiber originating from the psyllium plant, which absorbs liquid, bulking up your stool and allowing it to pass through your system more comfortably. (Metamucil generally produces a laxative effect in twelve to seventy-two hours.)

- **Noxzema.** To soothe hemorrhoids, apply a dab of Noxzema around the affected area. Originally developed as a sunburn cream, Noxzema soothes the burning pain.

- **Vaseline Petroleum Jelly** and **Q-Tips Cotton Swabs.** To soothe hemorrhoids and help your bowels operate with less effort, lubricate the tail end of your anal canal with a dab of Vaseline Petroleum Jelly applied with a Q-Tips Cotton Swab approximately one-half inch into the rectum.

- **Vicks VapoRub.** To soothe hemorrhoids, apply a dab of Vicks VapoRub on the outside of the anus.

Doctor's Orders

Come from behind! If you discover bloody stools, black stools, or blood on toilet paper, consult a doctor to rule out a more serious ailment or condition.

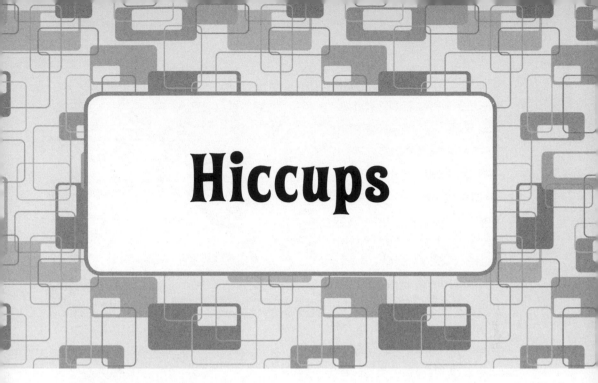

Hiccups

- **Aunt Jemima Original Syrup.** To put a stop to the hiccups, eat one tablespoon Aunt Jemima Original Syrup. The act of swallowing and clearing the mouth of this sticky pancake syrup interrupts breathing patterns, realigning the diaphragm, and the fructose in the corn syrup seems to stop the nerve impulses in the mouth from instructing the muscles in the diaphragm to spasm.

- **Birds Eye Frozen Peas** and **Bounty Paper Towels.** To cure the hiccups, wrap a bag of Birds Eye Frozen Peas with a sheet of Bounty Paper Towels, and place it over the diaphragm (just below the rib cage) for ten minutes. The bag of peas conforms to the shape of your body, and the frozen peas act like small ice cubes, numbing the muscles in the diaphragm to cease the spasms. The paper towel creates a layer of insulation to prevent frostbite. Refreeze the bag of peas for future ice-pack use, making sure to label the bag for ice-pack use only. If you want to eat the peas, cook them after they thaw the first time, never after refreezing.

- **Bounty Paper Towels.** To cure the hiccups, place a single sheet of Bounty Paper Towels over the top of a glass of water, and drink the water through

the paper towel. The strenuous gulping requires help
from your diaphragm, which
offsets the spasms.

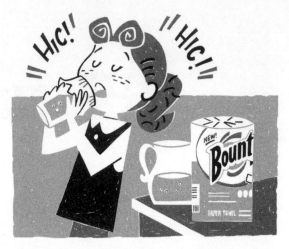

- **Dixie Cups.** Here's an
unusual way to relieve the
hiccups: Fill a Dixie Cup
with water, place it on a
countertop, and insert your
index fingers into your ears.
Using the thumb and pinkie
finger of each hand, pick up the cup, hold your breath, and gulp down the
water. This strange technique tames the spasms in your diaphragm by
increasing carbon dioxide levels, temporarily immobilizing the diaphragm,
and distracting your mind. The British medical journal the *Lancet* claims
that sticking your fingers in your ears temporarily short-circuits the vagus
nerve, which controls the hiccups.

- **Dole Pineapple Juice.** Drinking a glass of Dole Pineapple Juice relieves
the hiccups. Apparently, the acidic nature of the juice does the job.

- **Domino Sugar.** Eliminate a case of hiccups by taking one teaspoon Domino
Sugar and swallowing it dry. The sugar seems to inhibit the nerve impulses
in the mouth from instructing the muscles in the diaphragm to spasm
capriciously.

- **Heinz Apple Cider Vinegar.** To relieve the hiccups, swallow one teaspoon Heinz Apple Cider Vinegar.

- **Jif Peanut Butter.** Put an end to the hiccups by eating one heaping teaspoon
Jif Peanut Butter. The act of chewing, swallowing, and clearing the mouth of
this sticky food interrupts breathing patterns, recalibrating the diaphragm.

- **McCormick Dill Seed.** Chewing and swallowing one teaspoon McCormick Dill Seed seems to stimulate the vagus nerve, ceasing hiccups.

℞ STRANGE MEDICINE ℞

THE SOUND OF MUSIC

● No one knows for certain what causes the intermittent spasms of the diaphragm, the source of hiccups.

● Some doctors believe that hiccups are triggered by irritation or stimulation of the vagus nerve or phrenic nerve.

● To prevent hiccups, avoid drinking carbonated beverages such as soda and beer. The bubbles can trigger the muscles of the diaphragm to spasm.

● Eating rapidly causes you to swallow more air, increasing the likelihood of getting the hiccups.

● For a simple, surefire way to cure the hiccups, inhale deeply and hold your breath for ten seconds. Without exhaling, inhale more air and hold your breath for five seconds. Then without exhaling, inhale more air and hold your breath for another five seconds. This technique, developed by Dr. Luc G. Morris and his colleagues, cures the hiccups by increasing carbon dioxide levels, temporarily immobilizing the diaphragm, and expanding the lungs.

● Breathing into a small brown paper bag can be an effective hiccup remedy because doing so raises the carbon dioxide level in the blood.

● **Q-Tips Cotton Swabs.** To stop the hiccups, use a Q-Tips Cotton Swab to tickle the roof of the rear of your mouth. Triggering the gag reflex seems to disrupt the muscle spasms in the diaphragm.

● **ReaLemon.** Taking a spoonful of ReaLemon lemon juice can shock the nerves of the diaphragm enough to cease the spasms.

● **SueBee Honey.** Swallowing one teaspoon SueBee Honey seems to tickle the vagus nerve, bringing a halt to hiccups. (Do not feed honey to infants less than one year of age. Honey often carries a benign strain of

C. botulinum, and an infant's immune system requires twelve months to develop to fight off disease and infection.)

- **Swiss Miss Hot Cocoa.** Eating one teaspoon powdered Swiss Miss Hot Cocoa mix interrupts swallowing and breathing patterns, disrupting the muscle spasms in the diaphragm and ending the hiccups.

- **Tabasco Pepper Sauce.** Put a few drops of Tabasco Pepper Sauce on a spoon and swallow it. The burning sensation in your mouth diverts your body's attention away from creating spasms in your diaphragm.

- **Wonder Bread.** According to an article published in 1985 in the *Journal of Clinical Gastroenterology,* eating a slice of dry Wonder Bread cures the hiccups.

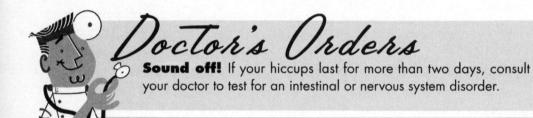

Doctor's Orders

Sound off! If your hiccups last for more than two days, consult your doctor to test for an intestinal or nervous system disorder.

High Blood Pressure

- **Chicken of the Sea Salmon, Chicken of the Sea Sardines,** or **Chicken of the Sea Tuna.** Eating salmon, sardines, or tuna once or twice daily adds the fatty acids commonly known as omega-3 oils to your diet, which can actually help lower blood pressure. These fatty acids also strengthen the immune system and increase resistance to stress.

- **Dannon Yogurt.** Eat one cup of Dannon Plain Nonfat Yogurt every day as part of a balanced diet. Each cup of yogurt contains more than 500 milligrams of potassium, 300 to 450 milligrams of calcium, and 43 milligrams of magnesium—all of which help reduce blood pressure. Also, the *Lactobacillus acidophilus* (probiotics) in yogurt convert the milk protein into tripeptides, which stop angiotensin-converting enzymes (ACE) from raising your blood pressure, the same way ACE-inhibitor drugs work.

- **Hershey's Special Dark Chocolate Bar.** Eating a small square of Hershey's Special Dark Chocolate daily helps lower blood pressure (particularly in people with hypertension), according to a 2011 study conducted at Harvard University. (Before you start eating chocolate daily, be aware that chocolate is high in saturated fat and calories.)

℞ STRANGE MEDICINE ℞

LOOKING HIGH AND LOW

● High blood pressure increases your risk for heart disease, kidney disease, and stroke. In response to high blood pressure, arteries thicken and harden, making the heart pump harder and raising the risk of blood clots.

● Obesity, smoking, a high-fat diet, a high-salt diet, alcohol abuse, stress, and lack of exercise cause high blood pressure, medically known as hypertension.

● Most people with high blood pressure can lower it to safe levels without medication by simply changing their diet and lifestyle.

● Many medications used to lower high blood pressure have dangerous side effects.

● Drinking fifteen 8-ounce glasses of water each day (one an hour) can significantly lower high blood pressure. Water relaxes the entire body, including the arteries.

● Taking 60 to 90 milligrams of coenzyme Q_{10} three times a day after each meal (for a total of 180 to 270 milligrams) can help lower high blood pressure. Found in every cell of your body, coenzyme Q_{10} helps the body produce ATP (adenosine triphosphate), the chemical that provides energy for physiological processes such as the muscular contraction of the heart.

● Walking for thirty minutes once a day provides sufficient exercise for a person with high blood pressure to relax artery walls and decrease stress, lowering high blood pressure.

● Hypertension caused by unresolved, unconscious, repressed feelings may be responsible for up to half of all cases of high blood pressure, according to doctors. Acknowledging your feelings by simply talking with a confidant, keeping a journal, sitting quietly to contemplate for twenty to thirty minutes each day, or listening to music can reduce hypertension—as can psychotherapy.

● **Jif Peanut Butter.** Magnesium can relax arteries, which helps lower blood pressure. While eating a wide range of legumes, nuts, whole grains, and vegetables will help you meet your daily dietary need for magnesium, you can quickly replace magnesium in your body by eating

Jif Peanut Butter (straight from the jar or in a sandwich). Four table-spoons of peanut butter contain 100 milligrams of magnesium (or 25 percent of the daily value).

- **McCormick Garlic Powder.** Cook your food with as much McCormick Garlic Powder as possible. A 2008 study at the University of Adelaide in Australia showed that garlic can help lower blood pressure.

- **Planters Dry Roasted Almonds, Planters Dry Roasted Cashews,** or **Planters Dry Roasted Peanuts.** Eating foods high in magnesium—like Planters Dry Roasted Almonds, Planters Dry Roasted Cashews, or Planters Dry Roasted Peanuts—can relax arteries, which helps lower blood pressure. One ounce of almonds provides 80 milligrams of magnesium, one ounce of cashews provides 75 milligrams, and one ounce of dry roasted peanuts provides 50 milligrams.

- **Quaker Oats.** To help lower your blood pressure, start each day with a bowl of Quaker Oats oatmeal. Studies show that oatmeal lowers both blood pressure and cholesterol levels, apparently due to the soluble fiber beta-glucan.

- **Sun-Maid Raisins.** Eat a small box of Sun-Maid Raisins every day. One 1.5-ounce box of raisins contains 220 milligrams of potassium, which helps to reduce blood pressure.

- **Welch's Grape Juice.** Drinking a twelve-ounce glass of Welch's Concord Grape Juice daily reduced both systolic and diastolic blood pressure measurements by nearly six points among hypertensive men, according to a study presented in 2003 at Experimental Biology in San Diego, California.

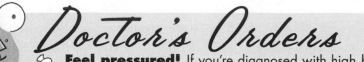

Doctor's Orders

Feel pressured! If you're diagnosed with high blood pressure, have your blood pressure screened regularly by your doctor.

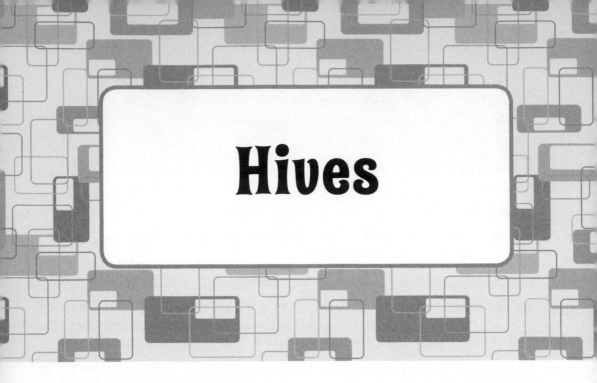

Hives

- **Arm & Hammer Baking Soda.** To relieve the itching and irritation of hives, mix one-half cup Arm & Hammer Baking Soda with enough water to make a thick paste, and spread the mixture on the affected areas. The alkaline baking soda soothes the skin.

- **Benadryl.** To relieve hives, take Benadryl (non-drowsy) according to the directions on the label. Diphenhydramine—the active ingredient in Benadryl—is an antihistamine that stops the mast cells in your body from producing histamine, the chemical that causes hives.

- **Chicken of the Sea Salmon, Chicken of the Sea Sardines,** or **Chicken of the Sea Tuna.** To help remedy hives, eat salmon, sardines, or tuna once or twice daily to add the fatty acids commonly known as omega-3 oils to your diet. The omega-3 fatty acids in these fish reduce inflammation and strengthen the immune system.

- **Desitin.** To remove the itch from hives, apply Desitin to the affected area. The active ingredient in Desitin is zinc oxide, an astringent that reduces blood supply to the skin.

- **Dickinson's Witch Hazel.** To subdue hives, use a cotton ball to apply

Dickinson's Witch Hazel to the affected areas. The astringent constricts blood vessels, reducing the amount of welt-causing histamine that the blood vessels can secrete.

- **Heinz Apple Cider Vinegar.** To soothe the itching, use a cotton ball to apply Heinz Apple Cider Vinegar to the affected areas.

- **Kingsford's Corn Starch** and **Heinz White Vinegar.** Blend three ounces Kingsford's Corn Starch with one ounce Heinz White Vinegar, and apply the paste to the hives. The antiseptic mixture stops the itching and helps dry up the hives.

- **Lipton Chamomile Tea.** To relieve the stress that may be causing or exacerbating your hives, drink a cup of Lipton Chamomile Tea, steeped for ten minutes. Chamomile acts like a sedative, calming your stress. (Coumarin, an anticoagulant in chamomile, may increase the likelihood of bleeding when taken in combination with the blood thinner Coumadin or other anticoagulant medications.)

- **Lipton Chamomile Tea** and **Stayfree Maxi Pads.** Place two Lipton Chamomile Tea bags in one cup of boiled water, cover with a saucer, and steep for fifteen minutes. Let cool until lukewarm, saturate a Stayfree Maxi Pad with the chamomile tea and apply to the hives for fifteen minutes. When applied externally to hives, chamomile soothes itchy skin and reduces the unsightly inflammation.

- **Lipton Peppermint Tea.** To soothe the hot, itchy bumps caused by hives, place a Lipton Peppermint Tea bag in a cup of boiling water, cover with a saucer, and steep for ten minutes. Let cool, and then use a cotton ball to apply the tea to the affected areas. The mint soothes the skin.

- **McCormick Basil Leaves.** To subdue itchy hives, place four heaping tablespoons McCormick Basil Leaves in a clean, empty glass jar, add one quart of boiling water, and seal the lid shut. Let cool to room temperature, strain out the basil leaves, and apply the liquid to the hives. The caffeic acid in basil tames the itching.

℞ STRANGE MEDICINE ℞

THINGS THAT GO BUMP IN THE NIGHT

● Hives are itchy, red bumps or welts on the skin caused by an allergy. Triggered by an allergen, mast cells in your connective tissue release histamine—a chemical that prompts blood vessels to ooze fluid into the skin.

● When suffering from hives, taking a warm shower (as warm as you can tolerate without inflicting any pain) for fifteen to twenty minutes triggers the mast cells in your body to release their entire supply of histamine, causing the itching to stop and the hives to subside. The body requires several hours to produce more histamine.

● Foods most likely to precipitate hives include berries, chocolate, eggs, fish, milk, nuts, shellfish, and tomatoes.

● A wide range of common medications can trigger hives—most notably aspirin, ibuprofen, naproxen, penicillin, and blood pressure medications.

● Applying a cold compress (a hand towel saturated with cold water) generally makes hives go away. The cold shrinks the blood vessels, reducing the amount of histamine released to the skin.

● Many cases of hives clear up within a few hours on their own. A mild case of hives typically does not necessitate treatment.

● To relieve intense itching, serious discomfort, or a persistent case of hives, take an over-the-counter antihistamine.

● **McCormick Cream of Tartar.** To relieve hives, mix one tablespoon McCormick Cream of Tartar with enough water to make a thick paste, and apply the mixture to the affected area.

● **Pepto-Bismol.** Using a cotton ball, dab the bumps with Pepto-Bismol. The alkalinity relieves the itching.

- **Phillips' Milk of Magnesia.** For another surefire way to soothe the itching of hives, use a cotton ball to dab the welts with Phillips' Milk of Magnesia. This alkaline solution stops the itching and cools the skin.

- **Quaker Oats.** To relieve hives, grind one cup uncooked Quaker Oats in a blender, add to tepid bathwater, and soak for fifteen minutes. Oats soothe itchy skin and the cool water reduces blood flow to the skin.

Doctor's Orders

Lump it! If you suffer from hives for more than six weeks, see an allergist or dermatologist to unearth the cause or multiple causes. If you develop hives around your eyes or mouth or start wheezing, seek emergency medical treatment.

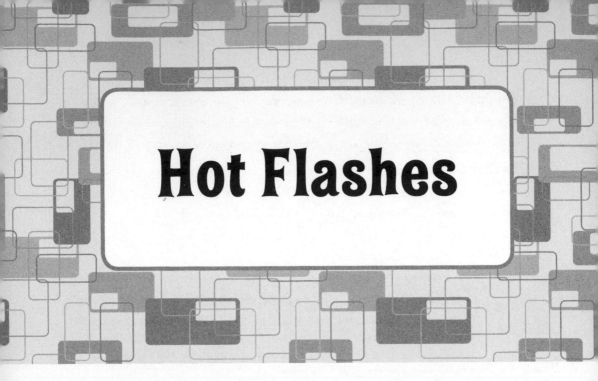

Hot Flashes

- **McCormick Ground Sage.** To reduce hot flashes and alleviate irritability, drink three cups of sage tea daily. Place a tea infuser filled with one tablespoon McCormick Ground Sage in a teacup, add boiling water, cover with a saucer, and steep for ten minutes. Let cool to room temperature and drink the soothing beverage.

- **Mott's Applesauce.** To decrease the intensity and longevity of hot flashes, eat one-half cup Mott's Applesauce every day. Applesauce contains a high concentration of phytoestrogens. Although the Mayo Clinic claims that most studies have found phytoestrogens ineffective at relieving hot flashes, many menopausal women insist that phytoestrogens in natural form cool them down.

- **Planters Sunflower Kernels** or **Planters Dry Roasted Almonds.** To help reduce the frequency and severity of hot flashes, eat one-quarter cup Planters Sunflower Kernels or Planters Dry Roasted Almonds every day. Sunflower seeds and almonds are packed with vitamin E, which helps minimize hot flashes. A study published in 2007 in *Gynecologic and Obstetric Investigation* showed that taking 267 milligrams of vitamin E daily relieves hot flashes. One-quarter cup of sunflower seed kernels provides 22.68 milligrams of vitamin E, or 143 percent of the recommended daily allowance. One-quarter cup of dry-roasted almonds provides 15 milligrams of vitamin E, or 100 percent of the recommended daily allowance.

- **Silk Soymilk.** To minimize hot flashes and other menopausal symptoms, add more soy foods to your diet, such as four 8-ounce glasses of Silk Soymilk

℞ STRANGE MEDICINE ℞

A FLASH IN THE PAN

- Two to twelve years before menopause, women experience a drop in estrogen, which, combined with other hormonal changes, causes hot flashes and night sweats.

- The typical hot flash lasts roughly three minutes, but hot flashes can last for up to thirty minutes.

- A night sweat is merely a hot flash that takes place during sleep, soaking the woman in perspiration.

- Drinking hot, caffeinated beverages tends to aggravate hot flashes—due to the combination of heat and caffeine.

- Heavy women experience more hot flashes than slim women.

- Exercising moderately (without building up a sweat), such as swimming, doing yoga or Pilates, or taking a brisk walk for thirty minutes three to five times a week minimizes the frequency of hot flashes and night sweats.

- Taking a hot bath for twenty minutes a day significantly reduces the severity of hot flashes. When the menstrual cycle diminishes or ceases, the body, needing another outlet to expel toxins from the body, intermittently sweats profusely. Taking a hot bath prompts the body to sweat and expel those toxins, eliminating the need for hot flashes.

every day. A 2012 study at the University of Minnesota demonstrated that women who consume 54 milligrams of soy isoflavones daily reduced the frequency of hot flashes by 20.6 percent and the severity by 26 percent, without any side effects. Four 8-ounce glasses of soymilk contain 50 milligrams of soy isoflavones.

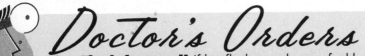

Doctor's Orders

Flash forward! If hot flashes make you feel horrible and prevent you from getting a good night's sleep for weeks, consult your doctor for a solution.

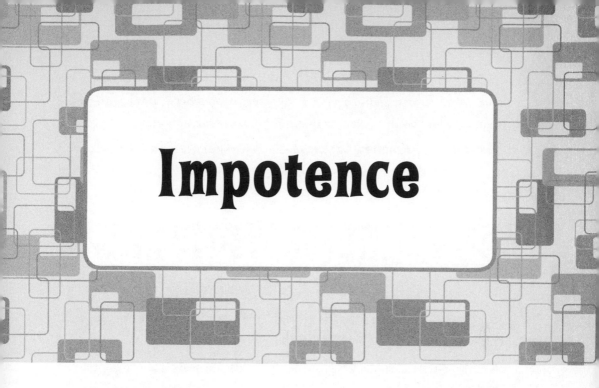

Impotence

- **Heinz Baked Beanz.** To strengthen your erections and boost your sperm count up to 74 percent, eat zinc-rich foods like Heinz Baked Beanz, according to the journal *Fertility and Sterility*.

- **Kleenex Tissues** and **Scotch Tape.** To determine whether you have an erection during your sleep (healthy men have several), take a Kleenex Tissue, cut a small strip, wrap it tightly around your flaccid penis, and use a small piece of Scotch Tape to secure the end of the tissue strip in place. In the morning, check the tissue. If it's torn, you most likely had an erection in your sleep, which rules out a physical problem (meaning the problem is psychological).

- **McCormick Pure Vanilla Extract.** Have your partner put a dab of McCormick Pure Vanilla Extract behind each ear as a perfume, or put a few drops in a tissue or cotton ball and inhale it. In a 1995 study, neurologist Alan Hirsch, founder of the Smell and Taste Treatment and Research Foundation in Chicago, found that the aroma of vanilla increases penile blood flow. The smells that evoke the security and pleasure of childhood, Hirsch concluded, sexually arouse men. Vanilla has been considered an aphrodisiac since Aztec times, and in a 1762 study, German physician Bezaar Zimmerman determined that a vanilla decoction cured male impotence.

- **Planters Dry Roasted Cashews.** Eat a handful of Planters Dry Roasted Cashews every day to ward off impotence. Zinc increases production of the

℞ STRANGE MEDICINE ℞

THE UPS AND DOWNS

- Impotence (also known as erectile dysfunction) occurs when a man becomes unable to get or maintain an erection firm enough for sexual intercourse.

- Having occasional difficulty maintaining an erection need not cause concern, but a persistent problem calls for medical attention.

- Impotence is generally caused by a physical problem, such as heart disease, atherosclerosis, high cholesterol, high blood pressure, diabetes, or obesity. A number of diseases can cause impotence, including Parkinson's disease and multiple sclerosis, as can smoking and substance abuse.

- Stress or psychological problems also cause or worsen impotence.

- Anything that causes insufficient blood flow to the penis can lead to impotence.

- Do not drink alcohol. Excessive consumption of alcohol correlates highly with impotence among men in their late forties and early fifties.

- If you smoke, quit. Smoking tobacco restricts blood flow to veins and arteries.

- Medications used to treat anxiety, depression, and high blood pressure can inhibit the ability to have an erection.

- Maintain a high level of HDL ("good") cholesterol by eating foods low in saturated and trans fats and high in fiber. Plaque lining the inner walls of the arteries in and leading to the penis can reduce blood flow.

male sex hormone testosterone. A handful of cashews provides 50 percent of the recommended daily allowance of zinc.

- **Planters Dry Roasted Peanuts.** To overcome erectile dysfunction, eat Planters Dry Roasted Peanuts. The amino acid arginine in peanuts helps the body produce nitric oxide in the blood vessel walls, which increases blood flow to the penis. One 3.5-ounce serving of peanuts contains more than 3,500 milligrams of arginine.

Doctor's Orders

Don't let me down! If you're unable to get or maintain an erection, consult your doctor to rule out heart disease or diabetes.

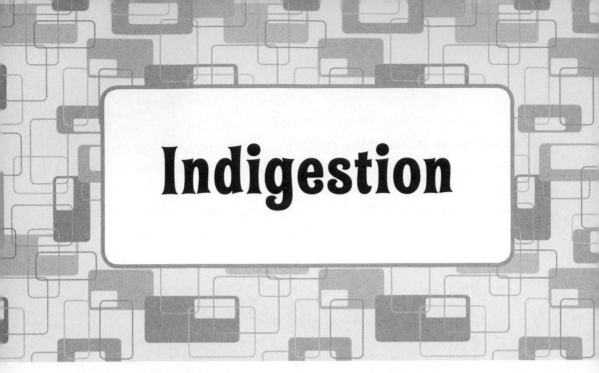

Indigestion

- **Arm & Hammer Baking Soda** and **ReaLemon.** To neutralize the stomach acid causing indigestion and relieve painful gas, dissolve one-half teaspoon Arm & Hammer Baking Soda in four ounces of warm water, add a few drops of ReaLemon lemon juice, and drink the solution. The alkaline baking soda neutralizes stomach acid and the lemon juice dispels some of the gas from the baking soda. (Do not use this remedy if you're on a sodium-restricted diet. Read the directions on the side of the box of baking soda before administering.)

- **Canada Dry Ginger Ale.** Drinking Canada Dry Ginger Ale—carbonated or flat—relieves an upset stomach. The ginger seems to relax the muscles in the stomach. Contrary to popular belief, Canada Dry Ginger Ale does indeed contain genuine ginger, included in the list of ingredients as "natural flavors." (Do not drink ginger ale if you have gallstones. Ginger can increase bile production.)

- **Coca-Cola.** Drinking flat Coca-Cola helps settle your queasy stomach. Pharmacies sell cola syrup that can be taken in small doses to relieve nausea. The concentrated sugars are believed to relax the gastrointestinal tract.

Letting the bubbles out of the soda prevents the carbonation from further upsetting your stomach.

- **Heinz Apple Cider Vinegar.** To soothe indigestion after eating a large meal, mix one teaspoon Heinz Apple Cider Vinegar in four ounces of water, and sip the tangy solution. Too little stomach acid causes as many cases of indigestion as too much stomach acid. Without an adequate supply of stomach acid, improperly digested food remains in the stomach, causing bloating. Apple cider vinegar aids in the overall digestive process by stimulating the stomach to secrete more hydrochloric acid.

- **Life Savers Pep-O-Mints.** Suck on a few Life Savers Pep-O-Mints to calm indigestion. Peppermint calms the stomach muscles and relieves nausea, and the menthol relaxes the lower esophageal sphincter (the valve at the bottom of the esophagus), allowing trapped gas to escape from the stomach.

- **Lipton Chamomile Tea.** To ease indigestion, place two Lipton Chamomile Tea bags in a cup, fill with boiling water, and cover with a saucer. Steep for ten minutes and drink. Chamomile doubles as an antispasmodic that relieves cramps and a mild sedative that calms the nerves. (Coumarin, an anticoagulant in chamomile, may increase the likelihood of bleeding when taken in combination with the blood thinner Coumadin or other anticoagulant medications.)

- **Lipton Ginger Tea.** To relieve indigestion, drink a cup of strongly brewed Lipton Ginger Tea (or as many cups as necessary until the indigestion subsides). The gingerol and shogaol in ginger reduce intestinal contractions and neutralize indigestion. (Do not drink ginger tea if you have gallstones. Ginger can increase bile production.)

- **McCormick Anise Seed, McCormick Caraway Seed, McCormick Dill Seed, McCormick Fennel Seed,** and **Ziploc Storage Bags.** To soothe indigestion, mix equal parts (one or two teaspoons each) of these four seeds in a Ziploc Storage Bag. When you feel indigestion or after

TURNING YOUR STOMACH

- Indigestion (commonly called an upset stomach) is vague discomfort in your stomach immediately after eating, caused by difficulty digesting food.

- The many possible causes of indigestion include overeating, eating too quickly, fatty or greasy foods, spicy foods, or too much coffee, alcohol, or carbonated beverages.

- To prevent indigestion, get regular exercise by going for a thirty-minute walk every day. Exercise enhances smooth digestion.

- Eating slowly allows you to chew your food into smaller pieces before swallowing and coat them with sufficient amounts of saliva to aid the digestive process.

- To help relieve indigestion and bloating, massage your belly and lower abdomen. Doing so helps trapped gas escape and helps waste move along its natural path.

- Stress and anxiety can cause indigestion. Keep mealtime stress-free by avoiding arguments and refraining from discussing work, school, or finances.

- Indigestion can be a sign of lactose intolerance—an inability to digest the milk sugar in dairy products.

- Antibiotics, aspirin, nonsteroidal anti-inflammatory drugs (NSAIDs), and other medications can cause indigestion.

- Recurring indigestion can be a sign of an underlying medical problem, such as gastroesophageal reflux disease, ulcers, or gallstones.

eating a big meal, chew and swallow one-half teaspoon of the blended seeds. Both anise and fennel contain anethole, a compound that doubles as an antiseptic and antispasmodic. Indian restaurants tend to put this mixture in bowls for patrons after they finish their meal. (Avoid anise during pregnancy.)

- **McCormick Fennel Seed.** Place a tea infuser filled with one tablespoon McCormick Fennel Seed in a teacup, add boiling water, cover with a saucer, steep for ten minutes, and then drink. As an antispasmodic, fennel aids the digestive process, dispersing gas from the intestinal tract. In India, fennel seeds are served after meals like after-dinner mints.

- **Nabisco Ginger Snaps.** To tame a bout of indigestion, eat a few Nabisco Ginger Snaps. The ginger in the cookies is one of the oldest remedies for nausea. (Do not use ginger if you have gallstones. Ginger can increase bile production.)

- **Pernod Anise.** To quell indigestion, sip a small glass of Pernod Anise. This after-dinner liqueur is made from anise, which settles the stomach. (Avoid anise during pregnancy.)

Doctor's Orders

Stop bellyaching! If indigestion lasts more than two weeks, consult your doctor. Nausea or heartburn pain accompanied by profuse sweating and chest pain could signal a heart attack; seek medical attention immediately.

Ingrown Toenails

- **Dr. Teal's Epsom Salt.** To soothe an ingrown toenail, dissolve a handful of Dr. Teal's Epsom Salt in a basin filled with warm water, and soak your foot in the solution for twenty minutes every day. The warm water softens the skin, enabling the Epsom Salt to fight the infection and relieve any inflammation.

- **Forster Toothpicks.** After soaking your foot in a warm bath (see Dr. Teal's Epsom Salt tip above), dry the toe, and then using a Forster Toothpick as a tool, insert a small piece of a cotton ball beneath the embedded edge of the nail to lift it just enough to grow over the skin.

- **Orajel.** To numb the pain of an ingrown toenail, squeeze a bead of Orajel along the cuticle and let sit for three minutes. The benzocaine in the ointment anesthetizes the spot, instantly blocking the pain.

- **Purell Instant Hand Sanitizer.** To disinfect the skin around an ingrown toenail, simply smear some Purell Instant Hand Sanitizer on the affected area. The alcohol in the hand sanitizer kills any germs.

- **Tabasco Pepper Sauce** and **Crisco All-Vegetable Shortening.** To relieve the pain of an ingrown toenail, mix one-quarter teaspoon Tabasco Pepper Sauce with two tablespoons Crisco All-Vegetable Shortening, and apply the spicy homemade ointment to the affected area up to five times a day. The capsaicin in the Tabasco Pepper Sauce relieves nerve pain. (Do not apply this salve on open sores and avoid contact with eyes and nose.)

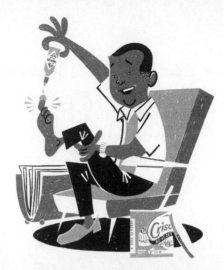

℞ STRANGE MEDICINE ℞

TOUGH AS NAILS

● An ingrown toenail occurs when the sharp edge at the corner of a toenail grows into the nearby skin, causing redness, pain, and possible infection.

● Trimming your toenails correctly averts ingrown toenails. Soak your feet in warm water to soften the nails before trimming them. Using a pair of nail scissors, cut the nails straight across, leaving sufficient nail protruding from each side. Then use an emery board to file the corners slightly, rounding them to eliminate sharp corners.

● Do not trim your toenails by picking and tearing off the excess toenail with your fingers. Doing so risks damaging the corners of the nail, leading to an ingrown toenail.

● To prevent ingrown toenails, wear shoes that fit comfortably without squeezing your toes. Buy your shoes in the afternoon, when your feet are most swollen. Be sure you buy a pair of shoes with plenty of room in the toe area. From the tip of the shoe, your longest toe should have space measuring the width of your thumb.

● Wearing tight socks that squeeze your toes together can cause the corners of toenails to grow into the skin. Instead, wear loose-fitting socks.

● Do not wrap an adhesive bandage around an ingrown toenail. Otherwise, the bandage presses the sharp edge of the nail close to the skin, perpetuating the problem.

- **Vicks VapoRub** and **Band-Aid Bandages.** Smear Vicks VapoRub under and around your ingrown toenail twice a day, and cover loosely with a Band-Aid Bandage to keep the balm on the nail. Repeat daily until the nail grows out. The menthol reduces the inflammation and lessens the pain, and the other ingredients soften the nail and the surrounding skin, allowing the embedded nail to grow out.

Doctor's Orders

Don't get nailed! If an ingrown toenail gets infected and starts oozing pus, see your doctor.

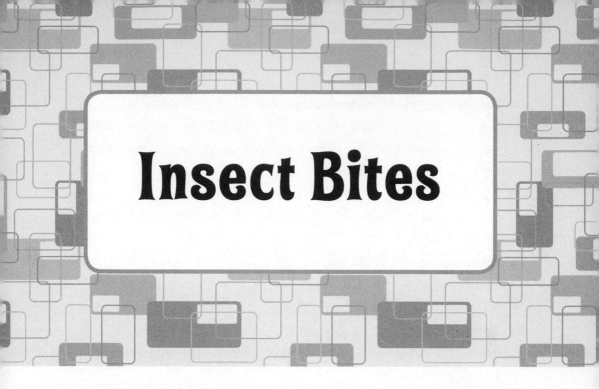

Insect Bites

- **Arm & Hammer Baking Soda.** To stop a bee, wasp, hornet, or fire ant sting from burning, mix one tablespoon Arm & Hammer Baking Soda with enough water to make a thick paste, and cover the affected area with the paste. The alkaline sodium bicarbonate neutralizes acidic bee, wasp, or fire ant venom.

- **Bayer Aspirin.** Using a mortar and pestle, crush one or two Bayer Aspirin tablets into a fine powder, add enough water to make a paste, and apply it to the sting. The salicylic acid in the aspirin neutralizes the insect venom, anesthetizing the pain.

- **Birds Eye Frozen Peas** and **Bounty Paper Towels.** To relieve the pain, swelling, and itch of an insect bite, cover a bag of Birds Eye Frozen Peas with a sheet of Bounty Paper Towels, and place the bag against the affected area for up to twenty minutes. The bag of peas conforms to the shape of your body, and the frozen peas act like small ice cubes, constricting the blood vessels and numbing the pain. The paper towel creates a layer of insulation to prevent frostbite. Refreeze the bag of peas for future ice-pack use. Be sure to label the bag for ice-pack use only. If you want to eat the peas, cook them after they thaw the first time, never after refreezing.

- **Colgate Regular Flavor Toothpaste.** To relieve fire ant, bee, wasp, or hornet stings, rub a dab of Colgate Regular Flavor Toothpaste into the affected area. No one knows why it works, although some people suspect the menthol in the mint, while others suspect the glycerin.

- **Dial Soap.** To quickly disinfect an insect sting, wash the affected area with Dial Antibacterial Soap to avoid infection. Triclosan, the antibacterial agent in the soap, kills bacteria.

- **Dickinson's Witch Hazel.** A few drops of Dickinson's Witch Hazel applied with a cotton ball to an insect bite or sting instantly relieves the pain. Witch hazel is an astringent.

- **Domino Sugar.** Mix one teaspoon Domino Sugar in enough water to make a thick paste, and apply it to the insect sting. The sugar neutralizes the poison from the sting.

- **Fruit of the Earth Aloe Vera Gel.** Slathering some Fruit of the Earth Aloe Vera Gel over the insect bites or stings soothes the pain and reduces the inflammation.

- **Heinz Apple Cider Vinegar.** After removing the stinger (see Visa tip on page 274), saturate a cotton ball with Heinz Apple Cider Vinegar and press it against the sting for five minutes. The acetic acid neutralizes the venom, soothes the pain, and reduces the inflammation.

- **Kingsford's Corn Starch** and **Heinz Apple Cider Vinegar.** Mix one teaspoon Kingsford's Corn Starch with enough Heinz Apple Cider Vinegar to make a thick paste, and apply it over an insect bite. The cornstarch sucks out venom from the bite, and the vinegar soothes the burning itch.

- **Lipton Chamomile Tea** and **Stayfree Maxi Pads.** Place two Lipton Chamomile Tea bags in one cup of boiled water, cover with a saucer, and steep for fifteen minutes. Let cool until lukewarm, saturate a Stayfree Maxi Pad with the chamomile tea, and apply to the insect bites or stings for fifteen minutes. When applied externally, chamomile soothes itchy skin, reduces inflammation, and speeds the healing of wounds.

- **Lipton Tea Bags.** To sterilize and soothe an insect bite, dampen a Lipton Tea Bag with warm water and press it against the sting. The tannin in the tea acts as an astringent, tightening the skin, reducing inflammation and irritation, and drawing infection from the skin.

- **Listerine.** After washing the bite with soap and water, use a cotton ball to dab on original formula Listerine antiseptic mouthwash. Listerine is an astringent.

- **McCormick Meat Tenderizer.** To desensitize insect stings, apply a mixture of one-half teaspoon McCormick Meat Tenderizer and two teaspoons of

℞ STRANGE MEDICINE ℞

SNUG AS A BUG IN A RUG

- Insect venom can trigger an allergic reaction, the severity of which depends on the individual's sensitivity.

- The stinger of a worker honeybee usually detaches when the insect attacks, and the honeybee dies a few hours later. A bumblebee retains its stinger, enabling it to sting repeatedly.

- When a bee injects its stinger into flesh, muscles still active in the stinger burrow it deeper into the wound, while other muscles continue pumping venom.

- Bees pollinate fruit trees, vegetable plants, and flowers. One simple way to get rid of an abundance of bees is to call a local beekeeper.

- Only the female mosquito "bites," and to do so, she inserts six needlelike stylets from her proboscis through the victim's skin, shoots saliva into the blood to prevent clotting, and then drinks the blood. Most people are allergic to mosquito saliva, which causes the swelling and itching.

- Mosquitoes spread some of the worst diseases known to man, including encephalitis, malaria, and yellow fever.

- According to entomologists, at least 95 percent of the insects in our yards and gardens are beneficial or harmless.

water to the affected area. Let sit for up to thirty minutes. The enzyme papain breaks down the proteins in the venom, reducing inflammation and pain.

- **McCormick Pure Vanilla Extract.** To repel mosquitoes, mix two teaspoons McCormick Pure Vanilla Extract and one cup of water in a trigger-spray bottle and mist yourself with the fragrant solution. Vanilla keeps mosquitoes away.

- **Noxzema.** Noxzema, the skin cream originally invented in 1914 as a sunburn remedy, relieves the itching of mosquito bites. The camphor, menthol, and eucalyptus oil in Noxzema do the trick.

- **Pepto-Bismol.** To soothe mosquito bites, use a cotton ball to apply Pepto-Bismol to the affected area. The alkalinity relieves the itching.

- **Scotch Tape.** If you brush against a hairy caterpillar and get those stinging hairs stuck in your skin, put a piece of Scotch Tape over the affected area, and peel it off gently to remove the imbedded hairs.

- **Sea Breeze.** To stop a mosquito bite from itching, saturate a cotton ball with Sea Breeze and dab it on the affected area. The camphor, eucalyptus, clove oil, eugenol, and peppermint oil stop the irritation.

- **Vicks VapoRub.** To numb mosquito or fire ant bites and alleviate the itching, smear a dab of Vicks VapoRub on the bites. The camphor, eucalyptus oil, and menthol in the balm soothe the itching.

- **Visa.** To prevent a honeybee's embedded venom sac from injecting more poison into your body, use the edge of a Visa credit card to scrape the stinger and attached venom sac out of the skin.

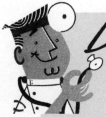

Doctor's Orders

Bite back! If the area around the bug bite or sting swells larger than four inches in diameter, or if you experience nausea, cramps, or diarrhea, see a doctor immediately. If the bug bite or sting triggers difficulty breathing, swelling of the lips or throat, dizziness, vomiting, hives, or rapid heartbeat, call 911 for emergency medical assistance.

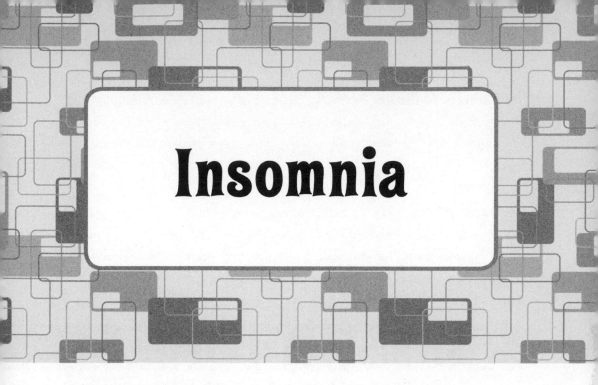

Insomnia

- **Dr. Teal's Epsom Salt.** To make yourself drowsy, fill the bathtub with warm water a few hours before bedtime, add a handful of Dr. Teal's Epsom Salt, and soak for ten minutes. The warm bath raises your body temperature, and as your temperature drops back down again, you'll feel increasingly tired. The Epsom Salt relaxes your muscles.

- **Lipton Chamomile Tea.** To lull yourself to sleep, drink one or two cups of Lipton Chamomile Tea before bedtime. Chamomile soothes the nerves. (Coumarin, an anticoagulant in chamomile, may increase the likelihood of bleeding when taken in combination with the blood thinner Coumadin or other anticoagulant medications.)

- **Lipton Peppermint Tea.** For restful sleep, drink one or two cups of Lipton Peppermint Tea before bedtime. Peppermint is a mild sedative that relieves stress and helps you drift off to sleep.

- **McCormick Tarragon Leaves.** Drinking a cup of tarragon tea before bedtime purportedly induces sleep. Place a tea infuser filled with one teaspoon McCormick Tarragon Leaves in a teacup, fill the cup with boiling water, cover with a saucer, and steep for thirty minutes.

- **Planters Sunflower Kernels.** To bring on sleep, eat a handful of Planters Sunflower Kernels approximately thirty minutes before going to bed every night. The body converts the amino acid L-tryptophan found in sunflower seeds to serotonin and melatonin, the calming neurotransmitters that sends you to sleep.

- **Quaker Oats.** An hour before going to bed, eat a bowl of Quaker Oats oatmeal cooked with milk. Oats calm the nerves and invite drowsiness, and milk, loaded with the amino acid L-tryptophan, helps the brain produce the neurotransmitters serotonin and melatonin, which promote sleep.

℞ STRANGE MEDICINE ℞

A DREAM COME TRUE

- Sleeping pills certainly induce sleep, but they can be addictive and make insomnia worse, plus they lose their effectiveness after a few weeks of nightly use. Sleeping pills also cause side effects and fail to address the root cause of the problem.

- If you've become reliant on sleeping pills, you can wean yourself off them by gradually lowering the dosage.

- Stress can cause insomnia, and learning techniques to reduce stress can effectively eliminate insomnia.

- To fall asleep easier at night, go for a brisk walk outdoors for twenty to thirty minutes every morning. The mild exercise reduces stress, sets your body clock to the presence of sunlight, and helps you sleep better at night.

- Do not consume coffee, caffeinated sodas, or chocolate after four o'clock in the afternoon. The caffeine can keep you awake at night.

- Drinking alcohol may help put you to sleep, but it also tends to disrupt your sleep, waking you up in the middle of the night.

- **SueBee Honey.** To overcome insomnia, drink one or two cups of non-caffeinated tea sweetened with two teaspoons SueBee Honey before bedtime. The calcium, magnesium, and B vitamins in honey have a calming effect on the nervous system. (Do not feed honey to infants less than one year of age. Honey often carries a benign strain of *C. botulinum*, and an infant's immune system requires twelve months to develop to fight off disease and infection.)

- **Tums.** To cure your sleeplessness, eat one Tums tablet after each meal. Your body can absorb only 500 to 600 milligrams of calcium at a time. A regular strength Tums tablet contains 500 milligrams of calcium carbonate. Sleep

- Use positive affirmations. Negative thoughts increase anxiety and inhibit sleep. Instead of telling yourself things like "I'll never fall asleep," replace those damaging thoughts with positive ones such as, "I always fall asleep eventually," "I'm going to have a wonderful night's sleep," or "I'm going to wake up feeling rested and refreshed."

- Wake up at the same time every day. Maintaining a regular sleep pattern helps you fall asleep faster.

- While lying in bed, occupy your mind with a repetitive task, like counting sheep, reciting song lyrics or poetry, or running through the multiplication tables. The boring activity distracts the mind, lulling you to sleep.

- If you can't fall asleep after twenty minutes, get out of bed, go to another room, sit quietly for fifteen minutes, and then return to bed.

- An hour or two before going to bed, write a list of all the things you need to do, put it aside, and sit quietly for ten minutes and reflect on the day you just experienced, putting all your problems in proper perspective to clear your mind.

- Turn the clock face away from you, so you can't look over to check the time. If you wake up in the middle of the night, refrain from looking at the clock. Doing so adds stress, making it more difficult to fall asleep.

disturbances can be related to a calcium deficiency. Calcium helps the brain use the amino acid L-tryptophan to manufacture the sleep-inducing neurotransmitters serotonin and melatonin. (If you've had calcium oxalate kidney stones, consult your doctor before taking Tums.)

- **Uncle Ben's Converted Brand Rice.** An hour or two before bedtime, eat one or two cups cooked Uncle Ben's Converted Brand Rice. The carbohydrates in rice can boost the production of serotonin and melatonin, the neurotransmitters that promote sleep and relaxation.

- **Welch's Grape Juice.** To sleep like a baby, drink an eight-ounce glass of Welch's Grape Juice before bedtime. The potassium brings on drowsiness.

- **Wonder Bread.** To help induce sleep, eat a few slices of Wonder Bread immediately before bedtime. The carbohydrates in bread can increase serotonin, a neurotransmitter that promotes sleep.

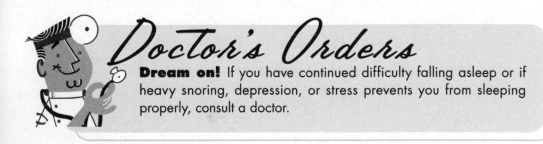

Doctor's Orders

Dream on! If you have continued difficulty falling asleep or if heavy snoring, depression, or stress prevents you from sleeping properly, consult a doctor.

Iron-Deficiency Anemia

- **Grandma's Robust Molasses.** To pump more iron into your body, eat one tablespoon Grandma's Robust Molasses every day. Dissolve the tablespoon of the blackstrap molasses in a cup of hot water, add it to a cup of tea, or spread it on a cracker. One tablespoon of blackstrap molasses provides 3.5 milligrams of iron (approximately 43 percent of the recommended daily allowance).

- **Heinz Baked Beanz.** To boost your iron levels and ward off anemia, eat Heinz Baked Beanz, an excellent source of iron. One serving of Heinz Baked Beans contains 22 percent of the recommended daily allowance of iron. One serving also provides more than half the recommended daily intake of folate, a key player in producing healthy red blood cells capable of carrying oxygen through the capillaries efficiently.

- **Kellogg's All-Bran, Kellogg's Special K,** or **Total.** To help your body produce healthy red blood cells, eat a bowl of Kellogg's All-Bran, Kellogg's Special K, or Total cereal every day to increase the amount of folate in your diet. A folate deficiency results in the production of fewer and larger red blood cells incapable of carrying oxygen or traveling through the capillaries as efficiently as normal red blood cells. One-half cup of Kellogg's All-Bran, Kellogg's Special K, or Total cereal contains 100 percent of the daily value of folate.

℞ STRANGE MEDICINE ℞

STRIKE WHILE THE IRON IS HOT

● Not getting enough iron in your diet or being a woman with heavy menstrual periods may lower the level of either red blood cells or hemoglobin, the protein that carries oxygen in red blood cells. The resulting low levels of oxygen in the blood makes you feel tired and weak.

● Aside from causing fatigue and lack of energy, iron-deficiency anemia may also cause abdominal pain, diarrhea, dizziness, or loss of appetite.

● Increasing iron intake relieves anemia.

● According to the National Institutes of Health, the recommended dietary allowance for iron is 8 milligrams daily for men between ages nineteen and fifty; 18 milligrams daily for women between ages nineteen and fifty; 27 milligrams daily for pregnant women; and 8 milligrams daily for men and women age fifty-one and older.

● Taking iron in the form of ferrous sulfate may irritate the stomach, lymphatic system, and liver. The body more easily digests and absorbs other forms of iron, such as ferrous gluconate, iron gluconate, and iron picolinate.

● Foods rich in iron include barley, beans and peas, sesame seeds, sunflower seeds, pistachios, pecans, almonds, sun-dried tomatoes, dried apricots, and fresh parsley.

● Consuming dairy products decreases iron absorption in women with anemia. If you're consuming less dairy, add more beans, leafy green vegetables, peas, soybeans, and sesame seeds to your diet to get sufficient calcium.

● Caffeine inhibits iron absorption, so if you're suffering from anemia, ease up on the coffee, tea, chocolate, and caffeinated soda.

● When suffering from anemia, reduce the amount of sugar, beer, wine, and other alcoholic beverages you consume. These deplete the body of B vitamins, making anemia worse.

- **McCormick Sesame Seed.** To increase your iron intake, sprinkle one tablespoon McCormick Sesame Seed into your cereal, oatmeal, yogurt, or other foods once a day. While not as easily absorbed by the body as the iron in meats, sesame seeds contain non-heme (plant-based) iron. One tablespoon of McCormick Sesame Seed contains 1.35 milligrams of iron (almost 17 percent of the daily value).

- **Minute Maid Orange Juice.** Drinking an eight-ounce glass of Minute Maid Orange Juice every day provides enough vitamin C to help your body absorb a sufficient amount of iron from other foods for your daily needs.

- **Planters Sunflower Kernels.** Sunflower seeds contain non-heme (plant-based) iron, which the body absorbs, though not as easily as the iron in meats. One-quarter cup of sunflower seed kernels contains 2.4 milligrams of iron (30 percent of the daily value of iron).

- **Quaker Oats.** While not as easily absorbed by the body as the iron in meats, oats contain non-heme (plant-based) iron. One serving of Quaker Oats oatmeal contains 11 milligrams of iron, or 61 percent of the daily value.

- **ReaLemon.** To help the body absorb non-heme iron in plant foods (such as Quaker Oats, Planters Sunflower Kernels, and McCormick Sesame Seed above), mix one tablespoon ReaLemon lemon juice in a glass of water, and drink the solution before meals. The vitamin C enhances absorption.

- **Sun-Maid Raisins.** While more difficult for the body to absorb than the iron in meats, Sun-Maid Raisins contain non-heme (plant-based) iron. One-half cup of raisins contains 1.6 milligrams of iron (9 percent of the daily value).

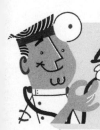

Doctor's Orders

Iron it out! If your energy levels decline and fail to return for four to six weeks, see a doctor to make certain the symptoms aren't being caused by a more serious problem.

Irritable Bowel Syndrome

- **Baker's Angel Flake Coconut.** To bring chronic diarrhea under control, eat two teaspoons Baker's Angel Flake Coconut. A 2010 study published in the *Journal of Ethnopharmacology* showed that coconut extract was just as effective as a leading antidiarrheal medication when tested on rats.

- **Dannon Yogurt.** To ease diarrhea caused by irritable bowel syndrome, eat a cup of Dannon Nonfat Yogurt once or twice a day. The beneficial *Lactobacillus acidophilus* (probiotics) in yogurt replace the helpful bacteria in your colon that the diarrhea may be depleting from your system, preventing the harmful bacteria from propagating beyond control.

- **Kellogg's All-Bran.** To conquer constipation caused by irritable bowel syndrome, eat one cup Kellogg's All-Bran cereal every morning for breakfast. Adding 20 to 35 grams of soluble fiber to your diet daily creates large, soft stools. One cup of Kellogg's All-Bran contains 20 grams of soluble fiber.

- **Lipton Ginger Tea.** Drink four to six cups of Lipton Ginger Tea every day to tame irritable bowel syndrome. Compounds in ginger suppress prostaglandins, the compounds believed to trigger intestinal contractions. The gingerol and shogaol in ginger relax the muscles to ease cramps. (Do not drink ginger tea if you have gallstones. Ginger can increase bile production.)

☙ STRANGE MEDICINE ☙

SHIRKING YOUR DUTY

● If you have irritable bowel syndrome, the muscles in the intestines no longer contract and relax rhythmically to send digested food smoothly through the colon. Instead, these contractions can be stronger and spasmodic, causing diarrhea, or weaker and shorter, causing constipation.

● No one knows precisely what causes irritable bowel syndrome, although suspected culprits are increased nerve sensitivity in the colon, malfunctioning muscles, abnormal serotonin levels, and a disproportionate amount of bad bacteria in the small intestine.

● With irritable bowel syndrome, bouts of diarrhea, constipation, and abdominal pain can be triggered by excess gas, certain foods and medications, stress, or hormonal changes.

● Learning to manage stress through yoga, meditation, or relaxation exercises can prevent irritable bowel syndrome from flaring up.

● Take note of the foods that trigger your irritable bowel and avoid them. Common culprits include coffee, caffeinated sodas, chocolate, and alcohol.

● Drink eight 8-ounce glasses of water or fluid every day to keep your bowels moving smoothly and regularly.

● Observe whether cramping and bloating occur primarily after eating dairy products. You may actually suffer from lactose intolerance rather than irritable bowel syndrome. Many people misdiagnosis themselves as having irritable bowel syndrome when, in fact, their symptoms result from an inability to digest milk sugar.

● Reduce the incidence of irritable bowel syndrome by reducing the amount of fat in your diet. Fat stimulates contractions in the colon.

● To avoid aggravating your delicate system, eat a healthy breakfast and have lunch and dinner at about the same time every day. Eating regularly prevents you from continually under- and overstimulating your digestive system.

● Consider counseling or therapy. Anxiety and worry can exacerbate irritable bowel syndrome and increase the frequency and severity of the symptoms. A psychologist or psychiatrist may help you unearth a subconscious conflict undermining your health.

- **Lipton Peppermint Tea.** To subdue irritable bowel syndrome, pour one cup of boiling water over two Lipton Peppermint Tea bags in a cup, cover with a saucer (to prevent the medicinal peppermint oil from evaporating), let steep for ten minutes, and drink the tea twice a day. The peppermint reduces spasms, calms your intestines, and clears up gas.

- **McCormick Ground Turmeric.** To help relieve the symptoms of irritable bowel syndrome, take one tablespoon McCormick Ground Turmeric daily by simply sprinkling it on your food or using the spice in recipes for rice, casseroles, soups, and stews. According to a 2004 study published in the *Journal of Alternative and Complementary Medicine,* people with irritable bowel syndrome who took a daily dose of turmeric showed significant improvement in abdominal discomfort and bowel patterns. (Turmeric may increase the likelihood of bleeding when taken in combination with the blood thinner Coumadin or other anticoagulant medications.)

- **Metamucil.** To reduce the severity of intestinal spasms caused by irritable bowel syndrome and minimize diarrhea, take one serving of Metamucil (as instructed on the package label) in or with eight ounces of water three times a day before meals. Metamucil contains psyllium seed husk, a natural dietary fiber originating from the psyllium plant, which absorbs liquid, bulking up your stool and allowing it to pass through your system more comfortably. (Metamucil generally produces a laxative effect in twelve to seventy-two hours.)

- **Quaker Oats.** To soak up liquid in your intestines and prevent irritable bowel syndrome from producing diarrhea, eat a bowl of Quaker Oats oatmeal every morning. Oats contain the mild sedative gramine; the complex carbohydrates seem to increase serotonin levels in the brain—relieving stress; and the fiber absorbs excess fluid in your intestines, generating soft, firm stools.

Doctor's Orders

Don't poop out! If diarrhea, constipation, or abdominal pain becomes severe or debilitating, or if you notice blood in your stool, consult your doctor.

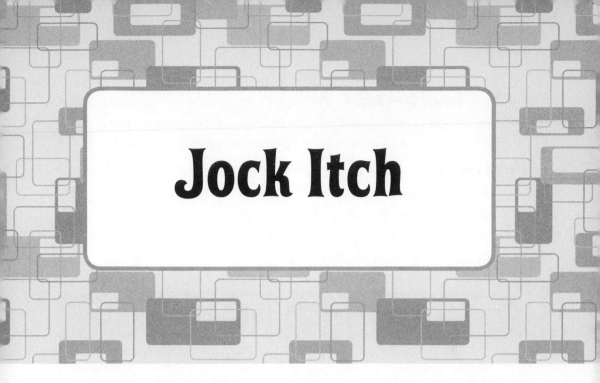

Jock Itch

- **Conair Hair Dryer.** After taking a shower or bath, set a Conair Hair Dryer on the coolest setting and hold it roughly twelve inches from your crotch to dry the moist area.

- **Desitin.** To put an end to jock itch, apply a thin coat of Desitin, the baby rash ointment, to the affected area after showering or bathing. The zinc oxide helps kill the fungus.

- **Head & Shoulders.** Anecdotal evidence shows that washing the groin with Head & Shoulders dandruff shampoo can wipe out jock itch. The anti-fungal properties of the shampoo apparently do the trick.

- **Heinz Apple Cider Vinegar.** To rid your crotch of jock itch, saturate a cotton ball with Heinz Apple Cider Vinegar and dab the affected area several times a day. The acetic acid in the vinegar turns your groin into an inhospitable environment for the fungus.

- **Johnson's Baby Powder.** To prevent jock itch, dust your groin with Johnson's Baby Powder when getting dressed or changing your clothes. The talc in the baby powder absorbs the moisture that provides a breeding ground for the fungus.

- **Kingsford's Corn Starch.** Powdering your groin with Kingsford's Corn Starch every time you get dressed or change your clothes helps prevent jock itch. The cornstarch absorbs moisture and keeps your private parts dry.

- **Lipton Ginger Tea.** Place two Lipton Ginger Tea bags in a cup of boiling water, cover with a saucer, steep for ten minutes, and let cool. Using a cotton ball, apply the tea to the affected area. The antifungal compounds in the ginger, particularly the caprylic acid, kill the fungus.

℞ STRANGE MEDICINE ℞

UP TO SCRATCH

- Jock itch, usually caused by the fungal infection tinea cruris, affects the warm, moist skin of your genitals, inner thighs, and buttocks, causing an itchy, red rash.

- The tinea fungus that causes athlete's foot also causes jock itch. If you have athlete's foot, wash your hands thoroughly after touching your feet to avoid infecting your crotch, and put on socks before putting on your underwear.

- Although named for athletes, jock itch can infect anyone.

- Overweight people have a greater risk of getting jock itch because they perspire more and have more folds in their skin. Losing weight lessens your chances of getting jock itch.

- To lessen your risk of getting jock itch, shower and wash well immediately after exercising, participating in sports, or sweating excessively; dry your groin thoroughly with a clean towel; and powder your crotch to absorb excess moisture.

- After exercising, change out of your workout clothes immediately and toss them in the hamper to be laundered.

- Tight-fitting underwear increases your susceptibility to jock itch. Instead of wearing briefs, try boxer shorts.

- To avoid contracting jock itch from others, do not share towels or clothes.

- **Listerine.** To eliminate jock itch, saturate a cotton ball with original formula Listerine antiseptic mouthwash and apply the mediciney mouthwash to the itchy area several times a day. The thymol in the mouthwash kills the fungus. (Do not put Listerine on open wounds; the alcohol stings.)

- **McCormick Thyme Leaves.** To eradicate jock itch, place two teaspoons McCormick Thyme Leaves in a cup, fill with boiling water, cover with a saucer, and let steep for twenty minutes. Strain out the leaves and let the tea cool to room temperature. Saturate a cotton ball with the thyme tea, and apply the solution to the itchy area three times a day. The thymol in thyme kills the fungus and also reduces inflammation.

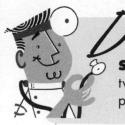

Doctor's Orders

Start from scratch! If a case of jock itch fails to improve within two weeks, consult a doctor to determine whether you need prescription medication.

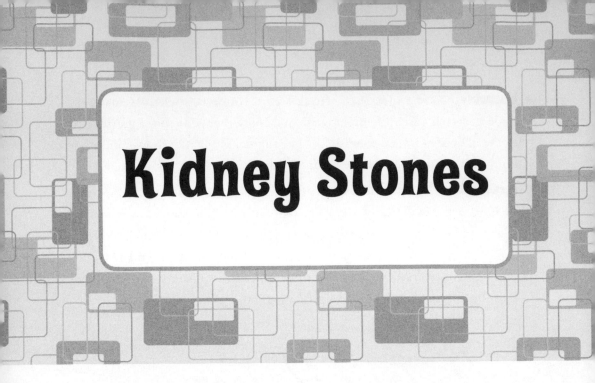

Kidney Stones

- **Budweiser.** Drinking an eight-ounce glass of Budweiser beer every day can lower the risk of kidney stones by approximately 25 percent, according to a 1996 study at the Harvard School of Public Health.

- **Lipton Tea.** Drinking a single eight-ounce cup of Lipton Tea (caffeinated or decaffeinated) every day can decrease the risk of kidney stones by approximately 14 percent, says a 1996 study at the Harvard School of Public Health.

- **Maxwell House Coffee.** Drinking a single eight-ounce cup of Maxwell House Coffee (caffeinated or decaffeinated) every day can decrease the risk of kidney stones by approximately 10 percent, according to a 1996 study at the Harvard School of Public Health. Substances in coffee cause the antidiuretic hormone in the kidney to produce more diluted urine, decreasing the risk of kidney stone formation.

- **Minute Maid Orange Juice.** To prevent kidney stones, drink two 8-ounce glasses of Minute Maid Orange Juice every day. A 2006 study published in the *Clinical Journal of the American Society of Nephrology* showed that orange juice increased levels of citrate in the urine and decreased urine acidity, which reduced the risk of kidney stones.

℞ STRANGE MEDICINE ℞

SET IN STONE

● A kidney stone is a small, grainy calcified deposit similar to a pebble that forms in your kidney when the concentration of calcium or oxalate rises too high in your urine. The stone travels down the ureter, a narrow tube, causing excruciating pain on its way to the bladder.

● Drink at least twelve 8-ounce glasses of water every day to help flush a kidney stone through your system.

● Although walking may be painful, the movement can help you pass a kidney stone by shaking it loose.

● Seventy-five to 80 percent of all kidney stone cases are calcium oxalate stones.

● Contrary to popular belief, drinking cranberry juice to prevent kidney stones may actually increase the risk for both calcium oxalate and uric acid stones. Cranberry juice raises the levels of citrate and magnesium in urine (which inhibit the formation of kidney stones) but simultaneously increases the amount of calcium and oxalate in the urine (two of the components of calcium oxalate kidney stones). Cranberry juice helps prevent urinary tract infections and helps reduce the risk for less common struvite and brushite stones.

● Eating foods high in magnesium decreases your risk of developing calcium oxalate kidney stones. A 1982 study published in the *Journal of the American College of Nutrition* found that supplementing the diet daily with 500 milligrams of magnesium reduced kidney stone formation by 90 percent. Magnesium keeps calcium dissolved in the blood, inhibiting it from forming kidney stones. While nuts provide high amounts of magnesium, they also contain high amounts of oxalates (one of the components of calcium oxalate stones).

● To reduce your chances of getting a kidney stone if you've already had one, drink enough liquid to pass 2.6 quarts of urine daily.

● If you've had a calcium oxalate stone, reduce the amount of oxalate-rich foods you eat, such as beets, blueberries, chocolate, grapes, okra, rhubarb, spinach, sweet potatoes, nuts, and soy products.

● Eating calcium-rich foods does not increase your risk of kidney stones, but taking calcium supplements can. Before doing so, consult your doctor.

- **ReaLemon.** To dissolve or dramatically reduce the incidence of calcium oxalate stones, drink four ounces of ReaLemon lemon juice every day (straight or diluted in water), and then brush your teeth well to prevent the lemon juice from damaging tooth enamel. The lemon juice doubles citrate levels in the urine, according to a 1996 study published in the *Journal of Urology*. The citrate binds to calcium in the urine, preventing the calcium from forming a stone by binding to other calcium in the urine.

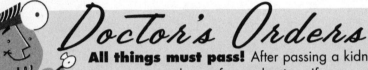

Doctor's Orders

All things must pass! After passing a kidney stone, bring the stone to your doctor for evaluation. If you can't pass the stone, experience severe pain, see blood in your urine, or have difficulty urinating, see your doctor.

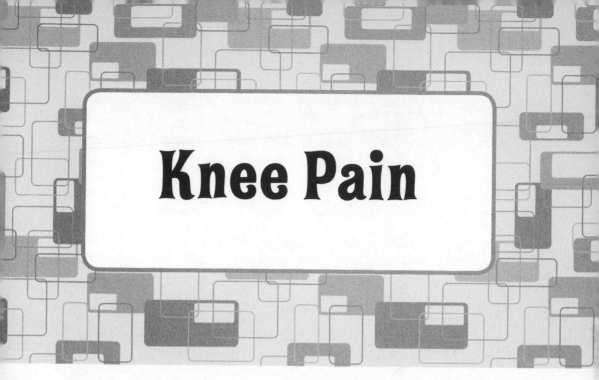

Knee Pain

- **Birds Eye Frozen Peas** and **Bounty Paper Towels.** To soothe knee pain, cover a bag of Birds Eye Frozen Peas with a sheet of Bounty Paper Towels, and apply to the affected area for fifteen minutes every hour. The frozen peas act like small ice cubes, reducing the inflammation causing the pain, and the bag of peas conforms to the shape of your knee. The paper towel creates a layer of insulation to prevent frostbite. Refreeze the bag of peas for future ice-pack use. Be sure to label the bag for ice-pack use only. If you want to eat the peas, cook them after they thaw the first time, never after refreezing.

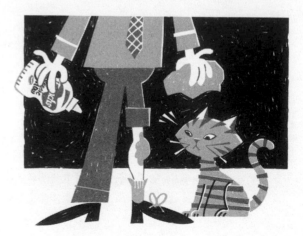

- **French's Mustard.** To relieve knee pain, smear French's Mustard on the affected area and cover with a washcloth dampened with warm water. The heat from the mustard soothes the pain.

WEAK AT THE KNEES

● Knees get injured from sports activities, falls, automobile accidents, overuse, daily wear and tear, kneeling, and squatting.

● If you're overweight, losing excess weight reduces the stress placed on your knees exponentially. Every pound you weigh places roughly six pounds of pressure on your knees.

● Knee pain can be caused by a medical condition, such as arthritis and gout.

● To relieve knee pain, sit down and prop up your injured leg. The elevation allows gravity to reduce the flow of blood to your legs, reducing inflammation.

● Rest helps speed healing of a knee injury. Taking your weight off the knee and minimizing the continual strain allows the injury to heal and avoids any further damage.

● To reduce the inflammation and lessen the pain of a knee injury, take aspirin, Advil (ibuprofen), or Aleve (naproxen). Tylenol (acetaminophen) will help relieve the pain, but it won't reduce the swelling, which is the cause of the pain.

● Prevent future knee injuries by doing exercises that strengthen your quadriceps and hamstrings, the muscles that support your knees.

● **Tabasco Pepper Sauce** and **Crisco All-Vegetable Shortening.** To relieve knee pain, mix one-quarter teaspoon Tabasco Pepper Sauce with two tablespoons Crisco All-Vegetable Shortening, and apply the spicy homemade ointment to the affected area up to five times a day. The capsaicin in the Tabasco Pepper Sauce relieves nerve pain. (Do not apply this salve on open sores and avoid contact with eyes and nose.)

● **Uncle Ben's Converted Brand Rice.** After relieving the inflammation for the first day or two with the Birds Eye Frozen Peas tip on page 291, fill a clean sock with Uncle Ben's Converted Brand Rice, tie a knot in the end, and heat in the microwave oven for ninety seconds. Making sure the sock isn't too hot, apply the heat pack to the affected knee. The rice-filled sock conforms to the shape of your knee and stays warm for roughly thirty minutes, allowing the soothing warmth to increase circulation to the area. The homemade heating pad is also reusable.

- **Vicks VapoRub.** To alleviate knee pain, rub Vicks VapoRub into your knee. The camphor and menthol in the balm reduce pain and inflammation.

- **Wilson Tennis Balls.** When the band of muscle running along the outer side of the thigh gets tight, it tends to pull on the knee, causing pain. To stretch out the band, lie down on floor on your side and place a Wilson Tennis Ball under the thigh. Bend your other leg forward so the weight presses your thigh into the tennis ball, causing a stinging sensation. Move the tennis ball to press into three different areas on your thigh (high, middle, and low), relieving the knee pain.

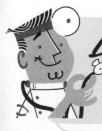

Doctor's Orders

Bend over backwards! If your knee swells or you notice weakness, ice the knee and see a doctor to rule out serious knee damage, like internal bleeding or torn cartilage.

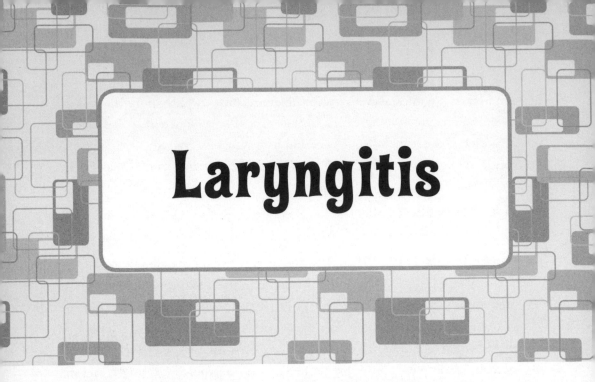

Laryngitis

- **Knorr Chicken Bouillon** and **McCormick Ground (Cayenne) Red Pepper.** To soothe the discomfort of laryngitis, dissolve a cube of Knorr Chicken Bouillon in a cup of boiling water, add one-quarter teaspoon McCormick Ground (Cayenne) Red Pepper, and drink the bouillon. The warmth of the broth provides relief, and the capsaicin in the cayenne pepper soothes pain like an analgesic.

- **Life Savers Pep-O-Mints.** To keep your throat moist, suck on Life Savers Pep-O-Mints. The volatile oils in peppermint increase saliva production, soothing your throat, and the menthol helps relax the larynx.

- **Lipton Chamomile Tea.** To alleviate and soothe laryngitis, fill a large bowl with boiling water and add three Lipton Chamomile Tea bags. Wearing a towel over your head to form a tent over the bowl, hold your face close to the steaming tea and breathe deeply for ten minutes. Keep a box of tissues nearby to blow your nose. The steam

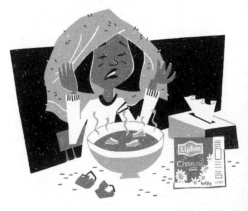

moisturizes your dry throat, and the chamomile reduces inflammation and speeds healing.

- **Lipton Tea, SueBee Honey,** and **ReaLemon.** To resuscitate your voice, savor a warm cup of Lipton Tea flavored with two or three teaspoons Sue-Bee Honey and one teaspoon ReaLemon lemon juice.

- **McCormick Ground Sage** and **SueBee Honey.** To relieve laryngitis and restore your voice, place a tea infuser filled with one tablespoon McCormick

☒ STRANGE MEDICINE ☒

LOOK WHO'S NOT TALKING

- Laryngitis is inflammation and irritation of the vocal cords, the bands of tissue stretched across the inside of the larynx. The swelling results from overuse, irritation, or an infection of the vocal cords.

- Normally your vocal cords open and close, making sounds when they vibrate. But with laryngitis, the swollen vocal cords distort the sounds, lowering the pitch of your voice, or fail to produce any sounds at all.

- Most cases of laryngitis clear up by themselves after a few days.

- Laryngitis can be caused by colds, the flu, allergies, sinusitis, smoking, dust, fumes, bronchitis, and even heartburn.

- To cure laryngitis, drink eight 8-ounce glasses of lukewarm water daily to help your body keep the larynx moist.

- Run a cold-air humidifier in your bedroom or office to keep your vocal cords moist.

- To regain your voice as quickly as possible, refrain from talking and avoid whispering (which puts more strain on your voice than speaking normally).

- To help laryngitis heal, avoid alcohol, caffeinated beverages, and decongestants— all of which dry out the throat.

Ground Sage in a teacup, fill the cup with boiling water, cover with a saucer, and steep for fifteen minutes. Sweeten with two teaspoons SueBee Honey. Sage, a mild astringent that kills bacteria and viruses, reduces the inflammation responsible for throat pain, and honey is a soothing antiseptic. (Do not feed honey to infants less than one year of age. Honey often carries a benign strain of *C. botulinum*, and an infant's immune system requires twelve months to develop to fight off disease and infection.)

- **Morton Salt.** To soothe laryngitis, dissolve one-half teaspoon Morton Salt in an eight-ounce glass of warm water, and gargle with the solution. This mild antiseptic solution helps soothe swollen vocal cords.

- **SueBee Honey, ReaLemon,** and **McCormick Ground (Cayenne) Red Pepper.** Sip a mixture of one tablespoon SueBee Honey, one-quarter teaspoon ReaLemon lemon juice, and a pinch of McCormick Ground (Cayenne) Red Pepper.

- **Tabasco Pepper Sauce.** If you don't have any McCormick Ground (Cayenne) Red Pepper for the Knorr Chicken Bouillon or SueBee Honey tips in this section, use a few drops of Tabasco Pepper Sauce instead. Like cayenne pepper, Tabasco Pepper Sauce contains capsaicin, which doubles as an analgesic to soothe laryngitis pain.

- **Wrigley's Spearmint Gum.** To help regain your voice, chew Wrigley's Spearmint Gum. The act of chewing prompts your salivary glands to produce more saliva, moistening your vocal cords, and the menthol in the mint relaxes the larynx.

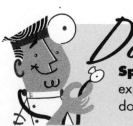

Doctor's Orders

Speak up! If your laryngitis lasts more than two weeks, or if you experience intense pain that impedes you from swallowing, call your doctor.

Memory Problems

- **Chicken of the Sea Salmon, Chicken of the Sea Sardines,** or **Chicken of the Sea Tuna.** To preserve your memory, eat salmon, sardines, or tuna three times a week to add the fatty acids commonly known as omega-3 oils to your diet. Eating these fish rich in eicosapentaenoic acid (EPA) and docosahexaenoic acid (DHA) helps prevent inflammation in brain cells, which destroys them. A 2011 study at Massey University in New Zealand revealed that DHA can boost memory function by 15 percent in healthy adults.

- **Jif Peanut Butter.** Magnesium enhances memory and prevents its impairment. In a 2010 study, neuroscientists from the Massachusetts Institute of Technology and Tsinghua University in Beijing found that magnesium improved short- and long-term memory in rats and increased the number of synapses in the brain. While eating a wide range of legumes, nuts, whole grains, and vegetables will help you meet your daily dietary need for magnesium, you can quickly replace magnesium in your body by eating Jif Peanut Butter (straight from the jar or in a sandwich). Four tablespoons of peanut butter contain 100 milligrams of magnesium (or 25 percent of the daily value).

RX STRANGE MEDICINE RX

A TRIP DOWN MEMORY LANE

● Occasional lapses of memory naturally occur with age and are rarely a sign of dementia or Alzheimer's disease.

● Drinking eight 8-ounce glasses of water each and every day keeps your body and brain properly hydrated.

● Maintain a high level of HDL ("good") cholesterol by eating foods low in saturated and trans fats and high in fiber. Plaque lining the inner walls of the arteries can reduce blood flow to the brain, reducing the supply of oxygen.

● To help reduce the risk of memory loss, exercise your brain by doing crossword and Sudoku puzzles, playing Scrabble, reading books, taking up a musical instrument, learning a second language, or undertaking any activity or pursuit that stimulates the mind.

● Listening to music frequently improves concentration and memory skills. A 2007 study at the Stanford University School of Medicine showed that music engages the areas of the brain involved with paying attention.

● Get eight hours of sleep every night, going to bed and waking up at the same time every day, even on weekends. During REM sleep in the eighth hour of sleep, the brain transfers short-term memory into long-term memory, according to James B. Maas, past chairman of the department of psychology at Cornell University. Eight hours of sleep dramatically increases memory retention, and people deprived of REM sleep experience significant difficulty retaining recently learned material.

● Contrary to popular belief, the supplement ginkgo biloba does not improve memory. A 2009 study published in the *Journal of the American Medical Association* found no evidence that ginkgo biloba prevents memory loss or slows the progression of cognitive decline in older adults.

● **Lipton Green Tea.** To prevent your memory from slipping, drink one or two cups of strongly brewed Lipton Green Tea daily. A study published in the *American Journal of Clinical Nutrition* in 2008 reported that drinking two cups of green tea a day made people (fifty-five and older) 54 percent less likely to exhibit signs of cognitive impairment or display a decline in mental acuity.

- **Maxwell House Coffee.** To prevent memory loss, drink three or four cups of Maxwell House Coffee every day. Studies show that elderly people who drink three or four cups of coffee a day experience up to 70 percent less memory loss than those who drink one cup a day or less. The caffeine in coffee also temporarily enhances your ability to concentrate.

- **McCormick Ground Cinnamon.** To boost your memory, strive to eat one-quarter to one-half teaspoon McCormick Ground Cinnamon daily by sprinkling the spice on toast, breakfast cereal, soups, and stews. A 2004 study at Wheeling Jesuit University in West Virginia showed that the taste or smell of cinnamon may boost your memory and cognitive skills. A potent antioxidant, cinnamon also reduces inflammation and lowers cholesterol and blood sugar levels.

- **McCormick Ground Turmeric.** To help ward off Alzheimer's disease, take one tablespoon McCormick Ground Turmeric daily by simply sprinkling it on your food or using the spice in recipes for rice, casseroles, soups, and stews. Curcumin, an antioxidant in turmeric, hinders the formation of amyloid plaques, sticky buildups in the brain that indicate Alzheimer's disease. People in India, where turmeric is plentiful in cooking, have relatively low rates of Alzheimer's disease. (Turmeric may increase the likelihood of bleeding when taken in combination with the blood thinner Coumadin or other anticoagulant medications.)

- **McCormick Rosemary Leaves** and **L'eggs Sheer Energy Panty Hose.** To boost your memory and increase alertness, place one teaspoon McCormick Rosemary Leaves in the foot cut from a pair of clean, used L'eggs Sheer Energy Panty Hose, tie a knot in the open end, and sniff the sachet

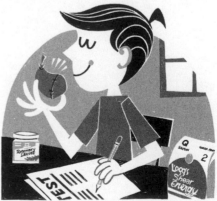

throughout the day. Studies show that the scent of rosemary enhances memory and prompts the brain to increase its production of beta waves.

- **Planters Sunflower Kernels.** To protect your memory, eat a handful of Planters Sunflower Kernels as a snack during the day or sprinkle them over a bowl of breakfast cereal or a salad. The magnesium in sunflower seeds increases the number of synapses in the brain. Sunflower seeds also contain omega-3 fatty acids that keep the membranes of brain cells flexible.

- **Sun-Maid Prunes.** To safeguard your memory, eat three or four Sun-Maid Prunes every day. Prunes absorb and neutralize large amounts of free radicals, molecules that can damage brain cells, expunging them from your system.

- **Wrigley's Big Red Cinnamon Gum.** Chew a stick of Wrigley's Big Red Cinnamon Gum to enhance your memory and pay better attention. A 2004 study at Wheeling Jesuit University in West Virginia showed that the taste or smell of cinnamon may boost your memory and cognitive skills.

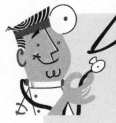

Doctor's Orders

Don't forget! If your memory rapidly deteriorates over a period of a few months, see a doctor to rule out a thyroid disorder, a medicinal side effect, a nutritional deficiency, high blood pressure, or a more serious ailment.

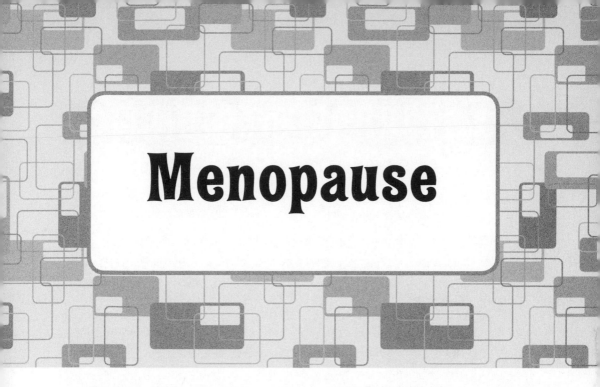

Menopause

- **Chicken of the Sea Salmon, Chicken of the Sea Sardines,** or **Chicken of the Sea Tuna.** To relieve the symptoms of menopause, eat salmon, sardines, or tuna three times a week to add the fatty acids commonly known as omega-3 oils to your diet. The drop in estrogen that occurs during menopause increases the risk of heart disease and osteoporosis. Eating these fish rich in omega-3 fatty acids lowers the risk of heart disease and osteoporosis. Also, one serving of Chicken of the Sea Chunk Light Tuna provides nearly 60 percent of the daily requirement for vitamin B$_6$, which can help alleviate menopausal mood swings.

- **Dannon Yogurt.** To offset the loss in bone mass that accompanies the onset of menopause, eat a cup of Dannon Plain Nonfat Yogurt every day to boost your calcium intake. Calcium strengthens the bones and can even increase bone mass.

- **Jif Peanut Butter.** Magnesium increases calcium absorption and helps build bones, which protects against osteoporosis during menopause. While eating a wide range of legumes, nuts, whole grains, and vegetables will help you meet your daily dietary need for magnesium, you can quickly replace magnesium in your body by eating Jif Peanut Butter (straight from the jar

TIME FOR A CHANGE

● During menopause, a woman's estrogen and progesterone levels drop, her ovaries gradually stop producing eggs, and menstruation eventually ceases.

● The Centers for Disease Control and Prevention reports that women typically enter menopause sometime between the ages of forty-five and fifty-five years old. According to the National Institute on Aging, the average woman completes menopause at age fifty-one.

● The sudden drop in estrogen levels increases the risk of heart disease and osteoporosis and can cause weight gain, vaginal dryness, hot flashes, emotional instability, and interrupted sleep.

● Menopausal symptoms can last up to five years with symptoms ranging from mild to severe. Menopause is complete when a woman has not had her period for one year.

● To relieve the symptoms of menopause, get at least thirty minutes of exercise every day by simply going for a walk. A 2008 study published in *Cancer Epidemiology, Biomarkers & Prevention* showed that moderate walking reduces menopausal symptoms including stress, anxiety, and depression.

● To prevent the weight gain that accompanies menopause and reduce other symptoms, eat a balanced diet that includes a variety of fruits, vegetables, and whole grains. And limit the amount of saturated fat, oils, and sugars you consume.

● Decreased estrogen production can cause women to lose up to 20 percent of their bone density in the five to seven years after menopause, making the women more susceptible to osteoporosis, according to the National Osteoporosis Foundation.

● Minimize the amount of alcohol you drink to avoid complications with osteoporosis. The National Osteoporosis Foundation reports that drinking heavily can reduce bone formation and may also affect the body's calcium supply.

or in a sandwich). Four tablespoons of peanut butter contain 100 milligrams of magnesium (or 25 percent of the daily value).

- **K-Y Jelly.** To compensate for the vaginal dryness caused by low estrogen levels, use a water-soluble lubricant like K-Y Jelly. Avoid oil-based lubricants like Vaseline Petroleum Jelly, which can cause further irritation.

- **Planters Dry Roasted Almonds, Planters Dry Roasted Cashews,** or **Planters Dry Roasted Peanuts.** Eating foods high in magnesium—like Planters Dry Roasted Almonds, Planters Dry Roasted Cashews, or Planters Dry Roasted Peanuts—increases calcium absorption and helps build bones, which protects against osteoporosis during menopause. One ounce of almonds provides 80 milligrams of magnesium, one ounce of cashews provides 75 milligrams, and one ounce of dry roasted peanuts provides 50 milligrams.

- **Silk Soymilk.** To minimize menopausal symptoms, add more soy foods to your diet, such as four 8-ounce glasses of Silk Soymilk once a day. A 2012 study at the University of Minnesota showed that women who consume 54 milligrams of soy isoflavones daily reduced the frequency of hot flashes by 20.6 percent and the severity by 26 percent, without any side effects. Four 8-ounce glasses of soymilk contain 50 milligrams of soy isoflavones.

- **Tums.** To make certain you're getting enough calcium, eat one regular Tums tablet after breakfast and a second tablet after dinner. Your body can absorb only 500 to 600 milligrams of calcium at a time. A regular strength Tums tablet contains 500 milligrams of calcium carbonate. (If you've had calcium oxalate kidney stones, consult your doctor before taking Tums.)

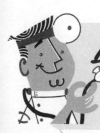

Doctor's Orders

Change your mind! If you experience changes in your menstrual cycle, unusual bleeding, urinary discomfort, or if you just feel lousy, consult a doctor to rule out a more serious medical problem.

Menstrual Cramps

- **Chicken of the Sea Salmon, Chicken of the Sea Sardines,** or **Chicken of the Sea Tuna.** To help reduce menstrual cramping, eat salmon, sardines, or tuna three times a week to add the fatty acids commonly known as omega-3 oils to your diet. Eating these fish rich in omega-3 fatty acids helps ease the cramping that accompanies menstruation. One serving of Chicken of the Sea Chunk Light Tuna provides nearly 60 percent of the daily requirement for vitamin B_6, which can help alleviate menstrual cramping and mood swings.

- **Dr. Teal's Epsom Salt.** To relieve menstrual cramps, fill the bathtub with warm water and add two cups Dr. Teal's Epsom Salt. Soak for twenty minutes, during which time the magnesium in the Epsom Salt passes into the body through osmosis and eases muscular aches.

- **Jif Peanut Butter.** Magnesium prevents cramps, boosts your mood, and curbs weight gain, bloating, and breast tenderness during your period. While eating a wide range of legumes, nuts, whole grains, and vegetables will help you meet your daily dietary need for magnesium, you can quickly replace magnesium in your body by eating Jif Peanut Butter (straight from the jar or in a sandwich). Four tablespoons of peanut butter contain 100 milligrams of magnesium (or 25 percent of the daily value).

- **Lipton Chamomile Tea.** To ease menstrual cramps, place two Lipton Chamomile Tea bags in a cup, fill with boiling water, and cover with a saucer. Steep for ten minutes and drink two or three cups a day. Chamomile doubles as an antispasmodic that relieves cramps and a mild sedative that calms the nerves. (Coumarin, an anticoagulant in chamomile, may increase

☥ STRANGE MEDICINE ☥

CRAMPING YOUR STYLE

- Fluctuating hormone levels during a woman's monthly menstrual cycle can cause anxiety, backache, bloating, cramps, depression, fatigue, headache, and irritability.

- To help ease the pain of menstrual cramps, get at least thirty minutes of exercise every day by simply going for a walk. Exercise prompts your body to produce endorphins, a natural painkiller.

- When it comes to relieving menstrual cramps, soaking in a soothing hot bath or using a heating pad on the affected area tends to work just as effectively as over-the-counter pain relievers.

- To alleviate menstrual cramps, get twenty minutes of daily exercise by going for a walk, riding a bicycle, running on a treadmill, or swimming. Exercise boosts circulation (diminishing the cramps) and increases endorphin levels in the brain, soothing stress and lifting your mood.

- Taking Advil or Motrin (ibuprofen) or Aleve (naproxen) according to the directions on the bottle may help relieve the pain of menstrual cramps. Before doing so, consult your doctor, who may prescribe a stronger nonsteroidal anti-inflammatory drug.

- To reduce the severity of menstrual cramps, ask your doctor for a prescription for birth control pills. The hormones in birth control prevent ovulation, minimizing the intensity of menstrual cramps.

- Wearing loose clothing that does not squeeze your abdomen helps reduce the intensity of menstrual cramps.

the likelihood of bleeding when taken in combination with the blood thinner Coumadin or other anticoagulant medications.)

- **Lipton Ginger Tea.** To relieve menstrual cramps, drink a cup of strongly brewed Lipton Ginger Tea two or three times daily. Compounds in ginger suppress prostaglandins, the compounds that trigger uterine contractions. The gingerol and shogaol in ginger relax the muscles. (Do not drink ginger tea if you have gallstones. Ginger can increase bile production.)

- **Planters Dry Roasted Almonds.** To quell the cramps that accompany menstruation, eat one-quarter cup Planters Dry Roasted Almonds daily. The almonds contain roughly 200 milligrams of magnesium, which prevents cramps, boosts your mood, and curbs weight gain, bloating, and breast tenderness during your period.

- **Planters Sunflower Kernels.** To alleviate cramping, eat one-quarter cup Planters Sunflower Kernels daily before and during your period. The sunflower seeds provide 0.82 milligrams of vitamin B_1 (54.7 percent of the recommended daily value). According to the American Congress of Obstetricians and Gynecologists, vitamin B_1 (thiamine) may help reduce painful cramping during periods.

- **Quaker Oats.** To reduce menstrual problems, eat a bowl of Quaker Oats oatmeal every morning. Oats contain the mild sedative gramine, the fiber absorbs excess estrogen, and the complex carbohydrates seem to increase serotonin levels in the brain, relieving stress.

- **Tums.** To alleviate the symptoms that accompany menstruation, eat one regular Tums tablet after each meal. Your body can absorb only 500 to 600 milligrams of calcium at a time. A regular strength Tums tablet contains 500 milligrams of calcium carbonate. Calcium relaxes the muscles, reducing the intensity of menstrual cramping. (If you've had calcium oxalate kidney stones, consult your doctor before taking Tums.)

- **Uncle Ben's Converted Brand Rice.** To relieve menstrual cramps, fill a clean sock with Uncle Ben's Converted Brand Rice, tie a knot in the end, and heat in the microwave oven for ninety seconds. Making sure the sock isn't too hot, apply the heat pack on your abdomen. The rice-filled sock conforms to the shape of your body, stays warm for roughly thirty minutes, and provides soothing heat. The homemade heating pad is also reusable.

Doctor's Orders

Feeling cursed? If you experience severe cramps, undergo heavy bleeding for more than a week, pass a blood clot larger than a quarter, or your cycles complete in less than three weeks, consult a doctor.

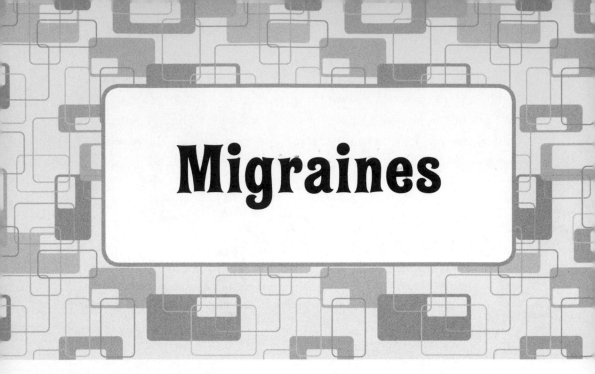

Migraines

- **Birds Eye Frozen Peas** and **Bounty Paper Towels.** To treat a migraine and reduce the pain, cover a bag of Birds Eye Frozen Peas with a sheet of Bounty Paper Towels, and apply as an ice pack on the back of your neck. The frozen peas act like small ice cubes, the bag of peas conforms to the contours of your neck, and the paper towel creates a layer of insulation to prevent frostbite. Refreeze the peas for future ice-pack use. Be sure to label the bag for ice-pack use only. If you want to eat the peas, cook them after they thaw the first time, never after refreezing.

- **Campbell's Tomato Juice.** Drinking juices that contain high doses of vitamin C helps alleviate a migraine headache. One cup of Campbell's Tomato Juice not only contains 46.6 milligrams of vitamin C but the chromium in tomato juice regulates blood sugar levels and helps subdue a migraine headache quickly.

- **Coca-Cola.** In 1886, Atlanta pharmacist John Pemberton invented Coca-Cola as a headache cure and marketed the soft drink as "a valuable Brain Tonic." Two years later fellow Atlanta pharmacist Asa Candler, convinced that drinking Coca-Cola relieved his migraine headaches, purchased the rights to the formula. The 45 milligrams of caffeine in a twelve-ounce can of Coke acts as a vasocon-strictor, reducing swelling of blood vessels that cause migraine headache pain.

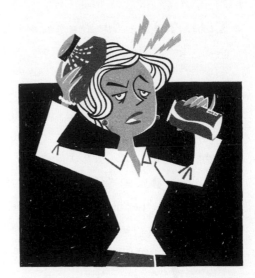

- **Dole Pineapple Chunks** or **Dole Pineapple Juice.** Eating a standard serving of Dole Pineapple Chunks once or twice a day (or drinking a glass of Dole Pineapple Juice) reduces the severity and incidence of migraine headaches. Bromelain, the enzyme found only in pineapples, seems to relieve the pain.

- **Dr. Teal's Epsom Salt.** To relieve a migraine headache, fill the bathtub with warm water and add two cups Dr. Teal's Epsom Salt. Soak for twenty minutes with your head partially submerged so you can still breathe. People who suffer from migraine headaches often have a magnesium deficiency, and soaking in an Epsom Salt bath allows the magnesium in Epsom Salt to pass into the body through osmosis.

- **Heinz Apple Cider Vinegar** and **SueBee Honey.** At the onset of a migraine headache, mix two tablespoons Heinz Apple Cider Vinegar and two tablespoons SueBee Honey in a glass of water, and drink the solution. (Do not feed honey to infants less than one year of age. Honey often carries a benign strain of *C. botulinum,* and an infant's immune system requires twelve months to develop to fight off disease and infection.)

- **Life Savers Pep-O-Mint.** To soothe a migraine headache, suck on one or two Life Savers Pep-O-Mint candies. Anecdotal evidence shows that pep-permint reduces migraine pain.

- **Lipton Tea** and **SueBee Honey.** Drinking coffee sweetened with sugar can trigger a migraine headache. Instead, switch to Lipton Tea and SueBee Honey. Within a month, the number of migraine headaches you typically experience will likely decrease dramatically. (Do not feed honey to infants less than one year of age. Honey often carries a benign strain of *C. botulinum,* and an infant's immune system requires twelve months to develop to fight off disease and infection.)

- **Maxwell House Coffee.** While drinking coffee triggers a migraine headache in some people, drinking coffee reduces the pain for many others. The 150 milligrams of caffeine in a nine-ounce cup of Maxwell House Coffee acts as a vasoconstrictor, reducing swelling of blood vessels that cause migraine headache pain.

- **Planters Dry Roasted Almonds.** For some people, eating almonds triggers a migraine headache. For others, eating almonds reduces the pain. Almonds contain two helpful ingredients: magnesium, which many migraine sufferers lack (a one-ounce serving of almonds contains 75 milligrams of magnesium); and salicin, which, when consumed, forms salicylic acid, the primary by-product of aspirin metabolization.

- **Uncle Ben's Converted Brand Rice.** Fill a clean sock with Uncle Ben's Converted Brand Rice, tie a knot in the end, and heat in a microwave oven for one minute. Place the homemade heating pack over your forehead for ten minutes to relieve the pain. If the heating pack is too hot, place a sheet of paper towel between your skin and the sock. The rice-filled sock can be reheated often and stored in a pantry closet for future use.

- **Vicks VapoRub.** Rub a dab of Vicks VapoRub on your temples and the back of your neck, lie down, and breathe deeply. The smell of menthol and eucalyptus reduces the intensity of migraine pain.

- **Wilson Tennis Balls.** For quick relief from migraine headache pain, place two Wilson Tennis Balls in a clean sock, tie a knot in the end, and stand with your back against a wall with the sock positioned between the wall and

℞ STRANGE MEDICINE ℞

HITTING THE NAIL ON THE HEAD

- No one knows for certain what causes migraine headaches.

- Avoid foods and scents that trigger migraine headaches.

- To minimize occurrences of migraine headaches, sleep and eat meals on a regular schedule and reduce stress by escaping or postponing any stressful situation that has previously triggered migraines.

- Regular exercise reduces stress and can help prevent migraines.

- Obesity is believed to be a factor in migraine headaches.

- If you're a woman and estrogen seems to trigger your migraine headaches or make them worse, consult your doctor to discuss alternatives to medications that contain estrogen, such as birth control pills and hormone replacement therapy.

- Treatments for migraine headaches include acupuncture, biofeedback, massage, and chiropractic therapy.

- Vitamin B_2 and the herbs feverfew and butterbur may prevent migraines or reduce their severity. Taking coenzyme Q_{10} or magnesium supplements may reduce the frequency of migraines as well. Consult a doctor to determine if these treatments are appropriate for you. Do not take feverfew or butterbur if you're pregnant.

- Taking a bath or shower typically reduces a migraine headache.

- Lying down in a dark, quiet room with your eyes closed can lessen the pain of a migraine headache. Bright or flashing lights tend to intensify a migraine headache.

- Massaging the muscle beneath the web of flesh between the thumb and index finger helps relieve headache pain.

- Applying a washcloth dampened with cold water to the back of the neck can bring instant relief and diminish migraine pain in a short space of time.

- Placing a cold compress on your forehead and soaking your feet in a tub of warm water tricks the brain, bringing quick relief from migraine pain.

your neck so that the two tennis balls apply pressure to the two pressure points located roughly two inches apart at the base of the skull. Slowly move your body up and down to allow the tennis balls to massage these two key pressure points.

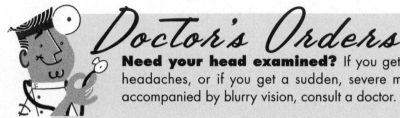

Doctor's Orders

Need your head examined? If you get frequent migraine headaches, or if you get a sudden, severe migraine headache accompanied by blurry vision, consult a doctor.

Morning Sickness

- **Canada Dry Ginger Ale.** Drinking flat Canada Dry Ginger Ale relieves morning sickness. The ginger seems to relax the muscles in the stomach. Contrary to popular belief, Canada Dry Ginger Ale does indeed contain genuine ginger, included in the list of ingredients as "natural flavors." (Do not drink ginger ale if you have gallstones. Ginger can increase bile production.)

- **Cheerios.** To prevent morning sickness or at least ease the nausea and vomiting, start your day by eating a bowl of dry Cheerios breakfast cereal. They're easy to digest and absorb the acids in your stomach.

- **Coca-Cola.** Drinking flat Coca-Cola helps settle your queasy stomach. Pharmacies sell cola syrup that can be taken in small doses to relieve nausea. The concentrated sugars are believed to relax the gastrointestinal tract. Letting the bubbles out of the soda prevents the carbonation from further upsetting your stomach.

- **Gatorade.** To help your body maintain the proper balance of electrolytes and calm the nausea of morning sickness, drink Gatorade, the sports drink that provides potassium, sodium, and glucose.

- **Life Savers Pep-O-Mints.** To counteract nausea, suck on a few Life Savers Pep-O-Mints. Peppermint calms the stomach muscles, and the menthol relaxes the lower esophageal sphincter (the valve at the bottom of the esophagus), allowing trapped gas to escape from the stomach.

- **Lipton Chamomile Tea** and **Lipton Peppermint Tea.** To soothe morning sickness, place one Lipton Chamomile Tea bag and one Lipton Peppermint Tea bag in the same cup, fill with boiling water, cover with a saucer,

℞ STRANGE MEDICINE ℞

A PREGNANT PAUSE

- Morning sickness is nausea that occurs during pregnancy, typically during the first trimester. Despite its name, morning sickness can strike any time of day.

- No one knows exactly what causes morning sickness, but scientists believe hormonal changes during pregnancy are responsible.

- Some women experience morning sickness throughout pregnancy.

- For some women, certain smells can trigger morning sickness. Avoiding those smells prevents making the nausea worse.

- Pregnant women who drink one eight-ounce glass of water every hour experience less morning sickness.

- To prevent morning sickness, eat several small meals throughout the day rather than three large meals. Doing so keeps your blood sugar levels constant. The fetus feeds on glucose around the clock, and keeping your blood sugar levels constant prevents sudden drops, making you less prone to nausea.

- Prenatal vitamins can trigger nausea. To prevent morning sickness, take the vitamins at night or with a snack, rather than first thing in the morning on an empty stomach.

- Avoid fried foods or any other food that may be difficult to digest. Instead, choose foods high in carbohydrates and low in fat.

steep for ten minutes, and drink. The plant compounds in chamomile seem to reduce the gag reflex, and peppermint eases digestion and prevents the spasms that cause vomiting. (Coumarin, an anticoagulant in chamomile, may increase the likelihood of bleeding when taken in combination with the blood thinner Coumadin or other anticoagulant medications.)

- **Lipton Ginger Tea.** To relieve the pangs of morning sickness, drink a cup of Lipton Ginger Tea (or as many cups as necessary until the nausea subsides). The gingerol and shogaol in ginger reduce intestinal contractions, neutralize indigestion, and prevent the brain from initiating the vomiting reflex. (Do not drink ginger tea if you have gallstones. Ginger can increase bile production.)

- **McCormick Fennel Seed.** To soothe an upset stomach, chew and swallow one-half teaspoon McCormick Fennel Seed. Fennel contains anethole, a compound that doubles as an antiseptic and antispasmodic.

- **Nabisco Original Premium Saltine Crackers.** Eating a few Nabisco Original Premium Saltine Crackers can ease the nausea of morning sickness. High in carbohydrates, the saltine crackers help settle your stomach and give you strength.

- **Planters Dry Roasted Almonds.** To tame morning sickness, eat a handful of Planters Dry Roasted Almonds throughout the day. Almonds settle queasiness and provide you with plenty of essential nutrients, like calcium, potassium, vitamin B_2, and vitamin E.

- **Popsicle.** If you can't keep any food down, suck on your favorite flavor Popsicle to rehydrate yourself and replace sugars lost through vomiting.

- **ReaLemon** and **SueBee Honey.** To calm your stomach, mix three tablespoons ReaLemon lemon juice and one teaspoon SueBee Honey in an eight-ounce glass of warm water, and sip the warm drink as needed. (Do not feed honey to infants less than one year of age. Honey often carries a benign strain of *C. botulinum,* and an infant's immune system requires twelve months to develop to fight off disease and infection.)

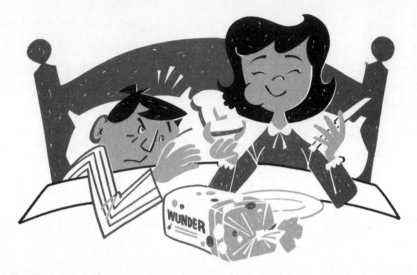

● **Wonder Bread.** Before you get out of bed in the morning, start your day with some slices of toasted Wonder Bread, which are easy to digest and absorb the acids in your stomach.

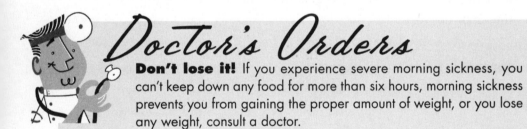

Doctor's Orders

Don't lose it! If you experience severe morning sickness, you can't keep down any food for more than six hours, morning sickness prevents you from gaining the proper amount of weight, or you lose any weight, consult a doctor.

Motion Sickness and Dizziness

- **Lipton Ginger Tea.** To relieve the nausea that accompanies dizziness, drink a cup of Lipton Ginger Tea (or as many cups as necessary until the nausea subsides). Ginger tames nausea. (Do not drink ginger tea if you have gallstones. Ginger can increase bile production.)

- **McCormick Ground Ginger.** To help prevent motion sickness, one hour before you commence your journey, mix a pinch of powdered ginger in a glass of water and drink the tangy liquid. The gingerol and shogaol in ginger reduce intestinal contractions, neutralize indigestion, and prevent the brain from initiating the vomiting reflex. Ginger works best preventing motion sickness rather than curing it. A study published in 1982 in the British medical journal the *Lancet* showed that ginger was more effective at relieving motion sickness than dimenhydrinate, the active ingredient in Dramamine. (Do not use ginger if you have gallstones. Ginger can increase bile production.)

- **McCormick Whole Cloves.** If you're susceptible to motion sickness, before boarding a boat, train, airplane, or car, chew on a few McCormick Whole Cloves. The eugenol in cloves helps stop the spasms.

$\underset{\text{Rx}}{\overset{}{\boxed{}}}$ STRANGE MEDICINE $\underset{\text{Rx}}{\overset{}{\boxed{}}}$

GOING THROUGH THE MOTIONS

● Motion sickness—caused by traveling in a car, boat, train, airplane, spacecraft, or amusement park ride—is believed to be triggered when the brain receives sensory signals regarding motion that do not match. For instance, if you're reading a book in the back seat of a moving car, your inner ear senses the motion of the car but your eyes do not, making motion sickness the likely result.

● Typically, the vestibular system—the organs of balance in the inner ear—accurately report information about motion to the brain. However, unusual motions exceed the rate that the vestibular system can relay information, causing the vestibular system to transmit false information that conflicts with information reported by the other senses. Scientists theorize that the brain presumes the vestibular system is providing false information because the body has been poisoned. The brain reacts by triggering vomiting as a defense mechanism.

● Motion sickness tends to subside after a day or so, once the traveler gets used to the motion and the brain grows accustomed to the contradictory input.

● To prevent or reduce motion sickness, minimize head movements and stare straight ahead at the distant horizon.

● **Nabisco Ginger Snaps.** To soothe the nausea that accompanies motion sickness, eat a few Nabisco Ginger Snaps. The ginger in the cookies is one of the oldest remedies for nausea. A study published in 1982 in the *Lancet* showed that ginger beats dimenhydrinate (Dramamine) for relieving nausea due to motion sickness. (Do not use ginger if you have gallstones. Ginger can increase bile production.)

● **ReaLemon** and **SueBee Honey.** To calm your stomach, mix three tablespoons ReaLemon lemon juice and one teaspoon SueBee Honey in an eight-ounce glass of warm water, and sip the warm drink as needed. (Do

- Traveling at night lessens the odds of motion sickness by lessening the conflicting visual input. If you do get motion sickness, lying down and closing your eyes can decease the severity.

- When you're feeling queasy, avoid smells that might trigger nausea, such as foods, engine fumes, or smoke.

- Doctors frequently diagnose dizziness as "benign positional vertigo."

- Conventional drugs used to treat dizziness and the resulting nausea typically leave the patient feeling sedated.

- To help prevent motion sickness, refrain from drinking any alcohol before or during your travels. Alcohol interferes with the communication between the eye, brain, and inner ear.

- To help avoid motion sickness, refrain from reading while traveling.

- To relieve feelings of nausea, identify the first crease on the inside of your wrist from the palm of your hand, measure two of your own thumb-widths up your arm from the center of that crease, and press that point with your thumb firmly, until it hurts slightly, for five to ten minutes. Repeat with your other wrist. Pressing this point on the wrist (known as the Pericardium 6 point in acupuncture) can relieve nausea.

not feed honey to infants less than one year of age. Honey often carries a benign strain of *C. botulinum*, and an infant's immune system requires twelve months to develop to fight off disease and infection.)

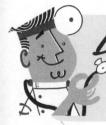

Doctor's Orders

Set things in motion! If you're frequently incapacitated by motion sickness, consult a therapist to conquer any underlying psychological problems.

Muscle Soreness

- **Birds Eye Frozen Peas** and **Bounty Paper Towels.** To soothe sore muscles, cover a bag of Birds Eye Frozen Peas with a sheet of Bounty Paper Towels, and apply to the affected area for fifteen minutes every hour. The frozen peas act like small ice cubes, reducing the inflammation causing the pain, and the bag of peas conforms to the shape of your body. The paper towel creates a layer of insulation to prevent frostbite. Refreeze the bag of peas for future ice-pack use. Be sure to label the bag for ice-pack use only. If you want to eat the peas, cook them after they thaw the first time, never after refreezing.

- **Dr. Teal's Epsom Salt.** Turn your bathtub into a rejuvenating mineral spring by adding two cups Dr. Teal's Epsom Salt to lukewarm bathwater and soaking for fifteen luxurious minutes. The magnesium in the Epsom Salt passes into the body through osmosis and eases muscular aches.

- **Lakewood Black Cherry Juice.** To soothe or prevent muscle soreness, drink one 8-ounce glass of Lakewood Black Cherry Juice every day until the pain subsides. Black cherry juice is packed with anti-inflammatory antioxidants, and a 2009 study at Oregon Health & Science University in Portland showed that people who drank tart cherry juice while training for a long distance run reported significantly less pain after exercise than those who did not drink cherry juice.

- **Maxwell House Coffee.** Thirty minutes before exercising or participating in a sports activity, drink a couple of cups of Maxwell House Coffee. A 2007 study at the University of Georgia found that a moderate dose of caffeine (the equivalent of two cups of coffee) can reduce post-workout pain by up to 48 percent.

- **McCormick Ground Turmeric.** To relieve sore muscles, take one tablespoon McCormick Ground Turmeric daily by simply sprinkling it on your food or using the spice in recipes for rice, casseroles, soups, and stews. Curcumin, an antioxidant in turmeric, reduces inflammation (just like nonsteroidal anti-inflammatory drugs such as aspirin, ibuprofen, and naproxen) and also inhibits the body from producing prostaglandins, the compounds that help signal pain. A 2010 study by endocrinologist Dr. Janet Funk at the University of Arizona College of Medicine showed that turmeric controls the formation of new blood vessels at the site of inflammation. (Turmeric may increase the likelihood of bleeding when taken in combination with the blood thinner Coumadin or other anticoagulant medications.)

- **Tabasco Pepper Sauce** and **Crisco All-Vegetable Shortening.** To relieve muscle soreness, mix one-quarter teaspoon Tabasco Pepper Sauce with two tablespoons Crisco All-Vegetable Shortening, and apply this spicy homemade ointment to the affected areas up to five times a day. The capsaicin in the Tabasco Pepper Sauce helps numb the pain. (Do not apply this salve on open sores and avoid contact with eyes and nose.)

- **Uncle Ben's Converted Brand Rice.** After relieving the inflammation for the first day or two with the Birds Eye Frozen Peas tip on the opposite page, fill a clean sock with Uncle Ben's Converted Brand Rice, tie a knot in the end, and heat in the microwave oven for ninety seconds. Making sure the sock isn't too hot, apply the heat pack to the affected area. The rice-filled sock conforms to the shape of your body and stays warm for roughly thirty minutes, allowing the soothing warmth to increase circulation to the area. The homemade heating pad is also reusable.

- **Vicks VapoRub.** To alleviate sore muscles, rub Vicks VapoRub into the affected area. The camphor and menthol in the balm soothe the pain and reduce the inflammation.

℞ STRANGE MEDICINE ℞

DON'T MOVE A MUSCLE

- After working out, playing sports, or doing housework, you can experience muscle soreness. Participating in a new activity or eccentric exercises, increasing the strenuousness of the activity, or lengthening your workout can cause tiny injuries called microdamage in the muscle fibers and connective tissue. Within twenty-four hours, your muscles will start feeling sore.

- If you repeat the same activity that caused the muscle soreness, your body will slowly get used to it as you strengthen the muscles involved.

- To relieve muscle soreness, apply ice for twenty minutes immediately after the activity to reduce inflammation, and then use heat later to increase blood flow to the affected area.

- To heal the sore muscle and reduce inflammation, after applying ice, refrain from any further athletic activity, avoid putting any weight on the affected area, wrap the injury with an elastic bandage, and elevate the injured limb above your heart (either by propping up your leg or putting your arm in a sling).

- Contrary to popular belief, stretching before a workout does not prevent sore muscles. Instead, warm up by starting with light exercises and gradually build to more strenuous ones. Stretch after your muscles warm up. Doing so reduces the risk of microtrauma to the muscles.

- A physical therapist or trainer can show you how to exercise safely and maintain good posture to avoid injuries.

- **Wilson Tennis Balls.** Insert three Wilson Tennis Balls into a sock, tie a knot in the open end of the sock, and have a partner roll it over your sore muscles. The tennis balls massage the affected area.

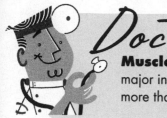

Doctor's Orders

Muscle in! Intense muscle pain that starts suddenly signals a major injury. If you feel severe pain or have moderate pain that lasts more than a few days, call your doctor.

Muscle Spasms

- **Canada Dry Tonic Water.** To prevent muscle cramps at night, try drinking a glass of Canada Dry Tonic Water before going to bed. Studies have shown that quinine, the essential ingredient in tonic water, can reduce the incidence of nocturnal leg cramps by up to 50 percent. (Never take quinine tablets to treat leg cramps. The Food and Drug Administration warns that the drug could cause severe side effects, including death.)

- **Dr. Teal's Epsom Salt.** Turn your bathtub into a rejuvenating mineral spring by adding two cups Dr. Teal's Epsom Salt to lukewarm bathwater and soaking for fifteen luxurious minutes. The magnesium in the Epsom Salt passes into the body through osmosis and relaxes the muscles.

- **French's Mustard.** To cease a leg cramp, eat one teaspoon French's Mustard. No one knows exactly why this remedy works, but some suspect the combination of turmeric and vinegar in the mustard.

- **Gatorade.** To relieve muscle cramps, drink two cups of Gatorade. Muscle cramps are often caused by dehydration, and the sports drink quickly replaces lost sodium and electrolytes.

- **Heinz Apple Cider Vinegar** and **SueBee Honey.** To relieve a nighttime leg cramp, mix two tablespoons Heinz Apple Cider Vinegar and one teaspoon SueBee Honey in a glass of water, and drink the tonic. No one knows why this folk remedy works, but perhaps the walk to the kitchen and the mental distraction are the actual cure. (Do not feed honey to infants less than one year of age. Honey often carries a benign strain of *C. botulinum*, and an infant's immune system requires twelve months to develop to fight off disease and infection.)

- **Jif Peanut Butter.** Magnesium relaxes muscles. While eating a wide range of legumes, nuts, whole grains, and vegetables will help you meet your daily dietary need for magnesium, you can quickly replace magnesium in your body by eating Jif Peanut Butter (straight from the jar or in a sandwich). Four tablespoons of peanut butter contain 100 milligrams of magnesium (or 25 percent of the daily value).

- **McCormick Rosemary Leaves.** Place one ounce McCormick Rosemary Leaves in a glass jar, add two cups of boiling water, seal the lid on the jar, and let steep for thirty minutes. Use a washcloth to apply the tea to the affected muscle two or three times daily, and, after doing so, drink three ounces of the tea (unless you're pregnant). Rosemary contains anti-inflammatory properties, and, when applied topically, the rosmarinic acid eases pain. A 2009 study published in *Pharmacology, Biochemistry and Behavior* demonstrated that rosmarinic acid is an anti-inflammatory that decreases sensitivity to painful stimuli.

- **Planters Dry Roasted Almonds, Planters Dry Roasted Cashews,** or **Planters Dry Roasted Peanuts.** Eating foods high in magnesium—like Planters Dry Roasted Almonds, Planters Dry Roasted Cashews, or Planters Dry Roasted Peanuts—relaxes muscles. In fact, a magnesium deficiency can cause leg cramps. One ounce of almonds provides 80 milligrams of magnesium, one ounce of cashews provides 75 milligrams, and one ounce of dry roasted peanuts provides 50 milligrams.

- **Tums.** To relieve a muscle cramp, eat one regular Tums tablet in the morning and a second tablet at night. Your body can absorb only 500 to 600 milligrams of calcium at a time. A regular strength Tums tablet contains 500 milligrams of calcium carbonate. The calcium in Tums helps loosen and relax your tense muscles. (If you've had calcium oxalate kidney stones, consult your doctor before taking Tums.)

- **Uncle Ben's Converted Brand Rice.** To tame the cramp and increase blood flow to the muscle, fill a clean sock with Uncle Ben's Converted Brand Rice, tie a knot in the end, and heat in the microwave oven for ninety seconds. Making sure the sock isn't too hot, apply the heat pack to the affected area. The rice-filled sock conforms to the shape of your body

℞ STRANGE MEDICINE ℞

A STRETCH OF THE IMAGINATION

- When one of your muscles abruptly hardens, tightens, and becomes inexplicably painful, you're experiencing a muscle cramp, caused by muscle spasms—an involuntary contraction of one or more muscles.

- Muscle spasms generally affect muscles in the foot, calf, front and back of the thigh, hands, arms, abdomen, and along the rib cage.

- A muscle spasm in the calf or thigh muscles is generally called a charley horse.

- Exercise-related muscle cramps are generally caused by overworking the muscle (from poor stretching or excessive exercising) or an electrolyte deficiency (from excessive perspiration).

- To ease a muscle cramp caused by overworking, massage, stretch, ice, or warm the affected muscle.

- Muscle cramps usually go away within a few minutes.

and stays warm for roughly thirty minutes, allowing the soothing warmth to increase circulation to the area. The convenient homemade heating pad is also reusable.

- **V8.** To prevent leg cramps, drink an eight-ounce glass of V8 Low Sodium Original Vegetable Juice every evening. A potassium deficiency frequently triggers leg cramps at night, but an eight-ounce serving of V8 Low Sodium vegetable juice contains 900 milligrams of potassium.

Doctor's Orders

Don't stretch the truth! If you get frequent or severe leg cramps, see a doctor to rule out circulation problems, blood clots, or a nerve injury.

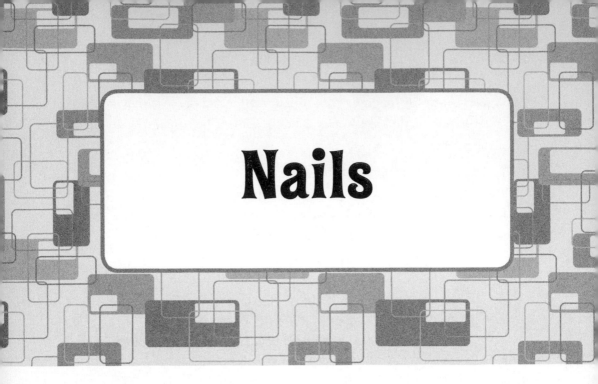

Nails

Biting

- **Heinz White Vinegar** and **Q-Tips Cotton Swabs.** Prevent fingernail biting by using a Q-Tips Cotton Swab to paint your fingernails with a quick dab of Heinz White Vinegar. Let dry. Should you absentmindedly put your fingernails in your mouth, the tart taste will quickly get your attention, reminding you to stop biting your nails.

- **Tabasco Pepper Sauce** and **Q-Tips Cotton Swabs.** To stop yourself from biting your fingernails, use a Q-Tips Cotton Swab to dab your fingernails with Tabasco Pepper Sauce. Let dry. If your fingernails unconsciously wander up to your lips, the spicy tang will quickly jolt your attention, compelling you to correct your behavior.

Breaks

- **Krazy Glue.** To fix a broken fingernail, apply a small drop of Krazy Glue, hold the nail in place for a few seconds, let dry, and then coat with the nail polish of your choice.

Brittleness

- **Chicken of the Sea Salmon, Chicken of the Sea Sardines,** or **Chicken of the Sea Tuna.** To rejuvenate brittle nails from within, eat salmon, sardines, or tuna three times a week. All these fish add the fatty acids commonly known as omega-3 oils to your diet, strengthening the immune system and giving you healthier nails.

- **Johnson's Baby Oil.** Rejuvenate brittle fingernails by warming a few tablespoons of Johnson's Baby Oil in a microwave oven, letting it cool to the touch, and then soaking your nails in warm oil for ten minutes.

- **Lubriderm.** To keep cuticles and nails looking healthy, slather Lubriderm on your fingertips several times a day. The moisturizer replenishes brittle nails and cracked cuticles.

- **Miracle Whip.** To fortify brittle fingernails, coat them with Miracle Whip, wait five minutes, and then wash clean.

- **Noxzema.** Soften fingernails by warming Noxzema and using the cold cream as a hot oil treatment.

- **ReaLemon, Heinz White Vinegar,** and **Oral-B Toothbrush.** Revitalize brittle fingernails, soften stiff cuticles, and whiten yellowed fingernails—by soaking your fingers for ten minutes in a mixture of equal parts ReaLemon lemon juice and Heinz White Vinegar. Use a clean, used Oral-B Toothbrush (or a regular nailbrush) to brush the mixture over your fingernails. Rinse clean. The citric acid bleaches fingernails naturally.

- **Silk Soymilk.** To strengthen brittle nails, all you need to do is add 5 grams of soy protein a day to your diet. Drinking one 8-ounce glass of Silk Soymilk daily adds 6 grams of soy protein to your diet, guaranteeing strong, healthy nails.

- **Star Olive Oil.** Apply warmed Star Olive Oil to your hands before bedtime, massage into the skin thoroughly, and wear a pair of cotton gloves or socks to bed. In the morning, massage your hands, wipe away excess oil with a tissue, rinse them, and pat dry with a towel.

- **Tums.** To strengthen your nails, eat one regular Tums tablet in the morning and a second tablet at night. Your body can absorb only 500 to 600 milligrams of calcium at a time. A regular strength Tums tablet contains 500 milligrams of calcium carbonate. A calcium deficiency is one cause of brittle nails, and taking 1000-milligrams of calcium daily can reverse that. (If you've had calcium oxalate kidney stones, consult your doctor before taking Tums.)

- **Vaseline Petroleum Jelly.** Before going to bed at night, rub a dab of Vaseline Petroleum Jelly into the nails and cuticles, put on a pair of cotton gloves or socks, and go to sleep. The petroleum jelly holds in moisture, reviving your nails.

Cuticles

- **Alberto VO5 Conditioning Hairdressing.** To soften dry cuticles, rub a dab of Alberto VO5 Conditioning Hairdressing into the cuticle of each finger. The five vital organic ingredients in the renowned hairdressing moisturize the cuticle.

- **Bag Balm.** To moisturize cuticles and soften brittle nails, massage Bag Balm around your fingernails before going to bed, put on a pair of white cotton gloves or socks, and go to sleep. By morning your cuticles will be soft and healthy.

- **Colgate Regular Flavor Toothpaste.** Use a dab of Colgate Regular Flavor Toothpaste on a toothbrush to gently scrub away excess cuticle and smooth rough edges.

- **Crisco All-Vegetable Shortening.** Moisturize cuticles by applying a thin coat of Crisco All-Vegetable Shortening.

- **Palmolive Dishwashing Liquid.** To soften your cuticles, fill a bowl with warm water containing one tablespoon Palmolive Dishwashing Liquid, mix well, and immerse your hands in the liquid for two minutes. Rinse clean with warm water and pat dry.

ALL FINGERS AND THUMBS

● Before trimming or shaping your nails, decide on a shape for them. Petite hands and fingers look best with almond-shaped nails; short and stocky fingers look best with squoval-shaped nails (squared-off oval); heavy-set hands (and fingers with wide nail beds) look best with squared-off ends. You can also match the shape of the cut end to the shape of the cuticle.

● To shape your nail with an emery board, use long, gentle strokes in a single direction (not a see-sawing stroke, which causes the keratin fibers to separate). Start at the outer corner of each nail, holding the emery board at a 45- to 90-degree angle against the edge of the nail, and move toward the center, repeating until you achieve the desired shape. Then repeat on the opposite edge of the nail.

● Shaping your fingernails so that the nail extends only slightly beyond the fingertip reduces the chances of breaking the nail.

● After shaping your nails, soak them in a bowl of warm water for two minutes, and then pat dry with a towel. Unless you're going to color your nails, apply a rich moisturizer to your hands, massaging well.

● To prevent nail biting, simply trim your fingernails and keep them short to remove the temptation.

● Nail fungus typically causes the nail to yellow, thicken, and develop crumbling edges. The fungus starts at the end of the nail and progresses to the root.

● Usually caused by a parasitic fungus called a dermatophyte, nail fungus can also be caused by yeasts or molds.

● You can contract a toenail fungus by walking barefoot in public gyms, shower stalls, or swimming pools.

● Nail fungus can spread from one nail to another. To avoid spreading the fungus, wash your hands after touching an infected nail.

Discoloration

- **Efferdent.** To whiten yellowed fingernails, dissolve two Efferdent tablets in a bowl of water, and then soak your fingernails in the denture cleansing solution for five minutes. Rinse clean.

- **Heinz White Vinegar.** If your nails develop a greenish tinge, soak them in a bowl of Heinz White Vinegar for five minutes several times a day. The acetic acid in the vinegar kills the bacterial infection causing the discoloration.

- **Hydrogen Peroxide.** Whiten yellowed fingernails by rubbing a cotton ball dampened with Hydrogen Peroxide over your fingernails.

- **Morton Salt and ReaLime.** Whiten yellowing fingernails by mixing one teaspoon Morton Salt and two teaspoons ReaLime lime juice in a bowl of warm water. Soak your fingernails for ten minutes.

- **ReaLemon.** Soak your fingernails in ReaLemon lemon juice to remove common stains.

Fungus

- **Heinz White Vinegar.** To help get rid of toenail fungus, mix two cups Heinz White Vinegar and four cups of warm water in a basin, and soak your feet in the mixture for twenty minutes every day until the fungus vanishes. Rinse thoroughly and pat dry.

- **Hydrogen Peroxide.** To kill toenail fungus, use a cotton ball to apply Hydrogen Peroxide to your toenails every day after showering until the fungus vanishes.

- **Listerine.** Soak your feet in original formula Listerine antiseptic mouthwash for twenty minutes a day for two weeks. The thymol and eucalyptol kill the fungus.

- **Vicks VapoRub.** To eliminate toenail fungus, slather Vicks VapoRub on your toes at night before going to bed and put on a pair of socks. The thymol, eucalyptol, and camphor in Vicks VapoRub are all antifungal compounds. Repeat nightly for two weeks.

Hangnails

- **Crisco All-Vegetable Shortening, Saran Wrap,** and **Scotch Tape.** To treat a hangnail, apply Crisco All-Vegetable Shortening on the affected area before going to bed, wrap the fingertip with a piece of Saran Wrap, and secure in place with Scotch Tape. The plastic wrap confines the moisture overnight, softening the cuticle by morning so the hangnail can be easily removed with a pair of nail scissors.

Manicure

- **Forster Toothpicks.** In a pinch, you can use a Forster Toothpick as a manicure tool to clean dirt from under fingernails.

- **Visa.** The corner of a Visa credit card works as a manicure tool to clean under your fingernails.

Doctor's Orders

Nail the problem! If your nails remain brittle after applying moisturizer for two weeks, consult a dermatologist.

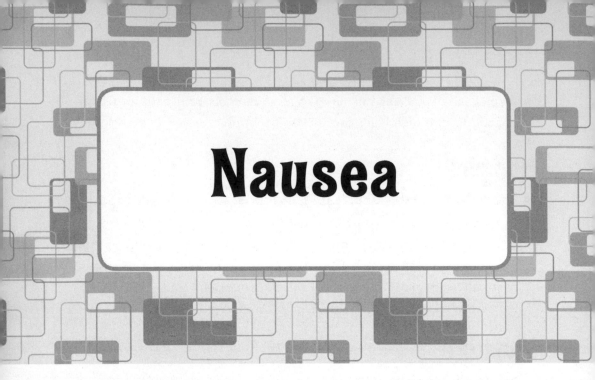

Nausea

- **Aunt Jemima Original Syrup.** To calm nausea, take one or two table-spoons Aunt Jemima Original Syrup. The corn syrup pacifies the gastro-intestinal tract.

- **Canada Dry Ginger Ale.** Drinking flat Canada Dry Ginger Ale relieves an upset stomach, taming nausea. The ginger seems to relax the muscles in the stomach. Contrary to popular belief, Canada Dry Ginger Ale does indeed contain genuine ginger, included in the list of ingredients as "nat-ural flavors." (Do not drink ginger ale if you have gallstones. Ginger can increase bile production.)

- **Coca-Cola.** To settle your queasy stomach, open a can of Coca-Cola, let it sit on the countertop at room temperature until it goes flat, and drink the defizzed Real Thing. Pharmacies sell cola syrup that can be taken in small doses to relieve nausea. The concentrated sugars are believed to relax the gastrointestinal tract. Letting the bubbles out of the soda prevents the car-bonation from further upsetting your stomach.

- **Dannon Yogurt, SueBee Honey,** and **McCormick Ground Carda-mom.** To quell an upset stomach, mix one-half cup Dannon Plain Nonfat

Yogurt, one-half teaspoon SueBee Honey, and one-quarter teaspoon McCormick Ground Cardamom. This traditional Indian recipe soothes nausea effectively. (Do not feed honey to infants less than one year of age. Honey often carries a benign strain of *C. botulinum,* and an infant's immune system requires twelve months to develop to fight off disease and infection.)

- **Domino Sugar.** To make your own elixir to subdue nausea, dissolve one-half cup Domino Sugar and one-quarter cup of water in a saucepan, and stir the ingredients over a medium heat to brew a clear syrup. Let cool to room temperature, take one to two tablespoons as needed, and store in an airtight container. The sugar calms the gastrointestinal tract.

- **Gatorade.** To relieve queasiness, drink Gatorade to quickly replace essential nutrients and electrolytes, preventing muscle spasms in your stomach.

- **Karo Corn Syrup.** Two tablespoons of Karo Corn Syrup tame nausea. The fructose calms the intestinal tract.

- **Life Savers Pep-O-Mints.** To counteract nausea, suck on a few Life Savers Pep-O-Mints. Peppermint calms the stomach muscles, and the menthol relaxes the lower esophageal sphincter (the valve at the bottom of the esophagus), allowing trapped gas to escape from the stomach.

- **Lipton Chamomile Tea.** To calm an upset stomach, drink a cup of Lipton Chamomile Tea, steeped for ten minutes. Chamomile seems to relax the muscles of the stomach and intestinal wall. (Coumarin, an anticoagulant in chamomile, may increase the likelihood of bleeding when taken in combination with the blood thinner Coumadin or other anticoagulant medications.)

- **Lipton Ginger Tea.** To relieve nausea, drink a cup of Lipton Ginger Tea (or as many cups as necessary until the nausea subsides). Ginger neutralizes nausea. (Do not drink ginger tea if you have gallstones. Ginger can increase bile production.)

- **Lipton Peppermint Tea.** To soothe nausea, drink a cup of Lipton Peppermint Tea. Peppermint relieves nausea by calming the stomach lining.

- **McCormick Anise Seed.** To settle your stomach, place a tea infuser filled with one tablespoon McCormick Anise Seed in a teacup, add boiling water, cover with a saucer, and steep for ten minutes. Let cool and sip. (Avoid anise during pregnancy.)

℞ STRANGE MEDICINE ℞

SICK TO YOUR STOMACH

- Nausea is a feeling of queasiness in the stomach, usually accompanied by an urge to vomit.

- Common problems that cause nausea include food allergies, food poisoning, gastro-esophageal reflux, medications or medical treatments (such as chemotherapy or radiation treatment), migraine headaches, morning sickness, motion sickness, and stomach viruses.

- To calm nausea, lie down and remain still. Doing so stabilizes the middle ear, which controls your equilibrium.

- To relieve feelings of nausea, identify the first crease on the inside of your wrist from the palm of your hand, measure two of your own thumb-widths up your arm from the center of that crease, and press that point with your thumb firmly, until it hurts slightly, for five to ten minutes. Repeat with your other wrist. Pressing this point on the wrist (known as the Pericardium 6 point in acupuncture) can relieve nausea.

- When trying to recover from nausea, steer clear of milk and other dairy products. The proteins and fats in milk prompt the human body to generate mucus, which exacerbates nausea.

- If stress is making you feel nauseous, saturate a washcloth in cold water and cover your face with it. Doing so may jolt the parasympathetic nervous system to slow your heart rate and kick the digestive system into gear.

- If you feel the urge to vomit, allow nature to take its course. Vomiting tends to end or diminish nausea.

- **McCormick Basil Leaves.** For yet another herbal tea to remedy nausea, place a tea infuser filled with one teaspoon McCormick Basil Leaves in a teacup, add boiling water, cover with a saucer, and steep for fifteen minutes. Sip the resulting tea. The camphor oil in basil soothes stomach upset.

- **McCormick Fennel Seed.** To ease nausea, place a tea infuser filled with one tablespoon McCormick Fennel Seed in a teacup, add boiling water, cover with a saucer, and steep for ten minutes. Fennel contains anethole, a compound that doubles as an antiseptic and antispasmodic.

- **McCormick Ground Cinnamon** and **McCormick Ground Ginger.** To combat nausea caused by food poisoning, mix one teaspoon McCormick Ground Cinnamon and one-half teaspoon McCormick Ground Ginger in a teacup, add boiling water, cover with a saucer, and steep for fifteen minutes. Strain and then sip the tea. The cinnamon can help kill the responsible bacteria, and the ginger tames nausea. (Do not use ginger if you have gallstones. Ginger can increase bile production.)

- **Mott's Applesauce.** Once you start to recover and regain your appetite, start with bland foods like Mott's Applesauce, which is easy to digest and filled with nutrients. The pectin in the applesauce is a soluble fiber that absorbs fluid in your intestine. Applesauce also contains malic acid and quercetin, which help inhibit harmful bacteria in your stomach.

- **Nabisco Ginger Snaps.** To allay nausea, eat a few Nabisco Ginger Snaps. The ginger in the cookies is one of the oldest remedies for nausea. (Do not use ginger if you have gallstones. Ginger can increase bile production.)

- **Nabisco Original Premium Saltine Crackers.** When you feel up to eating something, eat a few Nabisco Original Premium Saltine Crackers. High in carbohydrates, the saltine crackers help settle your stomach and give you strength.

- **Pernod Anise.** To quell indigestion, sip a small glass of Pernod Anise. This after-dinner liqueur is made from anise, which settles the stomach. (Avoid anise during pregnancy.)

- **7-Up.** Drinking flat 7-Up relieves an upset stomach.

- **Wonder Bread.** When you regain your appetite, eat a few slices of toasted Wonder Bread. The carbohydrates in bread help you regain energy.

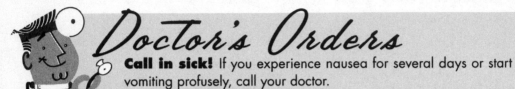

Doctor's Orders

Call in sick! If you experience nausea for several days or start vomiting profusely, call your doctor.

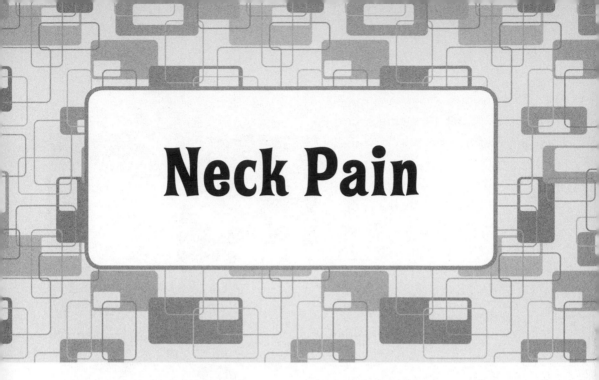

Neck Pain

- **Birds Eye Frozen Peas** and **Bounty Paper Towels.** To soothe neck pain, cover a bag of Birds Eye Frozen Peas with a sheet of Bounty Paper Towels, and apply to the affected area for fifteen minutes every hour. The frozen peas act like small ice cubes, reducing the inflammation causing the pain, and the bag of peas conforms to the shape of your neck. The paper towel creates a layer of insulation to prevent frostbite. Refreeze the bag of peas for future ice-pack use. Be sure to label the bag for ice-pack use only. If you want to eat the peas, cook them after they thaw the first time, never after refreezing.

- **Bubble Wrap, Oral-B Dental Floss,** and **Scotch Packaging Tape.** To make a lumbar support roll for your office chair to give you good back and head support, use a pair of scissors to cut a sheet of Bubble Wrap ten inches wide by fourteen feet long. Cut a piece of Oral-B Dental Floss forty inches long, center it along one of the ten-inch widths of Bubble Wrap, and starting at that end, roll up the sheet of Bubble Wrap into a tight cylinder. The resulting roll of Bubble Wrap will measure five inches in diameter and contain a length of dental floss threaded through the center. Secure the roll together with a few pieces of Scotch Packaging Tape. Position the roll horizontally to create lumbar support for your office chair and tie the ends of the dental floss together around the back of the chair to hold the roll in place. When you sit in the chair, the roll of Bubble Wrap should rest in the curve of your back, keeping your posture erect and your neck pain-free.

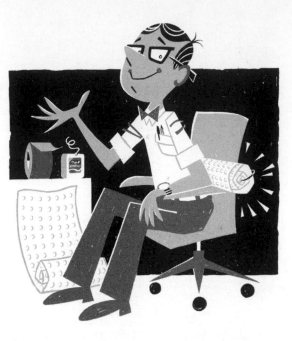

- **Conair Hair Dryer.** To relieve neck pain quickly, set a Conair Hair Dryer on warm and aim the nozzle at the back of your neck. The warm air helps relax the muscles and soothe the pain.

- **McCormick Ground Ginger.** Add one teaspoon McCormick Ground Ginger to salads or use it in recipes. Ginger, containing the active ingredient gingerol, is scientifically proven to reduce inflammation, mimicking nonsteroidal anti-inflammatory drugs such as aspirin, ibuprofen, and naproxen—but without the side effects. (Do not use ginger if you have gallstones. Ginger can increase bile production.)

- **McCormick Ground Turmeric.** Take one tablespoon McCormick Ground Turmeric daily by simply sprinkling it on your food or using the spice in recipes—until the neck pain subsides. Turmeric contains curcumin, an anti-inflammatory that reduces pain and inflammation, just like nonsteroidal anti-inflammatory drugs. (Turmeric may increase the likelihood of bleeding when taken in combination with the blood thinner Coumadin or other anticoagulant medications.)

℞ STRANGE MEDICINE ℞

A REAL PAIN IN THE NECK

● Neck pain generally results from poor posture, overuse, or wear and tear from age.

● To relieve neck pain, lie down intermittently throughout the day to give your neck a rest from holding up your ten- to twelve-pound head. Avoid too much inactivity, which can cause a stiff neck.

● Alleviate some of the pain by shrugging your shoulders up and down. Gently tilt your head toward one shoulder (keeping your shoulders down) and hold the position for thirty seconds. Then repeat toward the other shoulder. Turn your head to the right and hold it for thirty seconds. Then repeat to the left. Pull your shoulder blades together and then relax.

● If you get rear-ended in an automobile accident and feel severe pain in your neck, you most likely have whiplash, which should be treated immediately by a doctor. During a rear-end collision the head is jerked forward and then backward, stretching the soft tissues of the neck beyond their limits. Left untreated, whiplash can cause severe neck problems.

● To help prevent neck pain, maintain good posture to keep your head centered above your spine.

● If you work at a desk or drive long distances, take frequent breaks to stretch your neck muscles.

● To avoid straining your neck, never tuck your phone between your ear and shoulder when you talk. If you can't change that habit, get a headset or use speakerphone.

● Sleeping on your stomach puts stress on your neck. To sleep comfortably on your back, purchase a neck-support pillow that allows for the natural curve of your neck.

● **Noxzema.** Rub a dab of Noxzema into your neck to alleviate the pain. The camphor, menthol, and eucalyptus oil in Noxzema reduce inflammation and massaging the neck soothes the irritation.

- **Tabasco Pepper Sauce** and **Crisco All-Vegetable Shortening.** To relieve neck pain, mix one-quarter teaspoon Tabasco Pepper Sauce with two tablespoons Crisco All-Vegetable Shortening, and apply this spicy homemade capsaicin cream to the affected area up to five times a day. A 1996 study at Brooke Army Medical Center in San Antonio, Texas, demonstrated that topically applied capsaicin cream decreased neck pain. (Do not apply this salve on open sores and avoid contact with eyes and nose.)

- **Uncle Ben's Converted Brand Rice.** After relieving the inflammation for the first day or two with the Birds Eye Frozen Peas tip on page 339, fill a clean sock with Uncle Ben's Converted Brand Rice, tie a knot in the end, and heat in the microwave oven for ninety seconds. Making sure the sock isn't too hot, apply the heat pack to the affected area. The rice-filled sock conforms to the shape of your neck and stays warm for roughly thirty minutes, allowing the soothing warmth to increase circulation to the area. The homemade heating pad is also reusable.

- **Vicks VapoRub.** To alleviate neck pain, rub Vicks VapoRub into your neck muscles. The camphor and menthol in the balm reduce pain and inflammation.

Doctor's Orders

Save your neck! If you experience severe and persistent neck pain, see a doctor immediately.

Nicotine Dependency

- **Alka-Seltzer.** To get short-term relief from nicotine withdrawal, dissolve two Alka-Seltzer tablets in a glass of water and drink the solution at every meal—as long as you're not on a low-sodium diet or have peptic ulcers.

- **Dr. Teal's Epsom Salt.** To distract yourself from the urge to smoke, fill the bathtub with warm water, add two cups Dr. Teal's Epsom Salt, and soak for twenty minutes with your head partially submerged so you can still breathe. Soaking in an Epsom Salt bath relaxes you and allows the magnesium in the Epsom Salt to pass into the body through osmosis and relieve tension.

- **McCormick Cream of Tartar** and **Minute Maid Orange Juice.** To quit smoking cigarettes and minimize your cravings for nicotine, mix one-half teaspoon McCormick Cream of Tartar in a medium glass of Minute Maid Orange Juice, and drink the solution every night before bedtime for thirty days. The cream of tartar (potassium hydrogen tartrate) helps ease nicotine cravings by replacing the potassium that smoking robs from the cardio-vascular system. The orange juice replenishes the vitamin C that smoking

℞ STRANGE MEDICINE ℞

SMOKE SIGNALS

● Quitting smoking makes you feel healthier right away, increases your energy and focus, revives your senses of smell and taste, improves your breathing, gives you fresher breath, and allows stained teeth to get whiter.

● Quitting smoking reduces your risk for cancer, heart attacks, strokes, emphysema, early death, cataracts, and wrinkles.

● Nicotine is considered as addictive as heroin.

● Nicotine constricts blood vessels, impeding circulation, which forces your heart to work harder, increasing your risk of heart disease.

● Nicotine increases the release of dopamine, a neurotransmitter in the brain that makes you feel good. The brain develops a tolerance for nicotine, requiring more to achieve the same feeling, until the smoker is lighting a cigarette every thirty minutes.

● The most intense symptoms of nicotine withdrawal occur during the first week after you quit smoking.

● To distract yourself from nicotine cravings and reduce withdrawal symptoms, exercise for twenty to thirty minutes every day by going for a walk, bicycling, swimming, or working out.

● During nicotine withdrawal, cravings for a cigarette typically last less than five minutes. When you feel cravings, simply distract yourself for those five minutes by washing the dishes, eating a healthy snack, or going for a walk—until the symptoms pass.

● When you quit, throw out all your cigarettes, cigars, and lighters, and refuse to buy any more. If you don't possess any cigarettes, you can't smoke them.

● Avoid people, places, and situations that tempt you to smoke. Rearrange your activities to spend more time in places where smoking is banned.

cigarettes depletes from your body. Each cigarette you smoke depletes roughly 25 milligrams of vitamin C.

- **Tabasco Pepper Sauce.** To reduce cravings for nicotine, sprinkle Tabasco Pepper Sauce on your food at mealtime. Capsaicin, the substance in peppers that makes them spicy, desensitizes the taste receptors on your tongue and makes cigarette smoke taste repugnant.

Doctor's Orders

Don't go up in smoke! If you've made several attempts to stop smoking without success, ask your doctor to help you develop a treatment plan to conquer nicotine dependence.

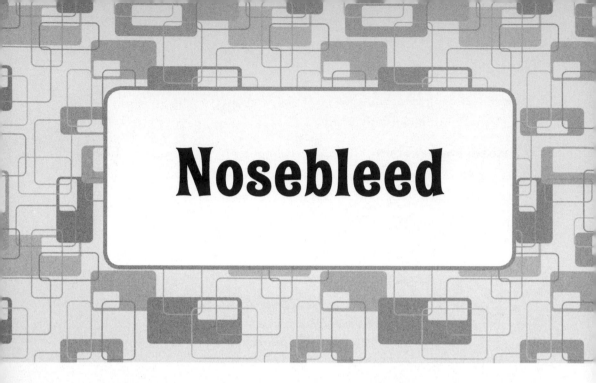

Nosebleed

- **Afrin.** A quick blast of Afrin nasal spray up your nostril stops a nosebleed. The oxymetazoline in the decongestant doubles as a vasoconstrictor, narrowing the blood vessels in the nose.

- **Arm & Hammer Baking Soda** and **Morton Salt.** To keep your nasal passages moist, dissolve one-quarter teaspoon Arm & Hammer Baking Soda and one-quarter teaspoon Morton Salt in one cup of boiled water. Let cool to room temperature, and use a bulb syringe or neti pot to flush your nostrils with the saline solution.

- **Birds Eye Frozen Peas** and **Bounty Paper Towels.** While gently squeezing the fleshy part of your nose just below the bridge, cover a bag of Birds Eye Frozen Peas with a sheet of Bounty Paper Towels, and place the bag against the bridge of your nose or the back of your neck. The bag of peas conforms to the shape of your face or neck, and the frozen peas act like small ice cubes, constricting the blood vessels to curb the bleeding. The paper towel creates a layer of insulation to prevent frostbite. Refreeze the bag of peas for future ice-pack use. Be sure to label the bag for ice-pack use only. If you want to eat the peas, cook them after they thaw the first time, never after refreezing.

℞ STRANGE MEDICINE ℞

AS PLAIN AS THE NOSE ON YOUR FACE

● Nosebleeds result from a punch to the nose, an object hitting the nose, irritated mucous membranes (from a cold, flu, or dry heat), high blood pressure, allergies, nose picking, and the side effects of various medications.

● To stop a nosebleed, hold your head up straight and gently squeeze the fleshy part of your nose just below the bridge for five minutes while breathing through your mouth.

● When trying to stop a nosebleed, do not tilt your head back. Doing so can cause you to swallow or inhale blood.

● To prevent the nose from bleeding again, keep your head above the level of your heart, refrain from blowing your nose, and do not insert anything into it.

● A ruptured blood vessel in your nose requires seven to ten days to heal.

● To prevent nosebleeds, drink eight 8-ounce glasses of water a day. Keeping your body well hydrated keeps your mucous membranes moist.

● If you live or work in a dry environment, run a humidifier that fills the air with a cool mist of distilled water to keep your mucous membranes moist and healthy.

● **Dickinson's Witch Hazel** and **Q-Tips Cotton Swabs.** To stop a nosebleed, saturate a Q-Tips Cotton Swab with Dickinson's Witch Hazel, and use it to coat the inside of the affected nostril. The astringent witch hazel constricts the blood vessels inside the nose.

● **Forster Clothespins.** If you don't have the patience or strength to pinch your nose to stop the bleeding, use a Forster Clothespin to gently squeeze the fleshy part of your nose just below the bridge for ten minutes.

● **Fruit of the Earth Aloe Vera Gel** and **Q-Tips Cotton Swabs.** To speed the healing of a clotted nosebleed, squeeze some Fruit of the Earth Aloe

347

Vera Gel on a Q-Tips Cotton Swab, and coat the inside of the affected nostril. The aloe vera gel soothes, heals, and moisturizes.

- **Heinz Apple Cider Vinegar.** To stop a nosebleed, mix two tablespoons Heinz Apple Cider Vinegar into an eight-ounce glass of water, and drink the tart solution.

- **McCormick Ground (Cayenne) Red Pepper.** To stop a nosebleed, put a pinch of McCormick Ground (Cayenne) Red Pepper on your palm and snort it into the affected nostril. Wash your hands afterward to avoid accidentally getting the pepper in your eyes. Cayenne pepper fosters blood clotting and soothes pain like an analgesic.

- **Star Olive Oil.** Keep your mucous membranes moist on dry days by lubricating the inside of your nostrils with a dab of Star Olive Oil.

- **Tampax Tampons.** To stop the bleeding, carefully insert a Tampax Tampon in the nostril, tilt your head slightly forward, and gently squeeze the fleshy part of your nose just below the bridge for ten minutes. The cotton tampon absorbs excess blood and helps stop the bleeding.

- **Vaseline Petroleum Jelly.** To prevent a nosebleed from recurring, lubricate the inside of your nostrils with a dab of Vaseline Petroleum Jelly. The lubricant helps stop the mucous membranes from drying and cracking, allowing the scab to heal.

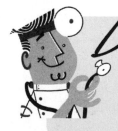

Doctor's Orders

Don't get your nose out of joint! If your nose continues bleeding after applying pressure for ten to fifteen minutes, seek immediate medical attention. If you experience frequent nosebleeds, consult your doctor to rule out a serious ailment.

Oily Hair

- **Budweiser.** Pour a can of Budweiser beer into a trigger-spray bottle, and keep it in your shower to use as a setting lotion after you shampoo and rinse. The beer gives hair plenty of body, and the alcohol dries the scalp.

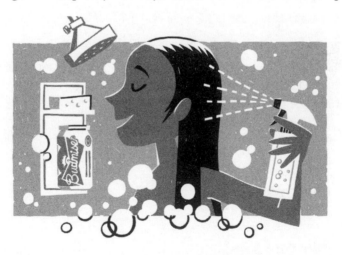

- **Heinz White Vinegar.** To cleanse excess oil from your hair, mix equal parts Heinz White Vinegar and water, and after shampooing, rinse with the acidic solution. Yes, your hair will smell like vinegar, but only until it dries.

℞ STRANGE MEDICINE ℞

OIL CAN HARRY

● Blonds tend to have more oil in their hair than brunettes, who have more oil in their hair than redheads. That's because blonds have more hair per square inch than brunettes, who have more hair per square inch than redheads. Each individual hair has its own oil gland.

● Hormones called androgens control the amount of oil secreted by the sebaceous glands, meaning people with oily hair also have oily skin. Stress increases the androgen level in the bloodstream, spurring the sebaceous glands to produce more oil.

● Shampooing your hair daily eliminates excess oil from hair.

● To shampoo your hair thoroughly, rinse your hair with water, lather in the shampoo, let sit for five minutes, and then rinse clean. Repeat if necessary.

● If you have oily hair, skip the conditioner, which adds more oil to your hair. If you have long hair and wish to prevent split ends, condition only the ends of your hair.

● Inexpensive shampoos tend to clean the hair and scalp more effectively than more costly shampoos.

● To avoid unnecessarily stripping your hair of all its sebum, massage shampoo into the first three inches of the hair closest to your scalp. When you rinse the shampoo from your hair, the runoff will lightly cleanse the remaining hair.

● Eating a low-fat diet can minimize oily hair. A high-fat diet of fried foods and saturated fat can cause the sebaceous glands in your scalp to produce excess oil, making your hair greasy and limp.

● **Kingsford's Corn Starch.** To remove excess oil from your hair with a dry shampoo, sprinkle a small amount of Kingsford's Corn Starch on your hair, work it into the scalp and through your hair, and then brush clean. The cornstarch absorbs the oil.

- **Listerine** and **Dickinson's Witch Hazel.** To reduce your scalp's production of oil, mix equal parts original formula Listerine antiseptic mouthwash and Dickinson's Witch Hazel, and after shampooing your hair and rinsing thoroughly, saturate a cotton ball with the solution and dab it directly on your scalp. The combination of the two astringents tightens the pores in your scalp, and the witch hazel dissolves oil.

- **McCormick Rosemary Leaves.** To slow the production of oil on the scalp, add two tablespoons McCormick Rosemary Leaves to one cup of boiling water, cover with a saucer, and steep for twenty minutes. Strain and let cool to room temperature. After shampooing and rinsing your hair, use the rosemary tea as a final rinse, massaging it into the scalp. Do not rinse out the rosemary solution. Rosemary impedes your sabaceous glands from producing excess sebum, the oil giving you that greasy look.

- **ReaLemon.** For oily hair, mix equal parts ReaLemon lemon juice and water, and after using your regular shampoo, rinse your hair with the lemon solution. Let sit for five minutes, and then rinse clean. The acidic lemon juice breaks down the oil.

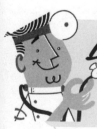

Doctor's Orders

No more greasy kid stuff! If none of these household remedies clear up your oily hair and you remain concerned, consult a doctor or dermatologist.

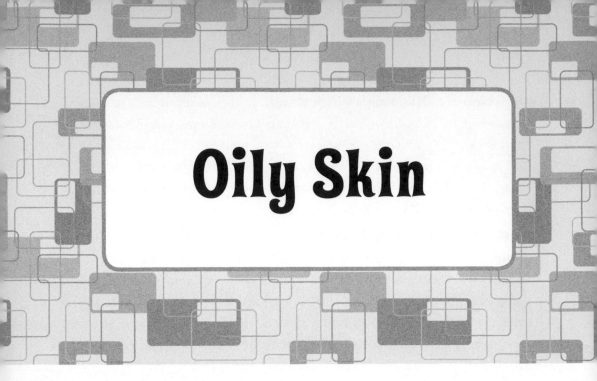

Oily Skin

- **Country Time Lemonade.** To cleanse and exfoliate oily skin, mix one tablespoon Country Time Lemonade powdered drink mix with enough water to make a thick paste. Massage the lemony paste over your face (avoiding your eyes), wait five minutes, then rinse clean. The gritty paste and citric acid help exfoliate dead skin, leaving your face smooth and soft. (Using citric acid on your skin makes you more prone to sunburn, so be sure to use sunscreen afterwards.)

- **Dickinson's Witch Hazel.** Using a cotton ball, apply Dickinson's Witch Hazel to oily skin on your face and neck. The tannins in witch hazel tighten the pores.

- **Huggies Baby Wipes.** To cleanse oil from your skin, wipe your face with a pre-moistened Huggies Natural Care Baby Wipe. These convenient, hypoallergenic, fragrance-free, alcohol-free wipes also contain soothing aloe and vitamin E.

- **Hydrogen Peroxide.** For oily skin, mix Hydrogen Peroxide with a little water and dab on the skin with a cotton ball.

- **Nestlé Carnation Nonfat Dry Milk.** To cleanse oily skin, mix one-quarter cup Carnation Nonfat Dry Milk powder with enough water to make a thick paste. Apply the milky paste to your face, let sit for ten minutes, and then wash off. The lactic acid in the milk helps exfoliate the dead skin cells, leaving your face smooth and soft.

- **Pepto-Bismol.** Use a cotton ball or a thin gravy brush to cover your face with Pepto-Bismol (avoiding your eyes), let dry, then rinse with warm water, followed by cool water. Pepto-Bismol absorbs oil from the skin and tightens the pores, leaving your skin looking smoother and feeling softer.

- **Purell Instant Hand Sanitizer.** Rub a dollop of Purell Instant Hand Sanitizer into your face, avoiding your eyes. The alcohol cuts through the oil, and the additional emollients moisturize your skin.

- **Quaker Oats** and **Dickinson's Witch Hazel.** To absorb excess oil from your face and exfoliate dead skin clogging pores, grind two tablespoons uncooked Quaker Oats in a blender, add enough Dickinson's Witch Hazel to make a thick paste, and apply to your face, massaging with your fingertips. Let sit for five minutes, and then rinse thoroughly with warm water, which opens the pores, followed by cool water, which closes the pores.

- **ReaLemon.** To cleanse oily skin and shrink the pores, add one teaspoon ReaLemon lemon juice to one cup of cold water, saturate a cotton ball with the solution, and apply to your face. Let dry, and do not rinse. Lemon juice, a natural astringent, removes any residue and refreshes your face.

- **Saco Buttermilk.** After washing your face, massage Saco Buttermilk, the only brand of buttermilk containing natural emulsifiers, into the skin. Let sit for a few minutes, and rinse clean. Do this two or three times a week. The lactic acid in buttermilk exfoliates the dead skin, cleanses the skin, and tightens pores.

- **Smirnoff Vodka.** For oily skin, clean and tighten your pores by applying Smirnoff Vodka to your face with a cotton ball.

℞ STRANGE MEDICINE ℞

BURNING THE MIDNIGHT OIL

● Oily skin is caused by the sebaceous glands, which, due to hereditary reasons, stress, or fluctuating hormone levels, produce excess sebum oil.

● Oily skin stays naturally moisturized, preventing wrinkles.

● Washing your skin helps remove dead cells and stimulates the development of new ones, making your skin look fresh and smooth. If you're under thirty, your skin cells renew themselves quickly. Unfortunately, the older you get, the longer the skin cells take to regenerate—and the resulting buildup of oil and dirt can make skin appear dull and flaky.

● A simple bar of soap with a pH value between 11 and 14 can be used to cleanse skin. If you have oily skin, use a non-greasy, milky skin cleanser that does not leave a sticky film on the skin.

● Washing your face with hot water dissolves more oil than washing with cool or lukewarm water.

● Drinking six to eight 8-ounce glasses of water a day replaces fluid in your body, flushes toxins from your system, and enhances your skin—for free.

● Splashing your face with water when you wake up first thing in the morning eliminates excess oils and revitalizes moisturizer applied the night before—negating the need to cleanse your face.

● If you enjoy wearing makeup, use water-based cosmetics rather than oil-based ones.

Doctor's Orders

Don't let it get under your skin! If your oily skin is causing acne or seems problematic, consult a dermatologist.

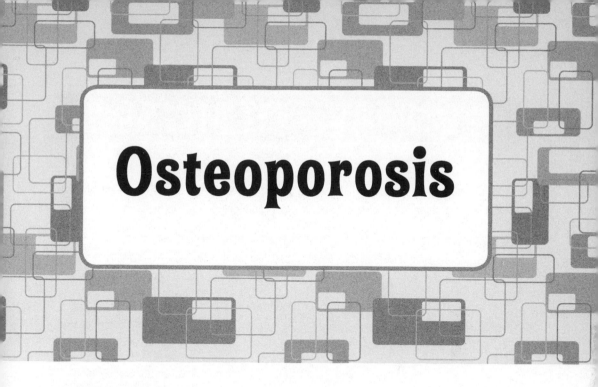

Osteoporosis

- **Dannon Yogurt.** To get calcium in your diet, eat one cup of Dannon Plain Nonfat Yogurt daily. One serving of Dannon Yogurt contains between 200 and 250 milligrams of calcium.

- **Jif Peanut Butter.** Magnesium increases calcium absorption and helps build bones, which protects against osteoporosis. While eating a wide range of legumes, nuts, whole grains, and vegetables will help you meet your daily dietary need for magnesium, you can quickly replace magnesium in your body by eating Jif Peanut Butter (straight from the jar or in a sandwich). Four tablespoons of peanut butter contain 100 milligrams of magnesium (or 25 percent of the daily value).

- **Total.** To get sufficient calcium in your diet, start each day by eating a bowl of whole grain Total, the breakfast cereal fortified with more calcium than any other cereal, according to the USDA. One cup of whole grain Total contains 1,472 milligrams of calcium.

- **Tums.** If you're not getting enough calcium in your diet, eat one regular Tums tablet after breakfast in the morning and a second tablet after dinner in the evening. Your body can absorb only 500 to 600 milligrams of

℞ STRANGE MEDICINE ℞

MAKE NO BONES ABOUT IT

● Osteoporosis is a disease that causes bones to become weak and brittle to the point where a simple fall can cause a fracture, most commonly in the hip, wrist, or spine.

● Bone is composed of active tissue, which is constantly regenerated as old cells are absorbed and replaced with new cells. When the absorption of old cells exceeds the creation of new cells, the bone becomes porous. The word osteoporosis means "porous bones."

● Osteoporosis develops silently over decades—painlessly and without any symptoms. You cannot feel your bones becoming weaker, and most people do not discover they have osteoporosis until they break a bone.

● Women are more prone to develop osteoporosis than men because the production of estrogen, a hormone that protects bones, drops sharply around the time of menopause.

● Osteoporosis can be treated with medication, dietary supplements, and weight-bearing exercise to help strengthen bones.

● Your bones and teeth store nearly all of your body's calcium. Calcium is added and withdrawn from your bones, based on your body's need for calcium. According to the National Institutes of Health, the recommended dietary allowance of calcium is 1,000 milligrams daily for men and women between ages nineteen and fifty; 1,000 milligrams daily for men between ages fifty-one and seventy; 1,200 milligrams daily for women between ages fifty-one and seventy; and 1,200 milligrams daily for men and women ages seventy-one and older.

● To help reduce your risk of developing osteoporosis, quit smoking. A Japanese study published in *Clinical Calcium* in 2005 found that smoking significantly decreased bone mineral density.

● Consuming more than two or three ounces of alcohol a day (especially during adolescence and the young adult years) increases your risk of osteoporosis.

● To slow the rate of bone loss and help increase bone density, go for a thirty-minute walk fives times a week. This simple weight-bearing exercise stimulates cells to generate new bone tissue.

calcium at a time. A regular strength Tums tablet contains 500 milligrams of calcium carbonate. (If you've had calcium oxalate kidney stones, consult your doctor before taking Tums.)

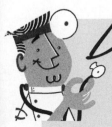

Doctor's Orders

Bone up! To determine whether you're at risk for osteoporosis, or if you notice that you are getting shorter or your upper back is curving forward, have a bone-density test. Women should be screened at the first signs of menopause. Men should be tested at age fifty.

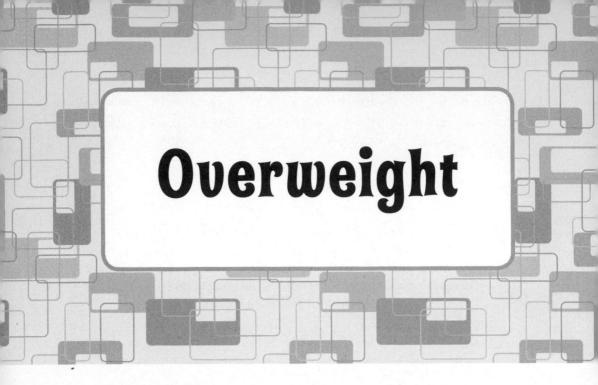

Overweight

- **Kellogg's All-Bran.** To reduce your weight, eat one-half cup Kellogg's All-Bran cereal for breakfast every day, sweetened with blueberries, strawberries, or sliced banana. A 1992 study at Vanderbilt University concluded that eating breakfast every morning helps reduce dietary fat and minimize impulsive snacking. One-half cup of Kellogg's All-Bran also contains 10 grams of fiber, which fills you up and helps remove excess cholesterol from the body.

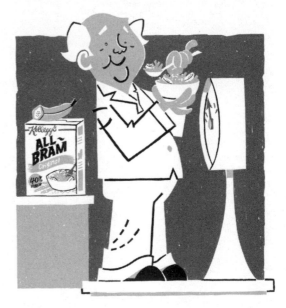

- **Metamucil.** To help reduce the number of calories absorbed by your body, take one serving of Metamucil (as instructed on the package label) in or with eight ounces of water three times

℞ STRANGE MEDICINE ℞

BATTLE OF THE BULGE

● To lose weight, you simply need to burn more calories than you consume. You can accomplish this by cutting extra calories from food and beverages, and burning more calories through physical activity.

● The best way to lose weight is to adopt a balanced daily diet of approximately 10 calories for every pound you weigh (50 percent from carbohydrates, 25 percent from protein, and 25 percent from fats and oils), and go for a twenty-minute walk at least three days a week (building up to thirty minutes daily).

● Eating three substantial meals a day and a small wholesome afternoon snack prevents you from binging to recover from a feeling of starvation. If you skip breakfast and have a small lunch, you'll inevitably consume a huge dinner because you're famished.

● Consider eating five or six smaller meals throughout the day rather than three large meals. By eating several smaller meals, you'll feel satisfied throughout the day, and your blood sugar stays level.

● Plan to lose no more than one-half to one pound per week to keep your expectations reasonable and prevent your body from rebelling against your weight-loss program.

● Set a reasonable goal of losing 10 percent of your body weight over a period of six months. When you reach that goal, maintain that weight for a few months to reassure yourself that doing so is possible before proceeding further.

● Learn to enjoy the foods you love in moderation.

● Weigh yourself on a scale daily to catch any weight gains before they accumulate and spiral out of control.

● To minimize cravings for food, drink at least eight 8-ounce glasses of water every day. Drinking water not only keeps your body hydrated and functioning properly, but the water fills your stomach, reducing hunger pangs.

a day before meals. Metamucil contains psyllium seed husk, a natural dietary fiber originating from the psyllium plant, which affects fat intake, absorbs liquid (bulking up your stool), and reduces feelings of hunger. (Metamucil generally produces a laxative effect in twelve to seventy-two hours.)

- **Nestlé Carnation Nonfat Dry Milk.** Rather than adding calorie-rich milk, cream, skim milk, or half-and-half to your coffee, add a pinch of Nestlé Carnation Nonfat Dry Milk.

- **Planters Dry Roasted Almonds.** To help lose weight, eat one handful (roughly one ounce) of Planters Dry Roasted Almonds every day. In a 2003 study at the City of Hope National Medical Center, participants who ate seventy almonds a day for six months, in conjunction with a reduced-calorie diet, dropped 18 percent of their body weight.

- **Quaker Oats.** To help you lose weight, start each day with a bowl of Quaker Oats oatmeal. With only 150 calories in a one-cup serving, oatmeal makes you feel full longer, minimizing the urge to snack. Studies show that oatmeal lowers both blood pressure and cholesterol levels, apparently due to the soluble fiber beta-glucan.

- **Tabasco Pepper Sauce.** Rather than seasoning your food with calorie-rich butter and sauces, sprinkle your meals with Tabasco Pepper Sauce. The capsaicin in the hot sauce suppresses your appetite and prompts your body to briefly burn more calories.

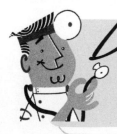

Doctor's Orders

Throw your weight around! If you have serious health problems due to your weight, consult your doctor to discuss the benefits and risks of weight-loss surgery or medications.

Panic Attacks

- **Chicken of the Sea Salmon, Chicken of the Sea Sardines,** or **Chicken of the Sea Tuna.** Eat salmon, sardines, or tuna three or four times a week to add omega-3 fatty acids to your diet. Omega-3 oils strengthen the immune system and increase resistance to stress. A 2011 study at the Ohio State University College of Medicine showed that omega-3 reduced stress levels by roughly 20 percent (compared to a placebo). Anxiety causes the body to produce inflammatory hormones, called cytokines, but omega-3 reduced production of cytokines by 14 percent.

- **Crayola Crayons.** To calm your fears and soothe a panic attack, simply open a box of Crayola Crayons and take a few whiffs. The scent of Crayola Crayons is among the twenty most recognizable fragrances to American adults, and the nostalgic aroma instantly catapults you back to happy childhood memories, inducing a reassuring sense of peace and security.

- **Kellogg's All-Bran.** To reduce the anxiety that produces panic attacks, eat a bowl of Kellogg's All-Bran cereal. A lack of vitamin B_{12} can cause anxiety, and a bowl of most breakfast cereals supplies 25 percent of the recommended daily value of vitamin B_{12}. One-half cup of Kellogg's All-Bran cereal contains 100 percent of the daily value of vitamin B_{12}.

☥ STRANGE MEDICINE ☥

HITTING THE PANIC BUTTON

● A panic attack is a sudden episode of overwhelming fear that occurs for no apparent reason and makes you feel a sense of impending doom, short of breath, dizzy, nauseous, or like you're having a heart attack.

● Research shows that panic attacks typically peak within ten minutes and last an average of thirty minutes.

● Taking prescription tranquilizers to relieve anxiety on a daily basis may lead to physical dependence within four weeks. Then, attempting to stop taking the tranquilizers produces withdrawal symptoms, which include anxiety, triggering the exact same nervous disorder you were trying to alleviate.

● Rather than relying on medication to control anxiety, use relaxation techniques and deep breathing.

● If your anxiety exceeds the level of concern required by a situation, you may have an anxiety disorder requiring professional care. Seek a therapist who specializes in anxiety disorders and uses cognitive-behavioral therapy, the most effective way to treat chronic anxiety and panic attacks.

● Use positive affirmations. If you feel anxious, you're likely repeating negative thoughts in your head. Instead, replace those thoughts with positive ones, such as, "I'll be done with this shortly, and I'll be very happy with myself," "Everything will work out fine, it always does," or "I just have to get this done, it doesn't have to be perfect."

● Use simple breathing techniques to calm yourself down. You may be bringing on a panic attack by unconsciously hyperventilating. When you get upset, you start taking short, quick breaths, which in turn make you faint, dizzy, numb, and nervous. You get the sense that you can't get enough air, because you're actually not getting enough air. To overcome this, simply breathe deeply, using your diaphragm.

● If you have experienced several panic attacks and you spend a great deal of time in constant fear of another attack, you may have a chronic condition called panic disorder.

- **Lipton Chamomile Tea.** To reduce the symptoms of a panic attack, pour one cup of boiling water over two Lipton Chamomile Tea bags in a teacup, cover with a saucer, let steep for ten minutes, and then drink the tea. Drink three cups a day to endure stressful times. Chamomile subdues tension, and a 2009 study at the University of Pennsylvania showed that taking chamomile reduces the symptoms of generalized anxiety disorder by 50 percent. (Coumarin, an anticoagulant in chamomile, may increase the likelihood of bleeding when taken in combination with the blood thinner Coumadin or other anticoagulant medications.)

- **McCormick Pure Vanilla Extract** and **Kleenex Tissues.** To help stop a panic attack, put a few drops of McCormick Pure Vanilla Extract on a Kleenex Tissue and sniff it. The aroma of vanilla triggers your pituitary gland and hypothalamus to produce endorphins, the neurotransmitters that produce a feeling of well-being. Studies show that the scent of vanilla significantly reduces anxiety.

- **McCormick Rosemary Leaves** and **L'eggs Sheer Energy Panty Hose.** To calm a panic attack, place one teaspoon McCormick Rosemary Leaves in the foot cut from a pair of clean, used L'eggs Sheer Energy Panty Hose, tie a knot in the open end, and sniff the sachet throughout the day. The aroma of rosemary has a calming effect.

- **SueBee Honey.** Instead of sweetening your foods and beverages with sugar, switch to SueBee Honey. Anecdotal evidence strongly suggests that honey may have antioxidant properties that reduce anxiety levels.

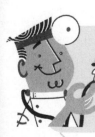

Doctor's Orders

Don't panic! If you have any panic attack symptoms (especially if panic attack symptoms mimic a heart attack), seek medical help as soon as possible. Left untreated, panic attacks may get worse.

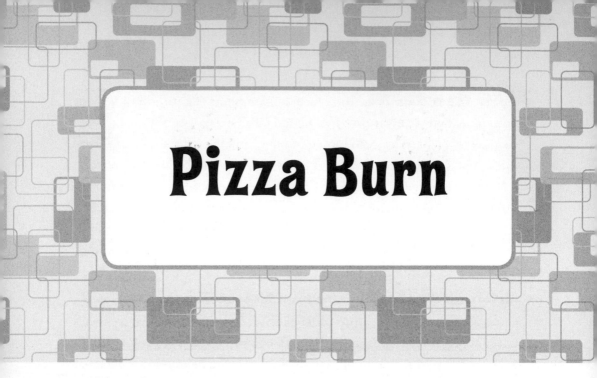

Pizza Burn

- **Cool Whip.** To quickly extinguish the searing pain of pizza burn on the roof of your mouth, place one tablespoon of Cool Whip on your tongue and press it against the affected area. The palm and coconut oils in the dessert topping soothe the burn.

- **Dannon Yogurt.** To alleviate the burning sensation on the roof of your mouth, take one tablespoon Dannon Plain Nonfat Yogurt and swish it around in your mouth.

- **Morton Salt.** Dissolve one-half teaspoon Morton Salt in an eight-ounce glass of warm water, and rinse with the salt water every hour to relieve the pain and speed healing.

- **Mott's Applesauce.** To relieve the burning sensation and speed healing, place one tablespoon Mott's Applesauce on your tongue and press it against the lesion. The applesauce soothes the irritation, and the pectin seems to promote healing.

- **Orajel.** To numb the pain, squeeze a dollop of Orajel on your tongue and press it against the roof of your mouth. The benzocaine in the ointment anesthetizes the spot, instantly blocking the pain.

- **Pepto-Bismol.** Swishing Pepto-Bismol around in your mouth coats the roof of it and soothes the burn.

- **Phillips' Milk of Magnesia.** Rinse your mouth with one tablespoon Phillips' Milk of Magnesia. The cool minty alkaline suspension of magnesium hydroxide, formulated by British pharmacist Charles Henry Phillips in 1880, is a soothing agent that appears to speed healing.

STRANGE MEDICINE
GOING THROUGH THE ROOF

- When the hot, melted mozzarella cheese on a pizza burns the delicate tissue lining the roof of your mouth, the resulting lesion blisters, requiring a week or more to heal on its own.

- Pizza burn is the generic term for a lesion on the roof of your mouth caused by any hot food or beverage.

- Other culprits that commonly singe the roofs of mouths include soups, sauces, coffee, hot chocolate, tea, and any melted cheese dish.

- To soothe the pain and reduce the inflammation of pizza burn, suck on an ice cube or drink an ice-cold glass of water.

- To help a pizza burn heal, avoid spicy or salty foods, which aggravate the lesion, and refrain from eating any food with sharp edges, such as potato chips, which can poke and tear the sore spot.

- To prevent pizza burn, let pizza cool to the touch before putting it in your mouth (obviously), and let microwaved food sit in the oven for two minutes after the timer sounds to cool down before eating it.

- **Popsicle.** To soothe pizza burn, press your favorite flavor Popsicle against the roof of your mouth. The Popsicle doubles as an ice pack, relieving the pain.

- **Reddi-Wip.** Spray some Reddi-Wip whipped cream into your mouth, and use your tongue to press it against the roof of your mouth. The coolness and creaminess soothe the burn.

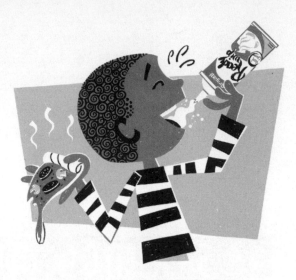

Doctor's Orders

Raise the roof! If the burning sensation on the roof of your mouth doesn't heal itself within a week to ten days, or if the lesion makes eating and drinking difficult, see your dentist to rule out a more serious problem.

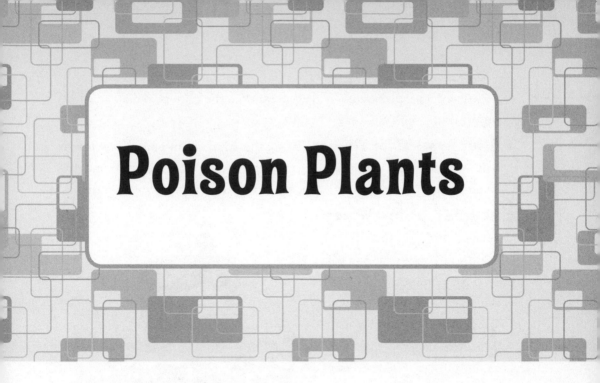

Poison Plants

- **Colgate Regular Flavor Toothpaste.** To soothe a poison ivy, poison oak, or poison sumac rash, apply Colgate Regular Flavor Toothpaste as an ointment to the affected area. The glycerin in the toothpaste provides a soothing cooling sensation and fast, temporary relief.

- **Dawn Dishwashing Liquid.** If your skin comes into contact with the urushiol clinging to you shoes, you can break out in a rash. Carefully remove your shoes and scrub them with Dawn Dishwashing Liquid and warm water. Dawn cuts through oily films, including urushiol.

- **Desitin.** To relieve the pain and itching of a rash caused by any poison plant, rub Desitin, the diaper rash remedy, on the affected area. The zinc oxide soothes the blisters and calms the itching.

- **Dr. Teal's Epsom Salt.** To relieve the inflammation caused by poison ivy, poison oak, or poison sumac, dissolve two tablespoons Dr. Teal's Epsom Salt in one cup of water, saturate a washcloth with the solution, and place the damp cloth over the affected area.

- **Fruit of the Earth Aloe Vera Gel.** Apply Fruit of the Earth Aloe Vera Gel to the rash caused by any poison plant. The anti-inflammatory and antibacterial properties of aloe vera gel soothe the blisters, reduce swelling, minimize the itch, and speed healing.

- **Heinz Apple Cider Vinegar.** To soothe a rash from poison ivy, poison oak, or poison sumac, mix equal parts Heinz Apple Cider Vinegar and cold water in a trigger-spray bottle, and mist the rash with the tangy solution.

- **Huggies Baby Wipes.** Immediately upon rubbing against poison ivy, poison oak, or poison sumac, wipe down the affected area with Huggies Baby Wipes. The alcohol in the wipe removes the toxic urushiol from the skin, preventing the itchy rash.

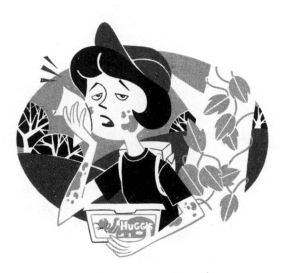

- **Ivory Soap.** After removing urushiol from the skin and within an hour of exposure, take a shower and use Ivory Soap to wash and rewash any urushiol from the skin, further minimizing your risk of breaking out with a painful rash.

- **Kiwi Shoe Whitener.** To soothe a rash from poison ivy, poison oak, or poison sumac, apply Kiwi liquid white shoe polish to the affected area. The pipe clay and zinc oxide in the shoe polish soothe the skin.

- **Morton Salt.** To relieve the itchy, blistery rash, wet the affected area with water and then cover it with a coat of Morton Salt. The highly absorbent salt helps dry out the blisters.

- **Nestea.** To relieve inflammation from poison ivy, poison oak, or poison sumac, pour one cup Nestea powder in the bathtub, fill with warm water, and soak in the tea for fifteen minutes. The tannin soothes the skin, calms the itching, and helps dry the blisters.

- **Nestlé Carnation Nonfat Dry Milk.** Mix one-half cup Nestlé Carnation Nonfat Dry Milk powder with enough water to make a thick paste, and spread it on the rash. The milky solution halts the itch.

- **Pepto-Bismol.** Using a gravy brush, paint Pepto-Bismol on a rash caused by any poison plant. The alkalinity relieves the itching and the pink solution helps dry the blisters.

℞ STRANGE MEDICINE ℞

ITCHING FOR TROUBLE

- Once you come into contact with poison ivy, poison oak, or poison sumac, you have fifteen minutes to wash off the urushiol—the sticky oil that adheres to your skin—before your body launches an allergic reaction.

- To avoid contact with poison plants, adhere to the adage: "Leaves of three, let it be."

- Urushiol adheres to clothes and shoes, and any skin that comes into contact with it can break out in a rash. Carefully remove your contaminated clothes and launder them in the washing machine with hot water and your regular detergent.

- The blistery rash from poison ivy, poison oak, or poison sumac, appearing anywhere from two hours to two weeks after contact with urushiol, generally lasts three weeks, but can linger for up to eight weeks.

- A poison ivy, poison oak, or poison sumac rash is not contagious nor can the fluid from a blister spread the rash.

- Inhaling smoke from burning poison ivy, poison oak, or poison sumac can irritate or injure your eyes or nasal passages. The smoke contains the urushiol oil.

- Although dogs and cats are immune to urushiol, their coats can get covered with the oil, which can then come into contact with you or others.

- To avoid getting poison ivy, poison oak, or poison sumac, learn how to recognize these poison plants before venturing into the wild, and, if necessary, wear long pants and a long-sleeved shirt.

- **Phillips' Milk of Magnesia.** For another surefire way to soothe the itching from poison ivy, poison oak, or poison sumac, use a cotton ball to dab the welts with Phillips' Milk of Magnesia. This alkaline solution stops the itching and cools the skin.

- **Purell Instant Hand Sanitizer.** The moment you come into contact with poison ivy, poison oak, or poison sumac, apply Purell Instant Hand Sanitizer to the affected area and then rinse clean. The alcohol dissolves the urushiol and cleanses it from the skin, averting or lessening the outbreak of painful blisters.

- **Quaker Oats.** To relieve the itching, grind one cup uncooked Quaker Oats in a blender, add to warm bathwater, and soak for fifteen minutes. Oats soothe itchy skin.

- **Quaker Oats.** To soothe the blisters from poison plants, cook up a bowl of Quaker Oats oatmeal according to the directions on the side of the canister, let cool, spread it on the affected area, cover with a clean, damp washcloth, and let sit for up to thirty minutes. Wash clean. Repeat whenever necessary. As an astringent, oatmeal soothes the itching and contains beneficial proteins.

- **Smirnoff Vodka.** To remove the resin from poison ivy, poison oak, or poison sumac from your skin immediately to prevent or minimize a reaction, pour Smirnoff Vodka over the affected area. The alcohol disperses the urushiol and removes it from the skin.

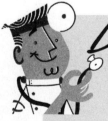

Doctor's Orders

Scratch that! If the rash covers a large area of your body and feels excruciating, or if the rash affects your eyes, mouth, or private parts, consult a doctor. Also seek medical attention if the blisters ooze (to prevent infection) or the rash lasts longer than three weeks.

Premenstrual Syndrome

- **Chicken of the Sea Salmon, Chicken of the Sea Sardines,** or **Chicken of the Sea Tuna.** To relieve the symptoms of premenstrual syndrome, eat salmon, sardines, or tuna three times a week to add the fatty acids commonly known as omega-3 oils to your diet. Eating these fish rich in omega-3 fatty acids helps ease the mood swings and cramping that accompany premenstrual syndrome. One serving of Chicken of the Sea Chunk Light Tuna provides nearly 60 percent of the daily requirement for vitamin B_6, which can help alleviate the unpleasant symptoms of premenstrual syndrome.

- **Dr. Teal's Epsom Salt.** To combat the mood swings that accompany premenstrual syndrome, fill the bathtub with warm water and add two cups Dr. Teal's Epsom Salt. Soak for twenty minutes, during which time the magnesium in the Epsom Salt passes into the body through osmosis and eases muscular aches, helping you relax.

- **Jif Peanut Butter.** Magnesium boosts your mood, prevents cramps, and curbs weight gain, bloating, and breast tenderness before and during your menstrual period. While eating a wide range of legumes, nuts, whole

℞ STRANGE MEDICINE ℞

SWINGING INTO HIGH GEAR

● Premenstrual syndrome causes mood swings, breast tenderness, fatigue, food cravings, irritability, and depression—starting a week or two before your menstrual period and ending at its onset.

● An estimated 75 percent of menstruating women experience one or more symptoms of premenstrual syndrome.

● Premenstrual syndrome typically affects women in their twenties and thirties.

● No one knows what causes premenstrual syndrome, but suspected culprits are hormone swings, fluctuations in serotonin levels, depression, stress, and poor eating habits.

● The symptoms of premenstrual syndrome fluctuate in intensity from month to month.

● To reduce the symptoms of premenstrual syndrome, exercise for thirty minutes every day by walking, bicycling, swimming, or working out. Exercise alleviates stress and boosts endorphin levels, lifting your mood.

● Altering your diet and eating habits can alleviate premenstrual syndrome symptoms. Minimizing the amount of salt and salty foods you eat decreases bloating and water retention. Eating five or six small meals throughout the day (rather than three large meals a day) also helps reduce bloating.

● Avoid caffeine and alcohol. Caffeine stimulates the production of stress hormones, making you more irritable, and alcohol can cause breast tenderness and lower your blood sugar level, exacerbating premenstrual syndrome symptoms.

● Drinking eight 8-ounce glasses of water a day flushes excess salt from your body, which reduces bloating and water retention.

● To balance your mood and bring irritability under control, avoid eating candy, cookies, and other snacks loaded with sugar. These foods send your blood sugar on a rollercoaster ride, increasing fatigue and irritability.

● Yoga, massage, meditation, and deep-breathing exercises help reduce the headaches, stress, and irritability that accompany premenstrual syndrome.

grains, and vegetables will help you meet your daily dietary need for magnesium, you can quickly replace magnesium in your body by eating Jif Peanut Butter (straight from the jar or in a sandwich). Four table-spoons of peanut butter contain 100 milligrams of magnesium (or 25 percent of the daily value).

- **Kellogg's All-Bran.** To stabilize your estrogen level and keep your mood even keeled, eat one cup Kellogg's All-Bran every day. One cup of Kellogg's All-Bran contains 20 grams of fiber. Eating 20 to 35 grams of fiber daily helps remove surplus estrogen from your body.

- **McCormick Rosemary Leaves.** To reduce the symptoms of premenstrual syndrome, frequently add McCormick Rosemary Leaves to foods, like chicken, lamb, and beans during the week before your period. Or make rosemary tea by placing a tea infuser filled with one teaspoon McCormick Rosemary Leaves in a teacup, adding boiling water, covering with a saucer, and steeping for fifteen minutes. Drink two cups a day. Compounds in rose-mary induce menstruation and are believed to help stabilize hormone levels. (Do not take rosemary if you're pregnant.)

- **Planters Dry Roasted Almonds.** To quell the mood swings that accom-pany premenstrual syndrome, eat one-quarter cup Planters Dry Roasted Almonds daily. The almonds contain roughly 200 milligrams of magne-sium, which boosts your mood, prevents cramps, and curbs weight gain, bloating, and breast tenderness associated with premenstrual syndrome.

- **Quaker Oats.** To reduce premenstrual syndrome symptoms, eat a bowl of Quaker Oats oatmeal every morning. Oats contain the mild sedative gramine, the fiber absorbs excess estrogen, and the complex carbohydrates seem to increase serotonin levels in the brain, relieving stress.

- **Tums.** To reduce headaches, mood swings, and muscle cramps, eat one regular Tums tablet after each meal. Your body can absorb only 500 to 600 milligrams of calcium at a time. A regular strength Tums tablet contains 500 milligrams of calcium carbonate. A 1998 study published in the *American Journal of Obstetrics & Gynecology* showed that taking 1,200 milligrams of calcium daily lowers the likelihood of suffering from premenstrual syndrome by approximately 48 percent. (If you've had calcium oxalate kidney stones, consult your doctor before taking Tums.)

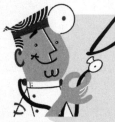

Doctor's Orders

Get into the swing of things! If you're unable to control premenstrual syndrome by changing your lifestyle, and if you find the symptoms debilitating, see your doctor.

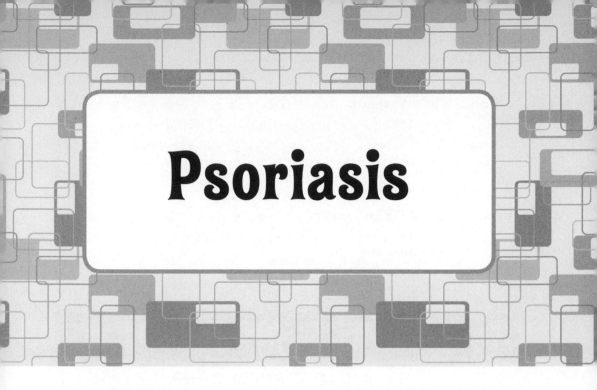

Psoriasis

- **Bag Balm.** To moisturize the dry, scaly patches of psoriasis on your skin, spread Bag Balm, the salve developed by Vermont farmers for use on cows' udders, on the affected areas. Bag Balm soothes dry, cracked skin.

- **Chicken of the Sea Salmon, Chicken of the Sea Sardines,** or **Chicken of the Sea Tuna.** To quell the inflammation caused by psoriasis, eat salmon, sardines, or tuna three times a week to add the fatty acids commonly known as omega-3 oils to your diet. These fish, rich in eicosapentaenoic acid (EPA) and docosahexaenoic acid (DHA), help reduce inflammation and pain, strengthen the immune system, and increase resistance to stress.

- **Dr. Teal's Epsom Salt.** Turn your bathtub into a rejuvenating mineral spring by adding two cups Dr. Teal's Epsom Salt to lukewarm bathwater and soaking for twenty luxurious minutes. The magnesium helps heal psoriasis, reduce itching, and remove scaly skin.

- **Fruit of the Earth Aloe Vera Gel.** To soothe psoriasis, apply Fruit of the Earth Aloe Vera Gel to the affected area. The anti-inflammatory and antibacterial properties of aloe vera gel speed healing, and the magnesium lactate in the aloe relieves the itching.

- **Heinz White Vinegar.** To relieve the itching of psoriasis, add one cup Heinz White Vinegar to a bathtub filled with cool water, and soak for fifteen minutes. No one knows why this remedy soothes psoriasis, but the acetic acid in vinegar does kill any bacteria that may be irritating the condition, and the cool water moisturizes the skin.

- **McCormick Ground Turmeric.** To reduce the inflammation caused by psoriasis, take one tablespoon McCormick Ground Turmeric daily by simply sprinkling it on your food or using the spice in recipes. Curcumin, an

℞ STRANGE MEDICINE ℞

IT'S ONLY SKIN DEEP

- Psoriasis is a common autoimmune skin disease that causes skin cells to renew themselves at a rapid pace, forming itchy, dry, red patches covered with white scales.

- Typically, psoriasis patches develop on the elbows, knees, and scalp.

- Psoriasis is a persistent, chronic disease that flares up (usually in the winter) and then goes into remission (for months or even years).

- Psoriasis is incurable.

- Applying an over-the-counter hydrocortisone cream to the affected area can reduce psoriasis symptoms.

- Sitting in sunlight for fifteen to thirty minutes every day for up to six weeks can significantly reduce the lesions caused by psoriasis. Be sure to wear sunscreen with a sun protection factor (SPF) of at least 15 on unaffected areas of the skin to avoid sunburn.

- Stress can trigger an outbreak of psoriasis. Yoga, massage, meditation, relaxation techniques, and deep-breathing exercises can help you reduce anxiety.

- In winter, run a humidifier in your bedroom or office to add moisture to dry indoor air to prevent an outbreak of psoriasis.

antioxidant in turmeric, speeds up healing and protects the skin by neutralizing free radicals. (Turmeric may increase the likelihood of bleeding when taken in combination with the blood thinner Coumadin or other anticoagulant medications.)

- **Miracle Whip.** To remedy dry, scaly patches of psoriasis on your skin, rub Miracle Whip into the affected area and let sit for fifteen minutes. The oil and vinegar in the Miracle Whip seem to moisturize and rejuvenate the dry skin and relieve the itch. To exfoliate dead skin, rub a dab of Miracle Whip into the affected area, let sit for a few minutes, and then massage with your fingertips. You can also give yourself a rejuvenating facial by applying Miracle Whip as a face mask. Leave it on for twenty minutes, and then wash off with warm water, followed by cold water. Miracle Whip cleanses the skin and tightens the pores.

- **Quaker Oats.** To relieve the itching of psoriasis, grind one cup uncooked Quaker Oats in a blender, add the fine powder to warm bathwater, and soak for fifteen minutes. Oats soothe itchy skin and bathing helps remove scales.

- **Saran Wrap** and **Playtex Living Gloves.** To boost the efficacy of prescription topical steroids to treat psoriasis on your feet and hands, after applying the ointment, wrap your feet in Saran Wrap and wear Playtex Living Gloves on your hands.

- **Star Olive Oil.** Soak for ten minutes in a warm bath, and then add one teaspoon Star Olive Oil to the water and soak for another five minutes. The warm water softens scaly patches of skin and soothes the itching, and the oil seals the moisture in your skin.

- **Star Olive Oil** and **Saran Wrap.** To loosen the scaly skin from your scalp, warm one-half cup Star Olive Oil, wet your hair (to prevent it from absorbing any oil), and use a gravy brush to apply the oil to your scalp. Wrap your head in Saran Wrap (above your eyes, nose, and mouth), and let sit for thirty minutes. Then shampoo and rinse thoroughly. Repeat daily until the psoriasis clears up.

- **Vaseline Petroleum Jelly.** To soften psoriasis patches and expedite healing, rub a few dabs of Vaseline Petroleum Jelly into the affected area. In 1859, Brooklyn chemist Robert Augustus Chesebrough learned from petroleum drilling workers in Titusville, Pennsylvania, that the jelly residue that gunked up oil drilling rods quickened healing when rubbed on a wound or burn.

Doctor's Orders

Don't jump out of your skin! If psoriasis causes you pain, spreads over a wide area, or covers your palms or soles, see a doctor for treatment.

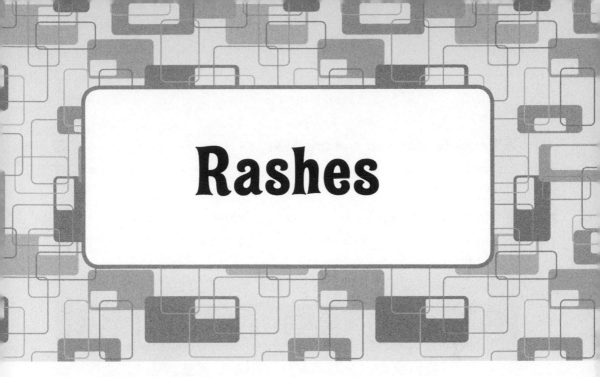

Rashes

- **Birds Eye Frozen Peas** and **Bounty Paper Towels.** To soothe the itching of a rash, cover a bag of Birds Eye Frozen Peas with a sheet of Bounty Paper Towels, and apply to the affected area for fifteen minutes every hour. The frozen peas act like small ice cubes, reducing the inflammation and irritation, and the bag of peas conforms to the shape of your body. The paper towel creates a layer of insulation to prevent frostbite. Refreeze the bag of peas for future ice-pack use. Be sure to label the bag for ice-pack use only. If you want to eat the peas, cook them after they thaw the first time, never after refreezing.

- **Chicken of the Sea Salmon, Chicken of the Sea Sardines,** or **Chicken of the Sea Tuna.** To soothe a burning rash, eat salmon, sardines, or tuna three times a week to add the fatty acids commonly known as omega-3 oils to your diet. These fish, rich in eicosapentaenoic acid (EPA) and docosahexaenoic acid (DHA), help strengthen the immune system and reduce inflammation and pain.

- **Heinz White Vinegar** and **Stayfree Maxi Pads.** Mix one ounce Heinz White Vinegar and two cups of water, saturate a Stayfree Maxi Pad with the solution, and apply the compress to the affected area. The vinegar soothes the rash and relieves inflammation.

- **Nestlé Carnation Nonfat Dry Milk.** Mix one-half cup Nestlé Carnation Nonfat Dry Milk powder with enough water to make a thick paste, and spread it on the rash. The milky solution soothes the itch.

- **Planters Walnuts.** To reduce a rash, eat Planters Walnuts. One ounce of walnuts contains 2.6 grams of omega-3 fatty acids, which decrease inflammation and strengthen the immune system.

℞ STRANGE MEDICINE ℞

MAKING YOUR SKIN CRAWL

● A rash (medically called contact dermatitis) is an itchy, red skin inflammation (sometimes with small bumps) caused by an irritant or allergen touching the skin.

● Identifying the cause of the rash and avoiding further contact with that particular substance alleviates the rash, which subsides in two to four weeks.

● Common causes of rashes include nickel (found in jewelry, zippers, and coins), cashews, soaps, detergents, cosmetics, fragrances, topical medicines, latex rubber, household cleansers, and poison plants.

● To soothe a rash without medication, dampen a washcloth with cool water and press it against the affected areas as a compress.

● Applying an over-the-counter hydrocortisone cream can help relieve the redness and itching of a rash.

● To relieve severe itching, take an over-the-counter antihistamine, such as Benadryl (diphenhydramine) or Claritin (loratadine).

● To avoid scratching a rash, which can break the skin and make it susceptible to infection, trim your nails and wear white cotton gloves (or a pair of socks over your hands) to bed at night.

- **Quaker Oats** and **L'eggs Sheer Energy Panty Hose.** To relieve a rash, grind one cup uncooked Quaker Oats in a blender, pour a few tablespoons of the fine powder into the foot cut from a clean, used pair of L'eggs Sheer Energy Panty Hose, and tie a knot in the open end. Fill a bathtub with lukewarm water, pour the remaining powdered oats into the tub, and, while soaking for fifteen minutes, saturate the panty hose sachet with water, and gently rub it over the affected area. The antioxidants in the oats reduce inflammation.

- **Revlon Clear Nail Polish.** To prevent allergic reactions and irritation from metal fasteners on jeans or dresses that come into contact with your skin, give them a coat of Revlon Clear Nail Polish.

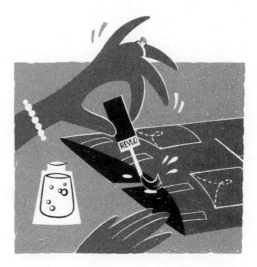

Doctor's Orders

Don't be rash! If a rash fails to heal within six days, consult a doctor for diagnosis.

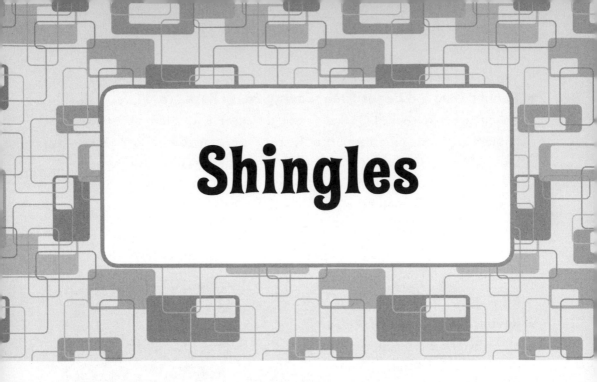

Shingles

- **Bayer Aspirin** and **Smirnoff Vodka.** To relieve the pain of shingles, use a mortar and pestle to crush two Bayer Aspirin tablets into a fine powder, mix it with two tablespoons Smirnoff Vodka, and apply the solution directly to the blisters. Applied topically, the salicylic acid and the alcohol in the vodka help alleviate the discomfort.

- **Clabber Girl Baking Powder.** To dry up the blisters and soothe itching, mix one-quarter cup Clabber Girl Baking Powder with enough water to make a paste, and apply it to the affected areas.

- **Dr. Teal's Epsom Salt.** Fill the bathtub with warm water, add two cups Dr. Teal's Epsom Salt, and soak for twenty minutes. The magnesium in the Epsom Salt soothes the itching and helps dry up the blisters.

- **Fruit of the Earth Aloe Vera Gel.** Applying Fruit of the Earth Aloe Vera Gel directly on the blisters helps soothe and heal the irritated skin.

- **Heinz Apple Cider Vinegar.** To mitigate the severe discomfort of shingles, apply full-strength Heinz Apple Cider Vinegar directly on the welts. Let air dry and repeat as often as necessary.

- **Heinz Baked Beanz.** To reduce the severity or duration of shingles, try eating one cup Heinz Baked Beanz every day. High in the amino acid lysine, baked beans may inhibit the herpes zoster virus from using other amino acids to construct the protein sheath that surrounds it, reducing and preventing the spread of shingles. One cup of baked beans contains 986 milligrams of lysine.

- **Hydrogen Peroxide.** If shingles blisters get infected, use a cotton ball to dab them with Hydrogen Peroxide. The bubbling solution disinfects the open sores.

- **Kingsford's Corn Starch.** To relieve the irritation of shingles, add a handful of Kingsford's Corn Starch to your bathwater, and soak for twenty minutes. The cornstarch helps soothe the itching.

- **Lipton Chamomile Tea** and **Stayfree Maxi Pads.** Place two Lipton Chamomile Tea bags in two cups of boiled water, cover with a saucer for twenty minutes, and then chill the tea in the refrigerator. Saturate a Stayfree Maxi Pad with the chamomile tea and apply to the blisters for fifteen minutes. When applied externally, chamomile soothes itchy skin, reduces inflammation, and speeds the healing of wounds.

- **Nestlé Carnation Nonfat Dry Milk.** Mix one-half cup Nestlé Carnation Nonfat Dry Milk powder with enough water to make a thick paste, and spread it on the affected areas. The milky solution soothes the pain and discomfort of shingles.

- **Quaker Oats.** To soothe the pain and reduce inflammation, cook up a bowl of Quaker Oats oatmeal according to the directions on the side of the canister, let cool, spread it on the affected areas, cover with a clean, damp washcloth, and let sit for up to thirty minutes. Wash clean. Repeat whenever necessary. As an astringent, oatmeal soothes the skin and relieves itching.

- **Quaker Oats** and **L'eggs Sheer Energy Panty Hose.** To relieve the pain of shingles, grind one cup uncooked Quaker Oats in a blender, pour a

☥ STRANGE MEDICINE ☥

HOT SPOTS

● Shingles—a painful band of short-lived blisters—are caused by the varicella-zoster virus, the same virus that causes chicken pox. If you've ever had chicken pox, you remain at risk of getting shingles any time during your life. After a chicken pox infection, some of the varicella-zoster virus tends to remain in your nerve cells, where it lies dormant. The virus may or may not reactivate many years later, resurfacing as shingles.

● Shingles usually appear as a single line of blisters that wraps around the left or the right side of your torso and causes tingling, burning pain, and numbness—ranging from mild to excruciating.

● Older adults and people with weakened immune systems stand the greatest risk of getting shingles.

● No one knows what triggers shingles, but the primary suspect is lowered immunity to infections that accompany age.

● Shingles are not contagious, but the varicella-zoster virus is to any person who lacks immunity to chicken pox. Infection, usually caused by direct contact with the open sores of the shingles rash, causes the person to develop chicken pox.

● Shingles can lead to postherpetic neuralgia—a condition in which the pain of shingles persists long after the blisters heal.

● If you have had chicken pox, the shingles vaccine can protect you from getting shingles. Approved by the FDA in 2006, the vaccine reduced the risk of shingles by 51 percent in clinical trials. It can also reduce the pain in people who still get shingles after being vaccinated. The Centers for Disease Control and Prevention recommends that adults sixty years and older get a single dose of the shingles vaccine.

● To soothe shingles, dampen a washcloth with cool water and press it against the affected areas as a compress.

few tablespoons of the fine powder into the foot cut from a clean, used pair of L'eggs Sheer Energy Panty Hose, and tie a knot in the open end. Fill a bathtub with lukewarm water, pour the remaining powdered oats into the tub, and, while soaking for fifteen minutes, saturate the panty hose sachet with water, and gently press it over the blisters. The antioxidants in the oats reduce inflammation.

- **SueBee Honey.** To alleviate the pain and speed healing, slather SueBee Honey on the shingles blisters several times a day. Anecdotal evidence confirms this folk remedy truly works.

- **Tabasco Pepper Sauce** and **Crisco All-Vegetable Shortening.** To relieve the lingering pain from shingles, mix one-quarter teaspoon Tabasco Pepper Sauce with two tablespoons Crisco All-Vegetable Shortening, and apply the spicy homemade ointment to the affected areas up to five times a day for up to a month. The capsaicin in the Tabasco Pepper Sauce relieves nerve pain. (Do not apply this salve on open sores and avoid contact with eyes and nose.)

Doctor's Orders

Hit the spot! At the first sign of shingles, see your doctor, who can prescribe an antiviral drug, which, when administered promptly, can shorten the duration of the awakened virus, reduce the intensity of the pain, and hasten healing. If you find the pain from shingles unbearable, let your doctor know.

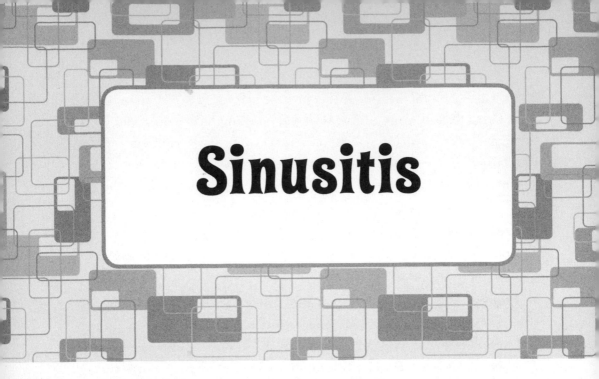

Sinusitis

- **Dr. Bronner's Eucalyptus Castile Soap.** To relieve a clogged nose, use Dr. Bronner's Eucalyptus Castile Soap in the shower or bath. The penetrating scent of eucalyptus clears congestion and opens nasal passages.

- **Gold's Horseradish** and **Nabisco Original Premium Saltine Crackers.** To clear up congested sinus passages, eat one teaspoon Gold's Horseradish spread on a Nabisco Original Premium Saltine Cracker. The pungent root flushes the sinuses.

- **Heinz Apple Cider Vinegar.** To help drain your stuffy sinuses, mix one teaspoon Heinz Apple Cider Vinegar in a glass of water, and drink the mildly tart concoction.

- **McCormick Garlic Powder.** To alleviate the symptoms of sinusitis and give your immune system a boost, use McCormick Garlic Powder in your cooking, or once a day eat a slice of lightly buttered bread sprinkled with one-half teaspoon McCormick Garlic Powder. Aside from being a natural antibiotic, garlic contains alliin, a chemical that makes mucus less sticky, clearing the sinuses.

- **McCormick Thyme Leaves** and **Lipton Peppermint Tea.** To decongest your sinuses, place three teaspoons McCormick Thyme Leaves and three

℞ STRANGE MEDICINE ℞

LOOKING DOWN YOUR NOSE

● Sinusitis is inflammation and swelling of the sinus cavities (located around your nasal passages), which impedes drainage and causes mucus to build up, making breathing through your nose difficult.

● Sinusitis frequently causes pressure and pain in the face around the eyes and nose, yellowish-green nasal discharge, and sinus headache.

● The most common causes of sinusitis include the common cold, bacteria, allergies, and fungal infections.

● Most cases of sinusitis improve on their own after a week.

● To speed recovery from sinusitis, get plenty of rest so your body can focus its energy on fighting the sinus infection.

● To liquefy blocked mucus and prompt drainage, drink eight 8-ounce glasses of water or juice daily.

● To hasten recovery from sinusitis, avoid caffeine and alcohol—diuretics that dehydrate the body, causing mucus to dry and thicken. Consuming alcohol also causes nasal and sinus membranes to swell.

● Taking a hot shower and breathing in the steam helps ease sinus pain and clear congested mucus.

● Placing a washcloth dampened with warm water on your closed eyes, nose, and cheeks helps ease sinus pain.

● To help your clogged sinuses drain and prevent postnasal drip at night, sleep with your head elevated.

● Running a humidifier in your bedroom or office helps prevent your nasal and sinus passages from drying out, thickening clogged mucus.

● Sinusitis that continues for more than twelve weeks or perpetually recurs is called chronic sinusitis.

Lipton Peppermint Tea bags into a large bowl and carefully add two cups of boiling water. Lean over the bowl and drape a towel like a tent over your head and the bowl. Inhale the rising steam for ten minutes, keeping your face roughly ten inches above the surface of the water. Repeat whenever needed. Thyme doubles as an antibacterial, and peppermint contains mint, a natural decongestant.

- **Morton Salt** and **Arm & Hammer Baking Soda.** To loosen mucus and reduce inflammation, make a saline nose wash to rinse your nasal passages. Purify eight ounces of water by boiling for three minutes, let cool to room temperature, and dissolve one-quarter teaspoon Morton Salt and one-quarter teaspoon Arm & Hammer Baking Soda in the purified water. Use a bulb syringe or neti pot to rinse each nostril.

- **Tabasco Pepper Sauce** and **Campbell's Tomato Juice.** To help clear sinuses and drain mucus, add ten to twenty drops Tabasco Pepper Sauce to a glass of Campbell's Tomato Juice, and drink this mixture several times a day. The capsaicin in the hot sauce doubles as a decongestant and helps liquefy mucus.

- **Vicks VapoRub.** For another way to decongest your sinuses, fill a large bowl with two cups of boiling water and add one teaspoon Vicks VapoRub. Lean over the bowl and drape a towel like a tent over your head and the bowl. Inhale the rising steam for ten minutes, keeping your face roughly ten inches above the surface of the water. Repeat whenever needed. The eucalyptus kills several strains of bacteria that cause sinus infections, and the menthol is a natural decongestant.

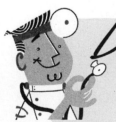

Doctor's Orders

Nose around! If sinusitis fails to respond to home treatments after a few days, consult a doctor to make sure the infection does not spread to your eyes (causing loss of vision) or the brain (causing meningitis).

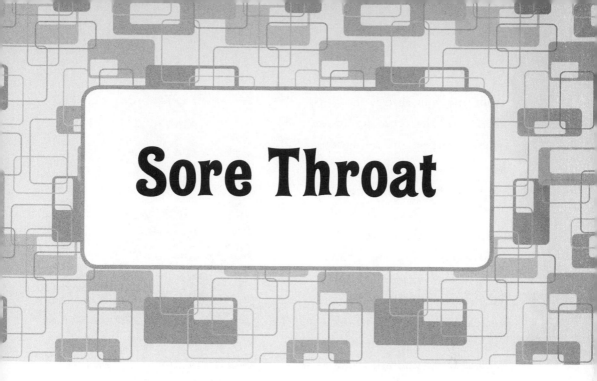

Sore Throat

- **Arm & Hammer Baking Soda.** Alleviate sore throat pain by dissolving one teaspoon Arm & Hammer Baking Soda in an eight-ounce glass of warm water, gargle with the solution several times a day, and spit out. Baking soda is a mild antiseptic.

- **Gold's Horseradish, SueBee Honey,** and **McCormick Ground Cloves.** Mix one tablespoon Gold's Horseradish, one teaspoon SueBee Honey, and one teaspoon McCormick Ground Cloves in an eight-ounce glass of warm water. Gargle with the concoction, or sip it slowly, stirring to keep the horseradish from sinking to the bottom. This Russian folk remedy soothes and relieves a sore throat.

- **Heinz Apple Cider Vinegar.** The moment you feel a sore throat coming on, mix equal parts Heinz Apple Cider Vinegar and warm water in a drinking glass, and gargle with the acidic solution every hour. The acetic acid in the vinegar kills the bacteria infecting your throat, potentially stopping the sore throat from gaining a foothold.

- **Life Savers Pep-O-Mints.** To keep your throat moist, suck on Life Savers Pep-O-Mints. The volatile oils in peppermint increase saliva production, soothing your throat, and the menthol helps relax the muscles, reducing inflammation and subduing the pain.

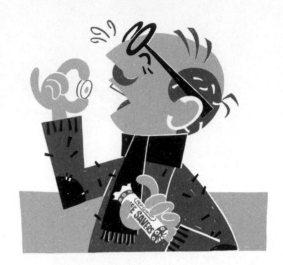

- **Lipton Chamomile Tea.** To tame the inflammation of a sore throat, place two Lipton Chamomile Tea bags in one cup of boiling water, cover with a saucer, and steep for ten minutes. Let cool until lukewarm, and gargle with the solution. Chamomile counters and soothes inflammation. (Coumarin, an anticoagulant in chamomile, may increase the likelihood of bleeding when taken in combination with the blood thinner Coumadin or other anticoagulant medications.)

- **Lipton Peppermint Tea.** To numb sore throat pain, place two Lipton Peppermint Tea bags in one cup of boiling water, cover with a saucer, and steep for ten minutes. Let cool until lukewarm, and gargle with the minty solution. The antiseptic and anesthetic compounds in mint kill germs, reduce inflammation, and provide quick, temporary relief from pain.

- **McCormick Ground Sage.** To relieve a sore throat, place a tea infuser filled with one tablespoon McCormick Ground Sage in a teacup, add boiling water, cover with a saucer, and steep for fifteen minutes. Let cool to a lukewarm temperature and gargle with the solution as frequently as necessary. Sage, a mild astringent that kills bacteria and viruses, reduces the inflammation responsible for throat pain.

- **McCormick Marjoram Leaves** and **SueBee Honey.** Fill a tea infuser with one teaspoon McCormick Marjoram Leaves, and brew a cup of tea with boiling water for five minutes. Add one teaspoon SueBee Honey, let cool to room temperature, and gargle with the solution. This herb doubles

℞ STRANGE MEDICINE ℞

THAT FROG IN YOUR THROAT

● While frequently a precursor to a cold or flu, a sore throat brings pain, scratchiness, or a burning sensation to the throat that tends to worsen when you swallow or talk. A sore throat frequently causes swollen glands in your neck or jaw, reddened and inflamed tonsils, and white spots on your tonsils.

● Commonly caused by a cold or flu, a sore throat usually goes away by itself within five to seven days without any medical attention. A sore throat caused by a bacterial infection—such as strep throat—requires treatment with antibiotics.

● As anyone who has ever shouted nonstop at a sporting event knows, overuse can cause a sore throat.

● To speed healing of a sore throat, get plenty of sleep and rest your voice so your body can focus its energy on fighting the infection.

● Relieve the pain of a sore throat by drinking eight 8-ounce glasses of water or juice daily to keep the throat tissue moist.

● Taking a hot shower and breathing in the steam helps ease sore throat pain.

● To help your sore throat heal, avoid secondhand smoke, and if you smoke, quit. Smoke irritates the throat.

● Running a humidifier in your bedroom or office helps keep your throat moist, expediting healing.

as an antibacterial pain reliever. (Do not feed honey to infants less than one year of age. Honey often carries a benign strain of *C. botulinum,* and an infant's immune system requires twelve months to develop to fight off disease and infection.)

● **Morton Salt.** To soothe a sore throat, dissolve one-half teaspoon Morton Salt in an eight-ounce glass of warm water, and gargle with the solution.

This mild antiseptic solution helps kill germs, dilute mucus, relieve the irritation, and rinse away phlegm.

- **SueBee Honey** and **ReaLemon.** To assuage a sore throat, dissolve three teaspoons SueBee Honey and one teaspoon ReaLemon lemon juice in a cup of boiled water and drink. As a mild antiseptic, honey soothes the irritated throat tissue, and the astringent lemon juice reduces the inflammation. (Do not feed honey to infants less than one year of age. Honey often carries a benign strain of *C. botulinum,* and an infant's immune system requires twelve months to develop to fight off disease and infection.)

- **Tabasco Pepper Sauce** and **Morton Salt.** Mix one-quarter teaspoon Tabasco Pepper Sauce and one-half teaspoon Morton Salt in one cup of warm water, and gargle with the spicy solution. The capsaicin from the capsicum peppers numbs the nerve endings in your throat, and the salt helps kill germs. Repeat several times daily as needed.

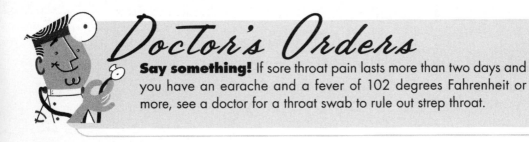

Doctor's Orders

Say something! If sore throat pain lasts more than two days and you have an earache and a fever of 102 degrees Fahrenheit or more, see a doctor for a throat swab to rule out strep throat.

Splinters

- **Dr. Teal's Epsom Salt.** To remove a wood splinter, dissolve one tablespoon Dr. Teal's Epsom Salt in one cup of warm water, and soak the area of skin where the splinter is embedded for ten minutes in this solution. The briny solution should cause the splinter to swell up, allowing you to remove it with ease.

- **Duck Tape.** To remove a wood splinter without the aid of tweezers, stick a strip of Duck Tape over the splinter, press down gently so the adhesive grabs the protruding sliver of wood, and lift the tape.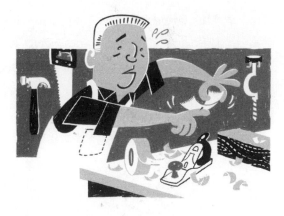

- **Elmer's Glue-All.** Cover the wood splinter with Elmer's Glue-All, let the glue dry, and peel off the glue. The glue should adhere to the protruding wood and lift it out.

- **Hydrogen Peroxide.** Saturating a splinter with Hydrogen Peroxide frequently bubbles the invader out of the skin. If this technique fails, you've merely sanitized the spot.

⚕ STRANGE MEDICINE ⚕

PRICK UP YOUR EARS

- Splinters are generally small slivers of wood, metal, or glass lodged in the skin that cause remarkable pain considering their minuscule size.

- To remove a splinter buried under the skin, sterilize a needle by holding it over a lit match for a few seconds (or dipping it in rubbing alcohol), let cool, and then use the pointed tip to gently lift the small piece of skin obstructing the end of the splinter. (Use a magnifying glass if necessary.) With the bit of skin raised, use a pair of tweezers to extract the splinter. Wash the spot with an antibacterial soap and put on a bandage.

- After removing a splinter, make sure no piece of it remains embedded in the skin. If it does, repeat the method above to remove the piece of splinter.

- If left embedded in the skin, a splinter almost always becomes infected.

- To prevent splinters, wear work gloves when handling lumber, plants, or broken glass. Wear shoes when walking outdoors or on wood decks, floors, or boardwalks.

- **Star Olive Oil.** Applying a drop of Star Olive Oil to the splinter softens the skin around it, enabling the sliver to slip out easily.

- **SueBee Honey** and **Band-Aid Bandages.** To excise a splinter, apply a dab of SueBee Honey over the shard, and wrap it with a Band-Aid Bandage to hold the honey in place. Check the splinter every three hours to see if the absorptive and hygroscopic honey has extracted it. If not, repeat the process.

Doctor's Orders

Look sharp! If a splinter is metal and you haven't had a tetanus shot within the last five years, or if it causes pain, pus, or swelling, consult your doctor.

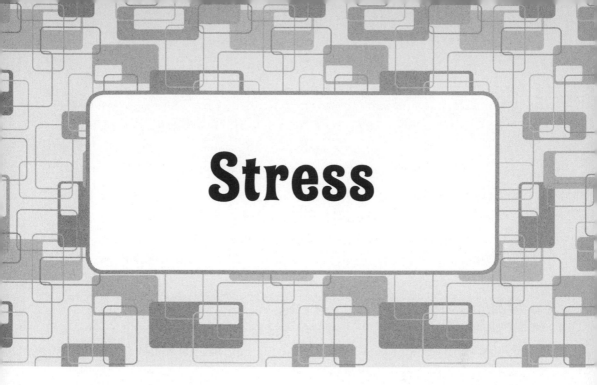

Stress

- **Dr. Teal's Epsom Salt.** Turn your bathtub into a rejuvenating mineral spring by adding two cups Dr. Teal's Epsom Salt to lukewarm bathwater and soaking for fifteen luxurious minutes. The magnesium in the Epsom Salt passes into the body through osmosis and eases muscular aches, helping you relax.

- **Heinz Baked Beanz.** To reduce stress and keep your energy level well balanced, eat one-half cup of Heinz Baked Beanz. Baked beans slow the release of blood sugar into your bloodstream, giving your body and brain a steady source of fuel, keeping you even keeled and uniformly energized. Beans also stabilize the adrenal glands, which regulate the body's stress response.

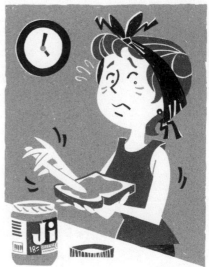

- **Jif Peanut Butter.** Magnesium helps relax tense muscles. While eating a wide range of legumes, nuts, whole grains, and vegetables will help you meet your daily dietary need for magnesium, you can quickly replace magnesium in your body by eating Jif Peanut Butter (straight from the jar or in a sandwich). Four tablespoons of peanut butter contain 100 milligrams of magnesium (or 25 percent of the daily value).

- **Kretschmer Wheat Germ.** To relieve stress and anxiety, add three teaspoons Kretschmer Wheat Germ to a cup of yogurt or bowl of cereal every day. Aside from containing magnesium, which relaxes muscles, wheat germ contains octacosanol, a phytonutrient that seems to help the body withstand tension.

- **Lipton Black Tea.** To calm your nerves, drink a cup of Lipton Black Tea four times a day. A 2010 study at the University College of London revealed that drinking four cups of black tea daily significantly reduces the level of the stress hormone cortisol in the blood after a stressful event.

- **Lipton Chamomile Tea.** To reduce stress, pour one cup of boiling water over two Lipton Chamomile Tea bags in a cup, cover with a saucer, let steep for ten minutes, and then drink the tea. Chamomile subdues tension, and a 2009 study at the University of Pennsylvania showed that taking chamomile reduces the symptoms of generalized anxiety disorder by 50 percent. (Coumarin, an anticoagulant in chamomile, may increase the likelihood of bleeding when taken in combination with the blood thinner Coumadin or other anticoagulant medications.)

- **Lipton Chamomile Tea** and **L'eggs Sheer Energy Panty Hose.** To give yourself soothing aromatherapy to reduce stress, place six Lipton Chamomile Tea bags in the foot cut from a pair of L'eggs Sheer Energy Panty Hose, tie the open end of the foot around the faucet in the bathtub, and fill the bathtub with warm water. Soak in the bath for fifteen minutes, savoring the calming scent of chamomile.

- **Planters Dry Roasted Almonds, Planters Dry Roasted Cashews,** or **Planters Dry Roasted Peanuts.** Eating foods high in magnesium— like Planters Dry Roasted Almonds, Planters Dry Roasted Cashews, or

℞ STRANGE MEDICINE ℞

WORRIED SICK

● Stress is that overwhelming feeling of physical, mental, or emotional duress when you feel that the demands being made on you exceed your ability to meet them.

● Stress can be a good thing, increasing your performance and motivating you to accomplish tasks. But stress overload can turn stress into distress, causing fatigue, exhaustion, illness, and a breakdown.

● If you're feeling stressed, avoid caffeinated products. Drinking coffee or caffeinated soda merely exacerbates the situation.

● Drinking alcohol, classified as a depressant, may seem like an effective way to reduce stress, but alcohol actually prompts your adrenal glands to produce more stress hormones. Alcohol also interferes with your sleep.

● Eating comfort foods like cake and cookies can increase stress. The sugar and carbo-hydrates intensify anxiety.

● Aside from weakening your immune system and causing headaches, backaches, and neck pain, stress can make you more susceptible to high blood pressure, heart attack, stroke, and a wide variety of diseases.

● Get thirty minutes of exercise—walking, bicycling, or swimming—at least three days a week. Exercise relieves stress.

● Yoga, massage, meditation, deep-breathing exercises, relaxation, listening to music, or taking a hot bath helps reduce stress.

● Use positive affirmations. If you feel stress, you're likely repeating negative thoughts in your head. Instead, replace those thoughts with positive ones, by chanting something like, "I can do this," "Everything will work out fine, it always does," or "I just have to get this done, it doesn't have to be perfect."

Planters Dry Roasted Peanuts—relaxes muscles, helping you relax. One ounce of almonds provides 80 milligrams of magnesium, one ounce of cashews provides 75 milligrams, and one ounce of dry roasted peanuts provides 50 milligrams.

- **Quaker Oats.** To reduce stress, eat a bowl of Quaker Oats oatmeal every morning. Oats contain the mild sedative gramine, and the complex carbohydrates seem to increase levels of serotonin, a neurotransmitter that promotes relaxation.

- **Wilson Tennis Balls.** Insert three Wilson Tennis Balls into a sock, tie a knot in the open end of the sock, and have a partner roll the sock over your back for a soothing massage to help relieve stress.

- **Wrigley's Spearmint Gum.** Chewing a stick of Wrigley's Spearmint Gum relieves anxiety, releases pent-up energy, and reduces stress. A 2008 study at Swinburne University of Technology in Melbourne, Australia, showed that gum chewing reduced levels of the stress hormone cortisol.

Doctor's Orders

Don't worry your pretty little head! If you feel overwhelmed by anxiety, have difficulty falling and staying asleep, experience severe headaches, contemplate suicide, or feel incapacitated by any other symptoms caused by stress, consult your doctor or a therapist.

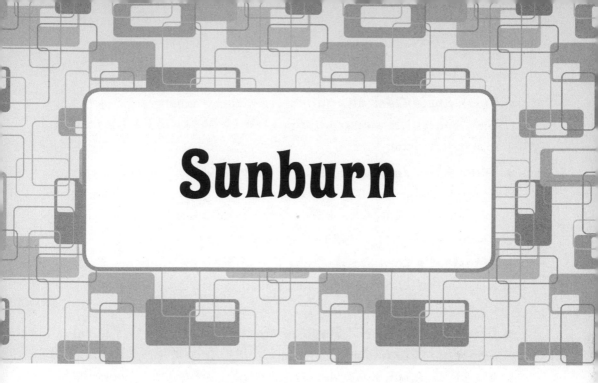

Sunburn

- **Arm & Hammer Baking Soda.** To soothe sunburn pain, mix one handful of Arm & Hammer Baking Soda in a bathtub filled with cool water and soak for twenty minutes. The sodium bicarbonate soothes inflammation and the cool water relieves the pain.

- **Bayer Aspirin.** Taking two Bayer Aspirin tablets every four hours helps relieve the pain and inflammation of a minor sunburn.

- **Colgate Regular Flavor Toothpaste.** To soothe a sunburn, apply Colgate Regular Flavor Toothpaste as an ointment to the affected area. The glycerin in the toothpaste provides a soothing cooling sensation and fast, temporary relief.

- **Dannon Yogurt.** To relieve sunburn pain, smear Dannon Plain Nonfat Yogurt over the affected area.

- **French's Mustard.** For instant relief from sunburn pain, slather French's Mustard on the burn to stop the stinging and prevent blistering. Let the mustard dry on the skin.

- **Fruit of the Earth Aloe Vera Gel.** To get soothing relief from sunburn pain, slather Fruit of the Earth Aloe Vera Gel over the affected area.

- **Heinz Apple Cider Vinegar.** To relieve itchy sunburn pain, pour two cups Heinz Apple Cider Vinegar in a bathtub filled with cool water, and soak in the solution.

- **Heinz White Vinegar** and **Bounty Paper Towels.** Saturate a few sheets of Bounty Paper Towels with Heinz White Vinegar and wrap them around the sunburned skin (avoiding the eyes). Let sit until the paper towels dry. The acetic acid in the vinegar helps relieve the pain and inflammation.

- **Kingsford's Corn Starch.** To relieve sunburn pain, mix one-half cup Kingsford's Corn Starch with enough water to make a paste, and apply it to the affected area.

- **Lipton Green Tea** and **Stayfree Maxi Pads.** To soothe a sunburn, brew a strong cup of Lipton Green Tea and let it cool. Saturate a Stayfree Maxi Pad with the liquid and apply it as a compress on the sunburn. The tannins in green tea soothe and strengthen the epidermis and reduce inflammation.

- **Lipton Tea.** If your eyelids get sunburned and swell, saturate two Lipton Tea bags with cool water, squeeze out the excess water, and place them over your closed eyes. The tannin in the tea reduces the inflammation and relieves the sunburn pain.

- **Nestlé Carnation Non-fat Dry Milk.** Mix one-half cup Nestlé Carnation Nonfat Dry Milk powder with enough water to make a thick paste, and spread it on the sunburned skin. The protein from the milk relieves the pain and soothes the itch.

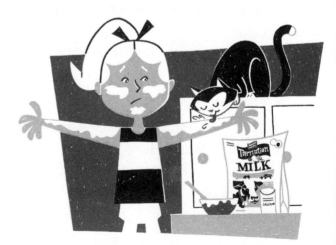

● **Quaker Oats** and **L'eggs Sheer Energy Panty Hose.** To relieve sunburn pain, grind one cup uncooked Quaker Oats in a blender, pour the fine powder into the foot cut from a clean, used pair of L'eggs Sheer Energy Panty Hose, tie a knot in the open end, and then tie the sachet to the bathtub faucet. Fill the bathtub with cool water, soak for fifteen

℞ STRANGE MEDICINE ℞

HERE COMES THE SUN

● To prevent sunburn, apply sunscreen with a sun protection factor (SPF) of 30 or higher to your skin at least thirty minutes before going outdoors, and limit the amount of time you spend in the sun. Reapply sunscreen every two hours.

● To protect yourself from sunburn, wear long pants, a long sleeved shirt, sunglasses, and a wide-brimmed hat.

● Stay out of the sun between 10 a.m. and 4 p.m., when the sun's rays are strongest.

● After swimming or perspiring heavily, reapply sunscreen.

● You can get a sunburn on cloudy, overcast days (the sun's ultraviolet rays penetrate clouds) and in the winter from sunshine reflected off snow and ice.

● Sunburned skin heals itself within a few days (or longer depending on the severity of the burn). The top layer of damaged skin peels off. The new layer of skin usually appears discolored for a short time.

● Sunburn can affect any part of you body, including your scalp, lips, ears, and eyes.

● You can relieve the pain and inflammation of sunburn by dampening a washcloth with ice cold water and applying it to the affected areas as a compress for ten minutes several times a day.

● To prevent dehydration and offset the desiccating effects of sunburn on the skin, drink plenty of water or juice to replenish lost fluid.

minutes or more, and let your body air-dry, so the gelatinous polysaccharides stay on your skin, forming a protective coat.

- **SunGuard.** To help stop ultraviolet (UV) rays from penetrating your clothing and causing sunburn, add SunGuard to your washing machine when laundering clothes. Clothes do not fully absorb the UV rays of the sun. A typical white t-shirt, for example, has an ultraviolet protection factor (UPF) rating of 5 or less. SunGuard infuses your clothes with a UV protectant that gives the fabric a UPF rating of 30, helping to prevent 96 percent of the sun's UV rays from reaching your skin. The protection lasts for up to twenty clothes washings.

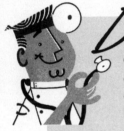

Doctor's Orders

Good day sunshine! If your sunburn blisters, you experience chills or a fever, or the pain becomes excruciating, consult your doctor. If your sunburn is accompanied by nausea, vomiting, headache, or fainting, seek immediate medical attention to rule out heat exhaustion or heat stroke.

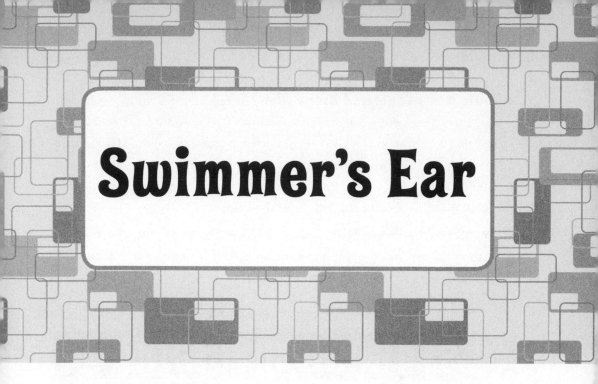

Swimmer's Ear

- **Conair Hair Dryer.** To avoid swimmer's ear, after getting out of the pool or shower and toweling dry, aim the nozzle of a Conair Hair Dryer set on low into your ear for thirty seconds to blow out any remaining water. Be sure to hold the hair dryer ten inches away from your ear.

- **Heinz White Vinegar.** To cure swimmer's ear, doctors recommend that you mix equal parts Heinz White Vinegar and water, and then use a dropper to fill the ear canal with the solution. Let sit for five minutes, and then tilt your head to the side to empty it out onto a hand towel. The vinegar raises the acidity in your ear canal, making it an inhospitable environment for bacteria and fungi.

- **Johnson's Baby Oil.** Use a dropper to place a few drops of Johnson's Baby Oil in each ear before swimming to prevent swimmer's ear. The oil repels the water.

- **Smirnoff Vodka.** To prevent swimmer's ear, after getting out of a pool or lake, use a dropper to fill the ear canal with Smirnoff Vodka, and then turn your head from side to side to let it run out. The alcohol dries the ear and kills bacteria and fungi.

- **Uncle Ben's Converted Brand Rice.** To relieve the pain of swimmer's ear, fill a clean sock with Uncle Ben's Converted Brand Rice, tie a knot in the end, and heat in the microwave oven for ninety seconds. Making sure the sock isn't too hot, apply the heat pack to one ear at a time. The rice-filled sock conforms to the shape of your head, stays warm for roughly thirty minutes, and the warmth eases the pain.

- **Vaseline Petroleum Jelly.** To replace the earwax worn away by the irritation of swimmer's ear, moisten a cotton ball with Vaseline Petroleum Jelly and insert it into your ear like an earplug.

℞ STRANGE MEDICINE ℞

WET BEHIND THE EARS

- Swimmer's ear is an infection of the outer ear canal. Water or perspiration trapped in the ear provides the perfect environment for bacteria (or occasionally a virus or fungus) to proliferate and invade the skin.

- Inserting fingers, cotton swabs, or foreign objects into your ears can cause small breaks in the thin layer of skin lining your ear canal, enabling a bacterial infection to cause swimmer's ear.

- Swimmer's ear makes the ear feel blocked and itchy, and if left untreated, the symptoms increase in severity and may include swelling and a discharge of fluid from the ear.

- To prevent swimmer's ear, simply make sure the insides of your ears are dry after swimming, bathing, or showering. Shake your head to remove the remaining water, and then tilt your head to one side to let gravity do the rest. Repeat with the other ear.

- Children tend to get swimmer's ear more frequently than adults because the narrow ear canal of a child is more prone to trap water.

- Wearing headphones, a hearing aid, or a bathing cap can increase the risk of swimmer's ear—as can swimming in a lake with high levels of bacteria.

- **Ziploc Storage Bags.** To soothe swimmer's ear, dampen a washcloth with warm water, fold it into quarters, and place it inside a Ziploc Storage Bag. Heat the unzipped bag in the microwave oven for fifteen seconds on a microwave-safe dish, and then zip the bag shut and place it on the sore ear for roughly twenty minutes.

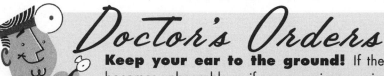

Doctor's Orders

Keep your ear to the ground! If the pain in your ear becomes unbearable or if you experience swimmer's ear for more than three days, consult a doctor.

Tartar and Plaque

- **Arm & Hammer Baking Soda.** Dampen your toothbrush bristles with water, dip them in an open box of Arm & Hammer Baking Soda, brush your teeth and along the gumline, and spit out. The mildly abrasive baking soda simultaneously cleans your teeth, removes unsightly stains, kills bacteria that cause gingivitis, neutralizes the acids emitted by bacteria, and deodorizes your breath.

- **Heinz Apple Cider Vinegar.** To prevent tartar and plaque, gargle with Heinz Apple Cider Vinegar before brushing your teeth in the morning. The acetic acid in the vinegar kills bacteria in your mouth and on your gums, whitens teeth, and removes stains.

- **Hydrogen Peroxide.** To augment your brushing and flossing, mix equal parts Hydrogen Peroxide and water, and rinse your mouth with the solution. The hydrogen peroxide kills the bacteria that excrete the chemicals that stimulate the proliferation of plaque.

- **Lipton Black Tea** or **Lipton Green Tea.** To prevent plaque from adhering to your teeth, drink one or two cups of Lipton Black Tea or Lipton Green Tea daily or use it as a mouthwash. The polyphenols in black and green teas are antioxidant compounds that inhibit plaque buildup, which leads to gum disease. A 2009 study at Kyushu University in Fukuoka, Japan, published in the *Journal of Periodontology*, found that men who drank a cup of green tea every day showed less risk and incidence of periodontal (gum) disease than those who did not.

Rx STRANGE MEDICINE Rx

STICKING AROUND

● Plaque, a sticky, colorless film of bacteria, constantly forms on your teeth above and below your gumline. The bacteria feed on sugars in foods and expel acids that etch into tooth enamel and cause cavities. The bacteria also excrete toxins that can irritate the gums and lead to periodontal (gum) disease.

● To remove plaque from your teeth, brush after each meal (or at least twice a day) and floss at least once daily.

● Plaque begins forming on your teeth between four and twelve hours after brushing.

● Plaque left on your teeth combines with minerals in your saliva to calcify and bond to your teeth, forming a rough, hard deposit called tartar (or calculus). Plaque bacteria cling to tartar, where they proliferate, leading to periodontal (gum) disease.

● Brushing and flossing cannot remove tartar from your teeth. Only a dentist or hygienist can remove tartar.

● Daily brushing and flossing and regular dental checkups for preventive care reduce tartar buildup and make periodontal (gum) disease less likely to develop.

● People vary greatly in their susceptibility to plaque and tartar, due to differences in the saliva, the types of plaque bacteria, and dietary factors.

● Brushing your teeth with tartar-control toothpaste accepted by the American Dental Association can help reduce the formation of tartar.

- **Listerine.** To ward off plaque buildup, rinse your mouth for thirty seconds two times daily with Listerine antiseptic mouthwash. A study reported by the *Journal of Clinical Periodontology* in 1993 showed that antibacterial Listerine prevents plaque from developing, reducing the incidence of gingivitis.

- **Ocean Spray Cranberry Juice.** Drinking cranberry juice, according to a 1998 study at Tel Aviv University School of Dental Medicine in Israel, prevents plaque-forming bacteria from adhering to teeth, thwarting gingivitis and periodontal (gum) disease.

- **Trident.** To inhibit plaque and prevent cavities, chew a piece of Trident sugarless gum for five minutes after every meal. Xylitol—an organic sugar substitute extracted from corn husks, birch, and various berries—inhibits the growth of the bacteria that cause tooth decay.

- **Visa.** To remove the bacteria and toxins festering on your tongue, use a clean, expired Visa credit card to scrape your tongue from back to front ten to fifteen times.

- **Wrigley's Big Red Cinnamon Gum.** To prevent plaque buildup and reduce the bacteria that cause bad breath, chew a stick of Wrigley's Big Red Cinnamon Gum for twenty minutes. A 2011 study at the University of Illinois at Chicago showed that the cinnamic aldehyde in the gum reduces the amount of oral bacteria in your saliva by 50 percent and kills 40 percent of the types linked to bad breath.

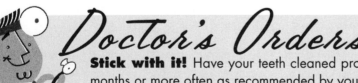

Doctor's Orders

Stick with it! Have your teeth cleaned professionally every six months or more often as recommended by your dentist or hygienist.

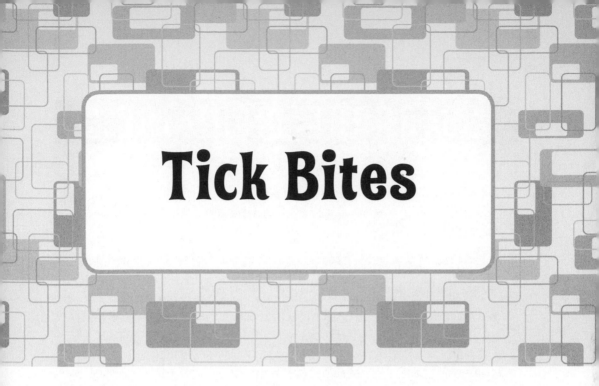

Tick Bites

- **Johnson's Baby Oil.** To remove an attached tick from your skin, wearing a pair of gloves, put a drop of Johnson's Baby Oil on the tick to loosen it from the skin, and then extract the tick with tweezers, grasping the tick at the skin line as close to the head as possible, and pulling gently but steadily. Loosening the tick with mineral oil helps remove the tick intact.

- **Listerine.** Place a few drops of original formula Listerine antiseptic mouthwash on the feeding tick's head, and use tweezers to grab the tick at the skin line and slowly pry it off. The antiseptic will prompt the tick to let go.

- **Neosporin.** After removing an engorged tick, dab the affected area with Neosporin. The antibiotic ointment provides extra protection against infection or tick-borne diseases.

- **Playtex Living Gloves.** Before removing a feeding tick, put on a pair of Playtex Living Gloves to avoid contact with your skin. Bacteria from the tick can penetrate through your skin.

- **Scotch Tape.** To kill ticks, use a strip of Scotch Tape to wrap up the tick, sealing it in plastic.

- **Ziploc Storage Bags.** After removing an engorged tick, place it in a jar of

℞ STRANGE MEDICINE ℞

WHAT MAKES THEM TICK

- Ticks—parasites related to mites and spiders—require blood to complete their life cycle and feed on warm-blooded animals. Their teeth, bent backwards, help the tick cling to its host.

- When gorging on a host's blood, ticks balloon up to fifty times their normal size.

- Ticks spread Lyme disease, Rocky Mountain spotted fever, and ehrlichiosis.

- Lyme disease often reveals itself within three days to a month as a small rash that looks like a bull's-eye target, flu-like symptoms, and Bell's palsy (paralysis on one side of the face). If left untreated, the disease can escalate to arthritis, meningitis, and neurological damage. If caught early, Lyme disease can be treated with antibiotics.

- Ticks live several feet off the ground on tall grass and weeds, lingering until a potential host passes by. Keeping your lawn cut minimizes this scenario.

- To remove a feeding tick, avoid squeezing the tick's body, which can inject the tick's blood or regurgitation into your body, causing infection.

- Place the tick in a small container filled with rubbing (isopropyl) alcohol. Mark the date on the container. The alcohol kills and preserves the tick so your doctor can identify and test it for diseases, should you start showing symptoms of a tick-borne disease.

alcohol to kill it, put the dead tick in a tightly sealed Ziploc Storage Bag, and write the date on the bag. Bring the tick to a doctor to have it analyzed at a lab for Lyme disease or any other tick–borne diseases.

Doctor's Orders

Get ticked off! If you are bitten by a tick and within a few weeks develop a fever, chills, aches and pains, or a rash, see a doctor immediately to determine whether you have a tick-borne disease.

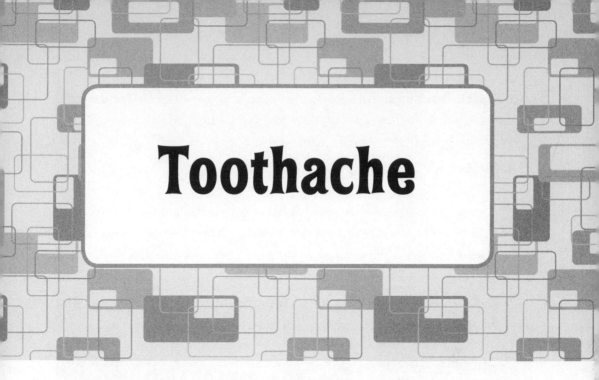

Toothache

- **Birds Eye Frozen Peas** and **Bounty Paper Towels.** To numb the nerves causing toothache pain until you can see a dentist, cover a bag of Birds Eye Frozen Peas with a sheet of Bounty Paper Towels, and press it against your cheek over the painful tooth for fifteen minutes every hour. The frozen peas act like small ice cubes, and the bag of peas conforms to the shape of your face. The paper towel creates a layer of insulation to prevent frostbite. Refreeze the bag of peas for future ice-pack use. Be sure to label the bag for ice-pack use only. If you want to eat the peas, cook them after they thaw the first time, never after refreezing.

- **Hydrogen Peroxide.** To temporarily relieve the pain of a toothache, rinse with Hydrogen Peroxide. The solution helps kill bacteria that might be exacerbating the pain.

- **Jif Peanut Butter** and **Colman's Mustard Powder.** To anesthetize toothache pain, place a dollop of Jif Peanut Butter on the tip of your index finger, sprinkle with Colman's Mustard Powder, and stick the glob with the mustard-side down on the affected tooth. The peanut butter holds the mustard in place, and the mustard numbs the nerve endings.

- **Lipton Tea Bags.** To soothe a toothache, dampen a Lipton Tea Bag with warm water, and press it against the affected tooth. The tannin in the tea is an astringent that helps reduce inflammation.

- **McCormick Ground Cloves.** To relieve toothache pain, dampen a cotton ball with water, sprinkle with a pinch of McCormick Ground Cloves, and place it against the affected tooth until the pain subsides. Eugenol, the main chemical compound in cloves, is a natural anesthetic that numbs the nerves. (Avoid letting the clove powder touch the tongue or sensitive gum tissue, which can increase the pain.)

- **McCormick Ground Ginger** and **McCormick Ground (Cayenne) Red Pepper.** To soothe a toothache, mix one-quarter teaspoon McCormick

℞ STRANGE MEDICINE ℞

A KICK IN THE TEETH

- A toothache can be caused by myriad problems, including tooth decay, a crack or fissure, a piece of food trapped between two teeth, a gum infection, or an abscessed tooth.

- Tooth decay is usually caused by poor dental hygiene, although susceptibility to tooth decay is also somewhat hereditary.

- To help relieve a toothache, cover an ice cube with a thin cloth and rub it on the back of your hand (belonging to the same side of the body as the toothache pain) on the muscle beneath the web of flesh between the thumb and index finger for five to ten minutes. A 1980 study at McGill University in Montreal, Canada, showed that doing so can reduce the intensity of toothache pain by half. The nerve pathways apparently stimulate an area of the brain that overrides the pain signals from the teeth.

- Rinsing your mouth vigorously with lukewarm water several times a day can help dislodge any trapped food debris from your teeth, alleviating the pain.

- To avoid exacerbating toothache pain or making the situation worse, refrain from poking at it with a toothpick or your tongue.

- Taking an over-the-counter pain reliever can help numb a toothache.

Ground Ginger, one-quarter teaspoon McCormick Ground (Cayenne) Red Pepper, and enough water to make a thick paste. Dampen a cotton ball with water, dip it into the mixture of spice, and place it against the affected tooth (avoiding the tongue and gums). Hold it in place until the pain subsides or you can no longer stand the burning sensation of the ginger and cayenne. The ginger and the capsaicin (in the cayenne) help numb the nerves. (Do not use ginger if you have gallstones. Ginger can increase bile production.)

- **Morton Salt.** To quell toothache pain, dissolve one teaspoon Morton Salt in a cup of boiled water, let cool, swish the simple mouthwash around in your mouth for thirty seconds, and then spit out. The salt water rinses out debris and helps reduce inflammation.

- **Oral-B Dental Floss.** If your toothache is caused by food particles lodged between your teeth or in the gum-line, after rinsing with salt water (see Morton Salt tip above), use Oral-B Dental Floss to floss the intruder free.

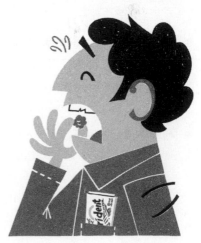

- **Trident.** To stop the pain caused by a cracked or broken tooth, seal the fissure or gap with a chewed piece of Trident Sugarless Gum. The temporary plug prevents air from triggering the nerve, reducing the pain until you can get to a dentist.

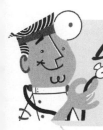

Doctor's Orders

That bites! If your toothache lasts longer than a day or two, you experience severe pain, or the toothache is accompanied by fever or an earache, see a dentist.

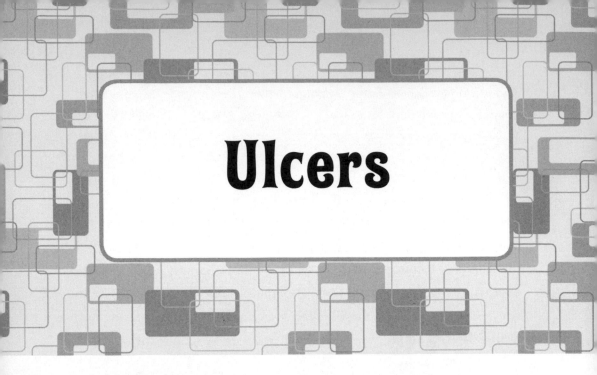

Ulcers

- **Chicken of the Sea Salmon, Chicken of the Sea Sardines,** or **Chicken of the Sea Tuna.** To prevent ulcers, eat salmon, sardines, or tuna three times a week to add linoleic acid, an omega-3 fatty acid, to your diet. Gastric ulcers have been linked to a deficiency of linoleic acid.

- **Dannon Yogurt.** To soothe an ulcer, eat a cup of Dannon Yogurt every day. The beneficial *Lactobacillus acidophilus* and *bulgaricus* (probiotics) in yogurt don't eliminate *Helicobacter pylori,* the bacteria responsible for most ulcers, but they may help inhibit them and heal the gastric mucosa.

- **Fruit of the Earth Aloe Vera Gel.** To heal an ulcer, drink one-quarter cup Fruit of the Earth Aloe Vera Gel three times a day. Fruit of the Earth Aloe Vera Gel is 100 percent pure aloe gel and edible. Studies show that drinking aloe vera gel reduces inflammation and helps heal gastric ulcers.

- **Lipton Chamomile Tea.** To eliminate an ulcer, place two Lipton Chamomile Tea bags in a cup of boiling water, cover with a saucer, and steep for ten to fifteen minutes. Drink three cups a day. Chamomile soothes inflammation, inhibits the growth of *Helicobacter pylori,* and reduces stress. (Coumarin, an anticoagulant in chamomile, may increase the likelihood of bleeding when taken in combination with the blood thinner Coumadin or other anti-coagulant medications.)

- **Lipton Ginger Tea.** To relieve the symptoms of an ulcer, drink a cup of strongly brewed Lipton Ginger Tea after each meal (or three times a day). A 2009 study at Jamia Hamdard University in India showed that ginger oil protects against ulcer formation in rats. (Do not drink ginger tea if you have gallstones. Ginger can increase bile production.)

- **McCormick Garlic Powder.** Spice your food by adding McCormick Garlic Powder to sauces, salads, and other foods to fight an ulcer. A 2001 study published in the *Journal of Nutrition* shows that the thiosulfinates in garlic act as a natural antibiotic to impede the growth of *Helicobacter pylori,* the bacteria responsible for ulcers.

- **Ocean Spray Craisins.** To prevent ulcers, eat a handful of Ocean Spray Craisins a couple of times a day. Dried cranberries contain flavonoids, and studies show that these flavonoids stop ulcers from forming.

- **Ocean Spray Cranberry Juice Cocktail.** To prevent or cure ulcers, drink one 8-ounce glass of Ocean Spray Cranberry Juice Cocktail daily. A 2005 study at the Beijing Institute for Cancer Research found that drinking one cup of cranberry juice daily eliminated *Helicobacter pylori,* the bacteria that cause stomach ulcers, in three times as many subjects as a daily placebo juice did. A 2000 study at Technion and Tel Aviv University found preliminary evidence that compounds in cranberry juice called proanthocyanidins inhibit *Helicobacter pylori* from attaching to the stomach lining and causing an ulcer. The findings also showed that cranberry juice could cause attached bacteria to release their grip on the stomach lining.

- **Phillips' Milk of Magnesia.** To stop ulcer pain, take one teaspoon Phillips' Milk of Magnesia. The antacid helps neutralize stomach acids.

- **Planters Walnuts.** Eating walnuts helps prevent ulcers. Walnuts contain linoleic acid, a deficiency of which has been linked to gastric ulcers.

STRANGE MEDICINE

A REAL HOLE IN THE WALL

● An ulcer is a sore in the lining of the stomach or duodenum (the upper part of the small intestine) that usually causes a burning pain in the stomach that flares up and subsides for a few days or weeks.

● Most ulcers are caused by an infection of the stomach with *Helicobacter pylori*, bacteria that eat through the thick layer of mucus lining the stomach or the duodenum (the uppermost section of the small intestine). Pepsin, a digestive enzyme, then seeps into the openings, digesting your own tissue, causing a burning pain.

● Ulcers tend to act up when your stomach is empty and subside again after you eat food.

● Long-term use of nonsteroidal anti-inflammatory drugs (such as aspirin and ibuprofen) can also cause ulcers.

● Contrary to popular belief, neither stress nor spicy food causes ulcers, but they can make ulcers worse.

● If you're suffering from an ulcer, stop drinking coffee and milk. Both of these beverages stimulate the production of more stomach acid, making the pain worse.

● If you smoke, quit. The National Institute of Diabetes and Digestive and Kidney Diseases reports that people who smoke cigarettes are more likely to develop an ulcer, and people with an ulcer who continue smoking may prevent that ulcer from healing.

● To reduce ulcer pain, drink eight 8-ounce glasses of water daily. Drinking a glass of water dilutes the acids in the stomach, lessening the discomfort.

● Eating five or six small meals a day (rather than two or three big meals) helps lessen ulcer pain by subduing stomach acids and increasing blood flow to the stomach walls.

● Yoga, massage, meditation, deep-breathing exercises, relaxation, listening to music, or taking a hot bath helps reduce stress that can exacerbate ulcers.

● Left untreated, ulcers get worse—possibly perforating the stomach or duodenum. A simple course of antibiotics can kill *Helicobacter pylori*, the bacteria most likely causing the problem.

- **SueBee Honey.** To remedy an ulcer, eat two tablespoons SueBee Honey daily until the ulcer disappears. Add the honey to a cup of tea, slather it on a slice of toast, or add it to a bowl of oatmeal. In a 1999 study published in *Pharmacological Research,* honey helped reduce ulcers up to 98 percent in rats. (Do not feed honey to infants less than one year of age. Honey often carries a benign strain of *C. botulinum,* and an infant's immune system requires twelve months to develop to fight off disease and infection.)

- **Tums.** To stop ulcer pain, chew one regular Tums tablet. The calcium carbonate helps neutralize stomach acids. (If you've had calcium oxalate kidney stones, consult your doctor before taking Tums.)

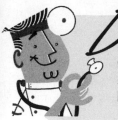

Doctor's Orders

Can't stomach it? If you feel a burning sensation in your stomach, have bad breath, or black stools (indicating digested blood from internal bleeding), see a doctor.

Urinary Tract Infections

- **Arm & Hammer Baking Soda.** The moment you feel the symptoms of a urinary tract infection, dissolve one-quarter teaspoon Arm & Hammer Baking Soda in an eight-ounce glass of water, and drink the solution. Repeat daily. The sodium bicarbonate increases the alkalinity in your bladder, lessening the ability of the bacteria to procreate. (Do not use this remedy if you're on a sodium-restricted diet. Read the directions on the side of the box of baking soda before administering.)

- **Dannon Yogurt.** To ward off a urinary tract infection, eat one cup of Dannon Yogurt every day. The *Lactobacillus acidophilus* (probiotics) may impede the *E. coli* bacteria from multiplying in the urinary tract. If you're taking an antibiotic to fight a urinary tract infection, eating a cup of yogurt daily replaces the beneficial bacteria wiped out by the drug.

- **Lipton Green Tea.** To help relieve bladder inflammation, drink two or three cups of Lipton Green Tea daily. A 2007 study at the University of Pittsburgh School of Medicine showed that the antioxidants in green tea protect bladder cells from inflammation.

THE WAY IT GOES

- The primary symptom of a bladder infection is painful, burning, frequent urination.

- Urinary tract infections are usually caused by bacteria that enter the urethra, typically from the anus. Women tend to get urinary tract infections more often than men because their urethra is shorter and closer to the anus, where bacteria thrive.

- Sexual intercourse can give a woman a urinary tract infection by introducing external bacteria into the urethra.

- Menopause also increases the risk of urinary tract infections because the increased thinness and dryness of the tissues in the vagina and urethra make them more vulnerable to infection.

- A bladder infection, medically known as cystitis, is usually caused by *Escherichia coli* (*E. coli*) bacteria that have migrated up the urinary tract to the bladder.

- To help flush bacteria from your urinary tract, drink eight 8-ounce glasses of water every day. The more water you drink, the more bacteria you flush out.

- Washing your genital area with soap and water before engaging in sex can help prevent bacteria from being inadvertently pushed into the urethra. And urinating immediately after sex washes any trespassing bacteria from the urethra.

- To prevent urinary tract infections, when using the bathroom, wipe from front to back to avoid pushing anal bacteria toward the urethra.

- If you are prone to urinary tract infections, use sanitary pads instead of tampons, and change the pad each time you use the bathroom. Some doctors believe tampons increase the likelihood of infections.

- Do not douche or use feminine hygiene sprays or powders. These products irritate the tissues in the urethra and vagina, creating the perfect environment for a urinary tract infection.

- To prevent bacteria from thriving, do not sit around in a wet bathing suit.

- **McCormick Garlic Powder.** Place one teaspoon McCormick Garlic Powder in a cup of boiling water, cover with a saucer, and steep for ten minutes. Sip the garlic tea. Garlic contains strong antibacterial compounds.

- **Ocean Spray Craisins.** To prevent urinary tract infections, eat one-third cup Ocean Spray Craisins daily. A 1998 study at Rutgers University showed that the antioxidants in dried cranberries hinder the growth of the tendrils that *E. coli* bacteria use to attach to the lining of the urethra.

- **Ocean Spray Cranberry Juice Cocktail.** To treat a urinary tract infection, drink an eight-ounce glass of Ocean Spray Cranberry Juice Cocktail three times a day. Components of cranberry juice—proanthocyanidins—inhibit the growth of the tendrils that *E. coli* bacteria use to attach to the lining of the urethra. To prevent a urinary tract infection, drink an eight-ounce glass of cranberry juice daily.

- **Uncle Ben's Converted Brand Rice.** Fill a sock with Uncle Ben's Converted Brand Rice, tie a knot in the end, and heat in the microwave for ninety seconds. Place the warm sock on your lower abdomen, allowing the heat to relieve cramping or pain from a urinary tract infection. The homemade heating pad can be reused repeatedly.

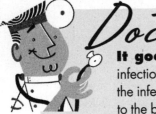

Doctor's Orders

It goes without saying! At the first sign of a urinary tract infection, see your doctor for a prescription for antibiotics to prevent the infection from spreading to the bladder and kidneys. If, in addition to the burning sensation and constant need to urinate, you get a fever, chills, or nausea, contact your doctor to rule out a kidney infection.

Vaginal Dryness

- **Chicken of the Sea Salmon, Chicken of the Sea Sardines,** or **Chicken of the Sea Tuna.** To reduce vaginal dryness, eat salmon, sardines, or tuna three times a week to add the fatty acids commonly known as omega-3 oils to your diet. These fatty acids help the body retain estrogen, which keeps vaginal tissues moist.

- **Corn Huskers Lotion.** This inexpensive hand lubricant, developed in Iowa to moisturize hands roughened by harvesting crops, doubles as a vaginal lubricant. (According to William Masters, Virginia Johnson, and Robert Kolodny in their 1995 book *Human Sexuality,* Corn Huskers Lotion is a water-based lubricant that can be used with a condom without weakening the latex rubber and causing it to break.)

- **Dynasty Sesame Seed Oil, Tampax Tampons,** and **Stayfree Maxi Pads.** Dampen a Tampax Tampon with Dynasty Sesame Seed Oil and insert it into the vagina overnight to relieve dryness. Wear a Stayfree Maxi Pad to absorb any oil that may seep out. Repeat nightly for one week until dryness subsides, and then repeat once a week or as needed.

- **Fruit of the Earth Aloe Vera Gel.** To alleviate vaginal dryness, apply Fruit of the Earth Aloe Vera Gel to the dry or inflamed skin around the vagina. Aloe vera gel is a soothing moisturizer.

- **K-Y Jelly.** To compensate for the vaginal dryness caused by low estrogen levels, use a water-soluble lubricant like K-Y Jelly. Avoid petroleum-based lubricants like Vaseline Petroleum Jelly, which can cause further irritation.

- **Silk Soymilk.** To ease vaginal dryness, add more soy foods to your diet, such as two 8-ounce glasses of Silk Soymilk every day. Soy isoflavones somewhat mimic the action of estrogen and may help alleviate vaginal dryness, according to the National Institutes of Health. Two 8-ounce glasses of soymilk contain 25 milligrams of soy isoflavones.

℞ STRANGE MEDICINE ℞

AN INSIDE JOB

- During and after menopause, reduced estrogen production causes physical changes in the vagina, most notably a decrease in natural lubrication, which can make intercourse painful.

- Other common causes of vaginal dryness are birth control pills, childbirth, breast-feeding, age, and vaginal infections.

- To increase vaginal lubrication, keep yourself well hydrated by drinking eight 8-ounce glasses of water every day.

- Douching can cause inflammation and dryness, exacerbating the problem.

- If you smoke, quit. Smoking depletes estrogen from the body, making vaginal dryness more pronounced.

- Remaining sexually active improves vaginal lubrication and keeps the tissues fit.

- **Star Olive Oil.** To use Star Olive Oil as a lubricant, apply topically to the vagina. The olive oil also moisturizes the dry tissues. (Do not use olive oil with a condom. Oil-based lubricants weaken the latex rubber of condoms and can cause them to break.)

- **Wesson Canola Oil.** Using one tablespoon Wesson Canola Oil in your food every day can help add lubrication to vaginal tissues. The omega-3 fatty acids in canola oil help the body retain estrogen. Canola oil can also be used as a topical lubricant. (Do not use canola oil with a condom. The oil weakens the latex rubber and can cause the condom to break.)

Doctor's Orders

Think outside the box! If vaginal dryness is accompanied by bleeding or severe itching, see a gynecologist to rule out more serious problems.

Varicose Veins

- **Dickinson's Witch Hazel.** To relieve the pain of varicose veins, chill a bottle of Dickinson's Witch Hazel in the refrigerator, saturate a clean dish towel or thin hand towel with the cold witch hazel, lie down with your legs elevated, and wrap the wet towel over the affected area. Let sit until the towel dries. Repeat as frequently as necessary. The astringent tannins in the witch hazel soothe the pain.

- **Heinz Apple Cider Vinegar.** A popular folk remedy for easing the pain of varicose veins calls for saturating a clean dish towel or thin hand towel with Heinz Apple Cider Vinegar, elevating your legs, wrapping them in the wet towel, and then soaking for thirty minutes—twice a day for six weeks.

- **Kellogg's All-Bran.** To help prevent varicose veins, eat one cup Kellogg's All-Bran every morning. One cup of Kellogg's All-Bran contains 20 grams of fiber, and consuming 20 to 35 grams of fiber daily helps prevent you from straining to pass a bowel movement, which puts pressure on the veins in your lower legs, promoting the gradual formation of varicose veins. Fiber absorbs water, making your stools softer, larger, and more regular. A daily minimum of five servings of fruits and vegetables, three servings of whole-

STRANGE MEDICINE

THROUGH THICK AND THIN

- Varicose veins are dark-blue, gnarled, enlarged veins that bulge through the skin, usually in the legs and feet.

- Varicose veins are usually painless, but if they do cause pain, common symptoms generally include achiness, burning, throbbing, and swelling.

- Spider veins are much smaller than varicose veins, appear closer to the skin's surface, and look like a spider's web (hence the name). Usually red and blue, spider veins typically occur on the legs and sometimes on the face.

- The common cause of varicose veins seems to be heredity and hormones. Age, weight, pregnancy, and working on your feet aggravate the condition.

- To ease the pain of varicose veins and prevent them from getting worse, exercise (to improve circulation), maintain a healthy weight (to avoid putting excess pressure on your legs), wear loose-fitting clothes (to avoid restricting circulation), elevate your legs (to reduce pressure on your veins), and avoiding standing or sitting for long periods of time (to encourage blood flow).

- If you or a loved one develops varicose veins during pregnancy, fear not. They generally go away without medical treatment within a year after delivery.

grain foods, and one serving of beans puts enough fiber in your diet to prevent constipation.

- **L'eggs Sheer Energy Panty Hose.** To prevent your varicose veins from swelling, put on a pair of L'eggs Sheer Energy Active Support Panty Hose in the morning. Support hose exert pressure along the entire length of the leg, pushing the blood away from the skin and into the deeper veins.
- **McCormick Rosemary Leaves.** To strengthen your veins and relieve the strain, frequently add McCormick Rosemary Leaves to foods, like chicken,

lamb, and beans. Or make rosemary tea by placing a tea infuser filled with one teaspoon McCormick Rosemary Leaves in a teacup, covering with boiling water, covering with a saucer, and steeping for fifteen to twenty minutes. Drink two cups a day (unless you're pregnant). Diosmin, a compound in rosemary, strengthens capillaries and is a synthetic ingredient in drugs prescribed for varicose veins.

- **Ocean Spray Craisins.** To help prevent varicose veins, eat one-third cup Ocean Spray Craisins daily. A 2006 study at Creighton University School of Medicine showed that the antioxidant compounds in dried cranberries prevent the growth of blood vessels.

Doctor's Orders

See yourself though it! If you're concerned about how your veins look or you're unable to ease the pain, see your doctor.

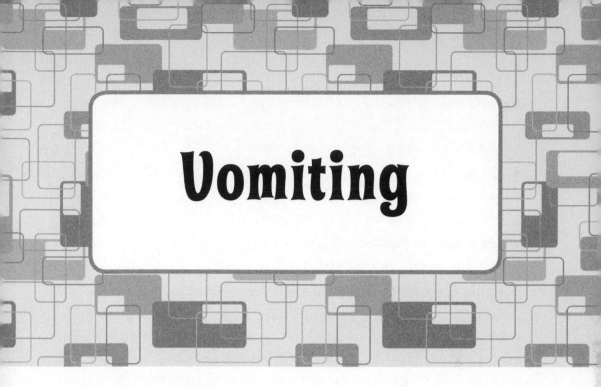

Vomiting

- **Canada Dry Ginger Ale.** After a bout of vomiting, drinking flat Canada Dry Ginger Ale helps settle your stomach. The ginger seems to relax the muscles in the stomach. Contrary to popular belief, Canada Dry Ginger Ale does indeed contain genuine ginger, included in the list of ingredients as "natural flavors." (Do not drink ginger ale if you have gallstones. Ginger can increase bile production.)

- **Coca-Cola.** Drinking flat Coca-Cola helps settle your queasy stomach. Pharmacies sell cola syrup that can be taken in small doses to relieve nausea. The concentrated sugars are believed to relax the gastrointestinal tract. Letting the bubbles out of the soda prevents the carbonation from further upsetting your stomach.

- **Domino Sugar** and **Morton Salt.** To replace the salts and fluid lost from vomiting and avoid dehydration, dissolve eight teaspoons Domino Sugar and one teaspoon Morton Salt in one quart of water, and drink the entire solution at your own pace. The rehydration cocktail replaces the electrolytes you've lost.

- **Gatorade.** To refortify your body with liquid and electrolytes after a bout of vomiting, drink Gatorade to quickly replace essential nutrients and minerals, preventing muscle spasms in your stomach.

- **Jell-O.** After reintroducing your shaky stomach to bland foods like crackers and toast, graduate onto more substantial (but equally tame) foods like Jell-O gelatin, which is high in carbohydrates.

- **Knorr Chicken Bouillon.** To replace the liquid, salts, and minerals depleted by vomiting, eat a cup of Knorr Chicken Bouillon.

- **Lipton Chamomile Tea** and **Lipton Peppermint Tea.** To prevent vomiting, place one Lipton Chamomile Tea bag and one Lipton Peppermint Tea bag in the same cup, fill with boiling water, cover with a saucer, steep for ten minutes, and drink. The plant compounds in chamomile seem to reduce the gag reflex, and peppermint eases digestion and prevents the spasms that cause vomiting. (Coumarin, an anticoagulant in chamomile, may increase the likelihood of bleeding when taken in combination with the blood thinner Coumadin or other anticoagulant medications.)

- **McCormick Ground Cinnamon** and **McCormick Ground Ginger.** To combat vomiting caused by food poisoning, mix one teaspoon McCormick Ground Cinnamon and one-half teaspoon McCormick Ground Ginger in a tea cup, add boiling water, cover with a saucer, and steep for fifteen minutes. Strain and then sip the tea. The cinnamon can help kill the responsible bacteria, and the ginger quells stomach spasms. (Do not use ginger if you have gallstones. Ginger can increase bile production.)

- **Mott's Applesauce.** Once the vomiting subsides, eat Mott's Applesauce. The pectin in the applesauce is a soluble fiber that absorbs fluid in your intestines and helps solidify soft bowel movements. Applesauce also contains malic acid and quercetin, which help inhibit harmful bacteria in your stomach that may be causing nausea.

- **Nabisco Original Premium Saltine Crackers.** When your stomach begins to settle, start with bland foods like Nabisco Original Premium

Saltine Crackers. The light carbohydrates give you energy, and the crackers absorb excess stomach acid.

- **Popsicle.** If you can't keep any food down after vomiting, suck on your favorite flavor Popsicle to replace lost sugars and rehydrate yourself.

- **Uncle Ben's Converted Brand Rice.** Once the vomiting subsides, eat small portions of plain, white Uncle Ben's Converted Brand Rice. The starch in rice helps absorb excess stomach acid.

℞ STRANGE MEDICINE ℞

ENDURING UPHEAVAL

- Vomiting forces the contents of the stomach—partially digested food or liquid mixed with digestive juices (gastric acid)—up through your esophagus to exit through your mouth. Vomit contains a high concentration of hydronium, a strong acid secreted by the stomach.

- Vomiting occurs naturally after nausea reaches an intolerable level. If you're feeling nauseous, do not use emetics or direct stimulation of the gag reflex to induce vomiting. Simply stop fighting the nausea, relax, breathe deeply, and let nature take its course.

- If you're feeling nauseous, drinking a glass of water or two may help trigger vomiting by giving the stomach something to regurgitate.

- Before stomach spasms trigger vomiting, the mouth salivates excessively. Hypersalivation allows saliva to coat the teeth to protect them from the acidity of vomit.

- Bile, which breaks down the food in the stomach, often gets pushed up with vomit. Produced by the liver, bile makes vomit taste bitter and gives it a greenish yellow color.

- Common causes of vomiting include food allergies, food poisoning, gastroesophageal reflux, medications or medical treatments (such as chemotherapy or radiation treatment), migraine headaches, morning sickness, motion sickness, and stomach viruses.

- After vomiting, do not eat or drink for one hour—to avoid a recurrent attack. After a few hours, drink fluids, and then gradually introduce gentle, easily digestible foods.

- **Wonder Bread.** To help yourself recover from a bout of vomiting, transition slowly to solid foods by starting with some slices of toasted Wonder Bread, which are easy to digest and provide starch.

- **Ziploc Storage Bags.** Need barf bags? Keep several gallon-size Ziploc Freezer Bags handy to use as barf bags. Afterwards, simply seal the bag shut and discard appropriately in the trash.

Doctor's Orders

Bring it up! If vomiting persists for more than twenty-four hours, or you have a fever or headache, consult a doctor. If your vomit contains digested blood (which looks like dark coffee grounds), contact your physician. If the vomit contains fresh blood, call 911 or get to an emergency room for immediate treatment.

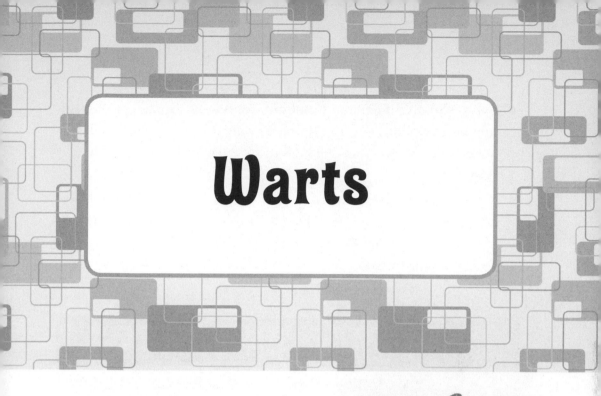

Warts

- **Crayola Chalk.** Rub a piece of Crayola Chalk on the wart once a day to create a thick coat. The chalk dries out the wart, killing the virus.

- **Duck Tape.** Cover the wart with a small piece of Duck Tape, and leave it alone for one week. Remove the Duck Tape, soak the affected area in warm water for five minutes, and gently file off the dead skin with an emery board. The next morning, cover the remaining wart with another small piece of Duck Tape, and repeat the process until it vanishes. The Duck Tape 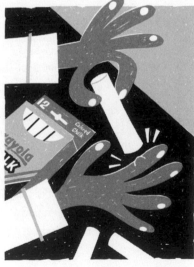 apparently irritates the skin just enough to trigger your immune system to combat the virus.

- **Fruit of the Earth Aloe Vera Gel.** To dissolve a wart, rub a dab of Fruit of the Earth Aloe Vera Gel on the protrusion. The malic acid in the aloe vera gel apparently does the trick.

- **Heinz White Vinegar** and **Band-Aid Bandages.** Saturate a cotton ball with Heinz White Vinegar, and tape it firmly over the wart with a Band-Aid Bandage for one hour. Do this daily until the acetic acid in the vinegar dissolves the wart.

- **Kretschmer Wheat Germ.** To prevent warts and help your immune system fight off existing ones, sprinkle a few tablespoons of Kretschmer Wheat Germ on your morning bowl of oatmeal. The vitamin E, B vitamins, magnesium, potassium, iron, and zinc in wheat germ boost the immune system.

℞ STRANGE MEDICINE ℞

A GROWING EXPERIENCE

- Warts—small, pale, benign skin tumors with a grainy surface—usually grow on the fingers or hands.

- Caused by the human papillomavirus, warts are transmitted by touch—from person to person, from used towel to person, or from you to yourself.

- Common warts tend to disappear on their own within two years.

- A dermatologist can remove warts by freezing them with liquid nitrogen or burning them off with a laser or an electric needle.

- To avoid spreading the virus that causes warts, do not brush, comb, or shave over a wart. If you use a nail file or pumice stone to reduce the size of a wart, do not use the same tools on other areas of your body. Do not pick at a wart with your fingers. If you do touch a wart, wash your hands with soap and water immediately afterwards.

- Warts do not have roots that grow deep into the skin.

- Plantar warts grow on the bottom of feet and can feel like you're stepping on a tack.

- To prevent plantar warts, wear flip-flops when using public showers, locker rooms, swimming pools, and other facilities to avoid foot contact with the virus.

- **Libby's Pumpkin.** To fight off warts, use canned Libby's Pumpkin to cook up pumpkin bread, pumpkin pie, or pumpkin muffins. The high amount of vitamin A in pumpkin boosts the ability of lymphocytes to fight off infections.

- **McCormick Garlic Powder, Vaseline Petroleum Jelly,** and **Band-Aid Bandages.** Mix one-half teaspoon McCormick Garlic Powder with enough water to make a thick paste, smear the skin surrounding the wart with a thin coat of Vaseline Petroleum Jelly, apply the paste to the wart, and cover with a Band-Aid Bandage. Replace with fresh paste and bandage daily. The wart will decompose within a week or two.

- **McCormick Meat Tenderizer** and **Band-Aid Bandages.** Mix one-half teaspoon McCormick Meat Tenderizer with enough water to make a thick paste, apply the paste to the wart, and cover with a Band-Aid Bandage. Replace with fresh paste and bandage daily. The enzyme papain in the meat tenderizer dissolves the dead skin.

- **Quaker Oats.** To fight warts, eat a bowl of Quaker Oats oatmeal every day for breakfast. The beta-glucan in oats boosts the immune system, prompting white blood cells to battle the infection.

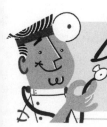

Doctor's Orders

Pluck up your courage! If you're over age forty-five and a wart suddenly appears on your skin, consult a doctor to rule out cancer.

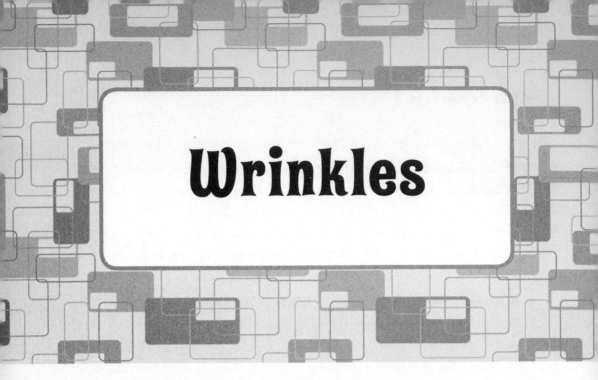

Wrinkles

- **Campbell's Tomato Soup** and **Gold Medal Flour.** To minimize wrinkles, mix together the contents of one can of Campbell's Tomato Soup with enough Gold Medal Flour to make a thick paste. Apply the paste to the face and neck, wait fifteen minutes, and then rinse clean with warm water. The acids from the tomatoes balance the pH level of the skin, exfoliate dead skin, and tighten pores.

- **Chicken of the Sea Salmon, Chicken of the Sea Sardines,** or **Chicken of the Sea Tuna.** To nourish your skin and prevent wrinkles, eat salmon, sardines, or tuna three times a week to add the fatty acids commonly known as omega-3 oils to your diet. These fatty acids help reduce inflammation, strengthen the immune system, and keep your skin moist and supple.

- **Country Time Lemonade.** Mix one tablespoon Country Time Lemonade powder with enough water to make a thick paste. Massage the lemony paste over your face (avoiding your eyes), wait five minutes, then rinse clean. The gritty paste and citric acid help exfoliate dead skin, leaving your face smooth and soft. (Using citric acid on your skin makes you more prone to sunburn, so be sure to use sunscreen afterwards.)

- **Crisco All-Vegetable Shortening.** Applying Crisco All-Vegetable Shortening as a salve on your face and hands every night before going to bed moisturizes the skin, keeping it soft, smooth, and healthy.

- **Fruit of the Earth Aloe Vera Gel.** To reduce the appearance of wrinkles, apply Fruit of the Earth Aloe Vera Gel to your face. The malic acid, a natural humectant, keeps the skin hydrated throughout the day, hiding wrinkles.

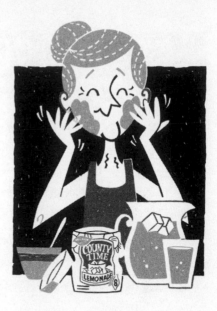

- **Gerber Carrots** and **SueBee Honey.** For normal or oily skin, mix five ounces (one small container) Gerber Carrots with five tablespoons SueBee Honey. Apply this antioxidant mask to your face, wait fifteen minutes, and then rinse clean.

- **Gerber Peaches, SueBee Honey,** and **Quaker Oats.** For normal skin, mix five ounces (one small container) Gerber Peaches, one tablespoon Sue-Bee Honey, and enough Quaker Oats to create a thick paste. Apply to your face, wait ten minutes, and then rinse well with cool water. Peaches contain large amounts of alpha-hydroxy acids, which gently exfoliate skin, accelerating cell renewal, leading to healthier skin tone. Alpha-hydroxy acids also help soften wrinkles.

- **Lubriderm.** To hide smaller wrinkles temporarily, rub Lubriderm into your face once a day. The moisturizer plumps up your skin by sealing in moisture, concealing small wrinkles.

- **McCormick Meat Tenderizer** and **Kingsford's Corn Starch.** To exfoliate the top layer of skin, mix two tablespoons McCormick Meat Tenderizer, one tablespoon Kingsford's Corn Starch, and enough water to make a paste,

READING BETWEEN THE LINES

● As people age, hormone levels decrease, causing the sebaceous glands to produce less sebum oil to nourish the skin, increasing fine lines and wrinkles.

● UVA rays from the sun penetrate the dermis, cracking and shrinking the collagen and elastin, causing the epidermis to prematurely wrinkle and sag. UVB rays penetrate the epidermis and cause most skin cancers.

● Moisturizers help keep skin soft and hydrated, and facial scrubs exfoliate dead skin cells and stimulate cell renewal.

● Drink eight 8-ounce glasses of water every day to help keep your skin cells hydrated.

● Eating fruits and vegetables helps fight off free radicals—molecules that destroy body tissue and cause wrinkling, sagging, and age spots.

● Vitamin C helps the body form collagen, the gluey fibers that hold skin taut. The best way to get vitamin C into the body is by eating fresh fruits and vegetables. The skin does not necessarily absorb topical applications of vitamin C deeply enough to affect collagen production. However, vitamin C is also an antioxidant, and stable topical formulations, applied directly to the skin, protect it from ultraviolet damage caused by prolonged sun exposure.

● If you smoke, quit. Smoking causes your skin to age faster.

● To prevent wrinkles, protect your skin from the sun. At least thirty minutes before going outdoors, apply sunscreen or a moisturizing product with a built-in sun protection factor (SPF) of at least 30 that blocks both UVA and UVB rays. Limit the amount of time you spend in the sun, and wear long pants, long sleeves, a wide-brimmed hat, and sunglasses.

● To prevent sun damage to your skin, stay out of the sun between 10 a.m. and 4 p.m., when the sun's rays are strongest.

● Steer clear of tanning beds, booths, or lamps. "Indoor tanning" increases the risk of wrinkles and leads to skin and eye cancer, according to a 2006 review by the International Agency for Research on Cancer of nineteen studies conducted over twenty-five years. The review also found that people who begin using tanning beds before age thirty-five increase their risk of melanoma by 75 percent.

and apply the mixture to your skin. Let sit for ten minutes, and then scrub clean with a washcloth. The enzyme papain in the meat tenderizer etches away the outer layer of skin, diminishing the appearance of wrinkles. The cornstarch helps remove debris from the skin.

- **Nestlé Carnation Nonfat Dry Milk.** Mix one-half cup Nestlé Carnation Nonfat Dry Milk powder with enough water to make a thick paste, and spread it on your face. Let sit for ten minutes, and then wash clean with warm water, followed by cool water. The alpha-hydroxy acids exfoliate dead skin cells, counteract free radicals, and encourage collagen growth.

- **Nestlé Carnation Nonfat Dry Milk** and **ReaLemon.** In a saucepan, mix three ounces Carnation Nonfat Dry Milk powder and one cup of water. Add two teaspoons ReaLemon lemon juice and stir well. Bring to a boil, then let cool until warm to the touch. Use a pastry brush to paint the mixture over your face and neck. Let dry, then rinse with warm water. The lactic acid in the milk and the alpha-hydroxy acids in the milk and lemon juice exfoliate dead skin, erasing wrinkles.

- **Preparation H.** Rub a small dab of Preparation H over wrinkles and puffy areas (avoiding the eyes) to tighten skin and make fine lines vanish for several hours. Once the hemorrhoid ointment dries, you can actually apply makeup over it.

- **SunGuard.** Clothes do not fully absorb the ultraviolet (UV) rays of the sun, which, over time, cause wrinkles. A typical white t-shirt, for example, has an ultraviolet protection factor (UPF) rating of 5 or less. To help stop UV rays from penetrating your clothing, add SunGuard to your washing machine when laundering clothes. SunGuard infuses your clothes with a UV protectant that gives the fabric a UPF rating of 30, helping to prevent 96 percent of the sun's UV rays from reaching your skin. The protection lasts for up to twenty washings.

Yeast Infections

- **Conair Hair Dryer.** To help combat a yeast infection, after taking a shower or bath, set a Conair Hair Dryer on the coolest setting and hold it roughly twelve inches from your crotch to dry the moist area.

- **Dannon Yogurt.** To help kill a yeast infection, eat a cup of Dannon Nonfat Yogurt daily. Studies show that *Lactobacillus acidophilus* or *bifidobacterium* (probiotics) in yogurt help replenish the beneficial bacteria in your digestive system that fight the parasitic *Candida albicans* fungus causing the yeast infection.

- **Dannon Yogurt** and **Tampax Tampons.** Applying *Lactobacillus acidophilus,* the live culture in yogurt, directly to a yeast infection can help cure the ailment. Dip a clean, unused Tampax Tampon in a cup of Dannon Plain Nonfat Yogurt, and insert the yogurt-coated tampon into the vagina. Remove after thirty minutes, and do this three or four times a day. The *Lactobacillus acidophilus* (probiotics) produce lactic acid, creating an inhospitable environment for the *Candida albicans* fungus.

- **Heinz White Vinegar.** To cure a yeast infection, mix two tablespoons Heinz White Vinegar in a quart of water, and douche with the solution twice a day for two days in a row. The vinegar increases the acidity in the vagina, creating an inhospitable environment for the fungus to thrive.

- **McCormick Cinnamon Sticks.** To fight off a yeast infection, break eight to ten McCormick Cinnamon Sticks in half, drop them into four cups of boiling water, cover, and let simmer for fifteen minutes. Remove from the heat and let steep, covered, for 45 minutes. Let cool, strain out the cinnamon sticks, and douche with the tea. The medicinal cinnamon oil is an antifungal that destroys *Candida albicans*.

- **McCormick Garlic Powder.** Spice sauces, salads, and other foods with McCormick Garlic Powder to battle a yeast infection. Garlic is an antifungal that can help eliminate *Candida albicans*.

- **Morton Salt.** To expedite the healing, reduce the itching, and minimize the pain of a yeast infection, dissolve one cup Morton Salt in a bathtub filled with warm water, and soak for twenty minutes daily.

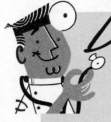

Doctor's Orders

Rise up! If you experience the symptoms of a yeast infection for the first time, see a doctor to rule out a more serious problem. If a yeast infection fails to go away after a few days of home treatment, or if the symptoms get worse, consult your doctor.

Acknowledgments

At Rodale, I am grateful to my editor, Karen Bolesta, for her passion, enthusiasm, and excitement for this book. I am also deeply indebted to my agent Stephanie Tade, researcher Debbie Green, senior project editor Hope Clarke, designer Chris Rhoads, and ace illustrator Glen Mullaly. A very special thank-you for my manager, Barb North, and the hundreds of people who visit my website and take the time to send me emails sharing their ingenious tips for brand-name products we all know and love.

Above all, all my love to Debbie, Ashley, and Julia.

Bibliography

- "Acne Vulgaris, Mental Health and Omega-3 Fatty Acids: A Report of Cases" by Mark G. Rubin, Katherine Kim, and Alan C. Logan, *Lipids in Health and Disease,* October 13, 2008, Volume 7, Number 36

- *Age-Defying Beauty Secrets* by Diane Irons (Naperville, Illinois: Sourcebooks, 2003)

- "Aged Garlic Extract Lowers Blood Pressure in Patients with Treated but Uncontrolled Hypertension: A Randomised Controlled Trial" by Karin Ried, Oliver R. Frank, and Nigel P. Stocks, *Maturitas,* October 2010, Volume 67, Number 2, pages 144–150

- "Almonds and Almond Oil Have Similar Effects on Plasma Lipids and LDL Oxidation in Healthy Men and Women" by Dianne A. Hyson, Barbara O. Schneeman, and Paul A. Davis, *Journal of Nutrition,* April 1, 2002, Volume 132, Number 4, pages 703–707

- "Almonds *vs.* Complex Carbohydrates in a Weight Reduction Program" by M. A. Wien, J. M. Sabaté, D. N. Iklé, et al., *International Journal of Obesity,* 2003, Volume 27, pages 1365–1372

- *Alternative Cures: The Most Effective Natural Home Remedies for 160 Health Problems* by Bill Gottlieb (Emmaus, Pennsylvania: Rodale, 2000)

- "Amelioration of Severe Migraine by Fish Oil (Omega-3) Fatty Acids" by T. McCarren, R. Hitzemann, C. Allen, et al., *American Journal of Clinical Nutrition,* April 1985, Volume 41, Number 4, page 874

- "Antioxidant Effects of Green Tea and Its Polyphenols on Bladder Cells" by Christian H. Coyle, Brian J. Philips, Shelby N. Morrisroe, et al., *Life Sciences,* July 4, 2008, Volume 83, Numbers 1–2, pages 12–18

- "Aspirin in the Management of Recurrent Herpes Simplex Virus Infection [Letter]" by Istavan Karadi, Sarolta Karpati, and Laszlo Romics, *Annals of Internal Medicine,* April 15, 1998, Volume 128, Number 8, pages 696–697

- "Bacteriologic Analysis of Infected Dog and Cat Bites" by D. A. Talan, D. M. Citron, F. M. Abrahamian, et al., *New England Journal of Medicine,* January 14, 1999, Volume 340, Number 2, pages 85–92

- "Baked Bean Consumption Reduces Serum Cholesterol in Hypercholesterolemic Adults" by Donna Winham and Andrea Hutchins, *Nutrition Research,* July 2007, Volume 27, Number 7, pages 380–386

- *Baking Soda Bonanza* by Peter A. Ciullo (New York: HarperPerrenial, 1995)

- *The Blood Pressure Cure: 8 Weeks to Lower Blood Pressure without Prescription Drugs* by Robert E. Kowalski (Hoboken, New Jersey: John Wiley & Sons, 2007)

- "Caffeine Attenuates Delayed Onset Muscle Pain and Force Loss Following Eccentric Exercise" by Victor Maridakis, Patrick O'Connor, Kevin K. McCully, and Gary A. Dudley, *Journal of Pain,* March 2007, Volume 8, Number 3, pages 237–243

- "Caffeine for Asthma" by Emma J. Walsh, Anna Bara, Elizabeth Barley, and Christopher J. Kates, *Cochrane Database of Systematic Reviews,* January 20, 2010, Number 1, CD001112

- "Calcium Carbonate and the Premenstrual Syndrome: Effects on Premenstrual and Menstrual Symptoms" by S. Thys-Jacobs, P. Starkey, D. Bernstein, and J. Tian, *American Journal of Obstetrics & Gynecology,* August 1998, Volume 179, Number 2, pages 444–452

- "Carvacrol, a Component of Thyme Oil, Activates PPAR-Gamma and Suppresses COX-2 Expression" by Mariko Hotta, Rieko Nakata, Michiko Katsukawa, et al., *Journal of Lipid Research,* January 2010, Volume 51, Number 1, pages 132–139

- "Chewing Gum Alleviates Negative Mood and Reduces Cortisol During Acute Laboratory Psychological Stress" by A. Scholey, C. Haskell, B. Robertson, et al., *Physiology & Behavior,* June 22, 2009, Volume 97, Numbers 3–4, pages 304–312

- "Childhood Asthma and Fruit Consumption" by B. J. Okoko, P. G. Burney, R. B. Newson, et al., *European Respiratory Journal,* June 1, 2007, Volume 29, Number 6, pages 1161–1168

- *Cholesterol Cures: More Than 325 Naturals Ways to Lower Cholesterol and Live Longer* by the editors of *Prevention* health books (Emmaus, Pennsylvania: Rodale, 2002)
- "Cinnamon Improves Glucose and Lipids of People with Type 2 Diabetes" by A. Khan, M. Safdar, M. M. Ali Khan, et al., *Diabetes Care*, December 2003, Volume 26, Number 12, pages 3215–3218
- "Coffee Drinking and Prevalence of Bronchial Asthma" by R. Pagano, E. Negri, A. Decarli, and C. La Vecchia, *Chest*, August 1988, Volume 94, Number 2, pages 386–389
- "Coffee, Tea, and Caffeine Consumption and Serum Uric Acid Level: The Third National Health and Nutrition Examination Survey" by Hyon K. Choi and Gary Curhan, *Arthritis Care & Research*, June 2007, Volume 57, Number 5, pages 816–822
- "A Comparative Study to Evaluate the Effect of Honey Dressing and Silver Sulfadiazine Dressing on Wound Healing in Burn Patients" by P. S. Baghel, S. Sukla, R. K. Mathur, and R.A. Rand, *Indian Journal of Plastic Surgery,* July–December 2009, Volume 42, Number 2, pages 176–181
- "Comparative Value of Orange Juice versus Lemonade in Reducing Stone-Forming Risk" by Clarita V. Odvina, *Clinical Journal of the American Society of Nephrology*, November 2006, Volume 1, Number 6, pages 1269–1274
- "Concentrated Red Grape Juice Exerts Antioxidant, Hypolipidemic, and Antiinflammatory Effects in Both Hemodialysis Patients and Healthy Subjects" by P. Castilla, R. Echarri, A. Dávalos, et al., *American Journal of Clinical Nutrition*, July 2006, Volume 84, Number 1, pages 252–262
- "Concord Grape Juice Reduces Blood Pressure in Men with High Systolic Blood Pressure" by D. Mark and K. Maki, presented at Experimental Biology, San Diego, California, April 11–15, 2003
- "Consumption of Cherries Lowers Plasma Urate in Healthy Women" by Robert A. Jacob, Giovanna M. Spinozzi, Vicky A. Simon, et al., *Journal of Nutrition*, June 1, 2003, Volume 133, Number 6, pages 1826–1829
- "Dark Chocolate May Lower Risk of Heart Disease" by Robert Preidt, *Philadelphia Inquirer*, April 25, 2012
- "Dietary Manipulation with Lemonade to Treat Hypocitraturic Calcium Nephrolithiasis" by M. A. Seltzer, R. K. Low, M. McDonald, et al., *Journal of Urology*, September 1996, Volume 156, Number 3, pages 907–909
- "Dietary N-3 Polyunsaturated Fatty Acids and Smoking-Related Chronic Obstructive Pulmonary Disease" by Eyal Shahar, Aaron R. Folsom, Sandra L. Melnick, et al., *New England Journal of Medicine*, July 28, 1994, Volume 331, Number 4, pages 228–233
- *The Doctors Book of Food Remedies* by the editors of *Prevention* magazine (Emmaus, Pennsylvania: Rodale, 1998)
- *The Doctors Book of Home Remedies: Quick Fixes, Clever Techniques, and Uncommon Cures to Get You Feeling Better Faster* by the editors of *Prevention* magazine (Emmaus, Pennsylvania: Rodale, 2009)
- *The Doctors Book of Home Remedies II: Over 1,200 New Doctor-Tested Tips and Techniques Anyone Can Use to Heal Hundreds of Everyday Health Problems* by Sid Kirchheimer and the editors of *Prevention* health books (Emmaus, Pennsylvania: Rodale, 1993)
- *Doctor's Guide to Natural Medicine: The Complete and Easy-to-Use Natural Health Reference from a Medical Doctor's Perspective* by Paul Barney (Pleasant Grove, Utah: Woodland Publishing, 1998)
- "Double Blind Cross-Over Study of the Efficacy of a Tart Cherry Juice Blend in Treatment of Osteoarthritis (OA) of the Knee" by H. Ralph Schumacher, Sally W. Pullman-Mooar, Smita R. Gupta, et al., *Arthritis & Rheumatism*, November 2011, Volume 63, Supplement 10, page 1092
- "Ear Candles—Efficacy and Safety" by D. R. Seely, S. M. Quigley, and A. W. Langman, *Laryngoscope,* October 1996, Volume 106, Number 10, pages 1226–1229
- "Effect of Physical Activity on Menopausal Symptoms of Urban Women" by Deborah B. Nelson, Mary D. Sammel, Ellen W. Freeman, et al., *Medicine & Science in Sports & Exercise*, January 2008, Volume 40, Number 1, pages 50–58
- "Effect of Plants Used in Mexico to Treat Gastrointestinal Disorders on Charcoal-Gum Acacia-Induced Hyperperistalsis in Rats" by F. Calzada, R. Arista, and H. Pérez, *Journal of Ethnopharmacology*, March 2, 2010, Volume 128, Number 1, pages 49–51

- "Effect of Rinsing Time on Antiplaque-Antigingivitis Efficacy of Listerine" by Norton M. Ross, Suru M. Mankodi, Karen L. Mostler, et al., *Journal of Clinical Periodontology*, April 1993, Volume 20, Number 4, pages 279–281

- "The Effect of Vitamin E on Hot Flashes in Menopausal Women" by S. Ziaei, A. Kazemnejad, and M. Zareai, *Gynecologic and Obstetric Investigation*, November 2007, Volume 64, Number 4, pages 204–207

- "Effects of Apple Cider Vinegars Produced with Different Techniques on Blood Lipids in High-Cholesterol-Fed Rats" by N. H. Budak, D. Kumbul Doguc, C. M. Savas, et al., *Journal of Agricultural and Food Chemistry*, June 22, 2011, Volume 59, Number 12, pages 6638–6644

- "The Effects of Grapefruit Pectin on Patients at Risk for Coronary Heart Disease without Altering Diet or Lifestyle" by J. J. Cerda, F. L. Robbins, C. W. Burgin, et al., *Clinical Cardiology,* September 1988, Volume 11, Number 9, pages 589–594

- "Effects of Magnesium Hydroxide in Renal Stone Disease" by G. Johansson, U. Backman, B. G. Danielson, et al., *Journal of the American College of Nutrition*, 1982, Volume 1, Number 2, pages 179–185

- "The Effects of Odors on Penile Blood-Flow—A Possible Impotence Treatment" by Alan R. Hirsch and J. J. Kim, *Psychosomatic Medicine*, 1995, Volume 57, Number 1, page 83

- "The Effects of Tea on Psychophysiological Stress Responsivity and Post-Stress Recovery: A Randomised Double-Blind Trial" by Andrew Steptoe, E. Leigh Gibson, Raisa Vounonvirta, et al., *Psychopharmacology*, January 2007, Volume 190, Number 1, pages 81–89

- "Effects of Walnut Consumption on Blood Lipids and Other Cardiovascular Risk Factors: A Meta-Analysis and Systematic Review" by Deirdre K. Banel and Frank B. Hu, *American Journal of Clinical Nutrition*, May 20, 2009, Volume 90, Number 1, pages 56–63

- "Efficacy of Cranberry Juice on *Helicobacter Pylori* Infection: A Double-Blind, Randomized Placebo-Controlled Trial" by L. Shang, J. Ma, K. Pan, et al., *Helicobacter*, April 2005, Volume 10, Number 2, pages 139–145

- "The Efficacy of Topical 2% Green Tea Lotion in Mild-to-Moderate Acne Vulgaris" by M. L. Elsaie, M. F. Abdelhamid, L. T. Elsaaiee, and H. M. Emam, *Journal of Drugs in Dermatology*, April 2009, Volume 8, Number 4, pages 358–364

- "Enhancement of Learning and Memory by Elevating Brain Magnesium" by Inna Slutsky, Nashat Abumaria, Long-Jun Wu, et al., *Neuron*, January 28, 2010, Volume 65, Number 2, 165–177

- "Extracted or Synthesized Soybean Isoflavones Reduce Menopausal Hot Flash Frequency and Severity: Systematic Review and Meta-Analysis of Randomized Controlled Trials" by Kyoko Taku, Melissa Melby, Fredi Kronenberg, et al., *Menopause,* July 2012, Volume 19, Number 7, pages 776–790

- *The Fatigue Solution: Increase Your Energy in Eight Easy Steps* by Eva Cwynar with Sharyn Kolberg (Carlsbad, California: Hay House, 2012)

- "Favourable Impact of Low-Calorie Cranberry Juice Consumption on Plasma HDL-Cholesterol Concentrations in Men" by Guillaume Ruel, Sonia Pomerleau, Patrick Couture, et al., *British Journal of Nutrition*, August 2006, Volume 96, pages 357–364

- "Flavonoid-Rich Cocoa Consumption Affects Multiple Cardiovascular Risk Factors in a Meta-Analysis of Short-Term Studies" by M. G. Shrime, S. R. Bauer, A. C. McDonald, et al., *Journal of Nutrition*, November 2011, Volume 141, Number 11, pages 1982–1988

- *Folk Remedies That Work* by Joan Wilen and Lydia Wilen (New York: HarperCollins, 1996)

- *Food: Your Miracle Medicine* by Jean Carper (New York: HarperTorch, 1998)

- "For Muscle Cramps, There's No Good Cure" by Thomas H. Maugh II, *Los Angeles Times*, February 23, 2010

- "Ginkgo Biloba for Preventing Cognitive Decline in Older Adults: A Randomized Trial" by Beth E. Snitz, Ellen S. O'Meara, Michelle C. Carlson, et al., *Journal of the American Medical Association*, December 23, 2009, Volume 302, Number 24, pages 2663–2670

- *The Green Pharmacy: New Discoveries in Herbal Remedies for Common Diseases and Conditions from the World's Foremost Authority on Healing Herbs* by James A. Duke (New York: St. Martin's Press, 1997)

- "HDL-Cholesterol-Raising Effect of Orange Juice in Subjects with Hypercholesterolemia" by Elzbieta M. Kurowska, J. David Spence, John Jordan, et al., *American Journal of Clinical Nutrition*, November 2000, Volume 72, Number 5, pages 1095–1100

- *The Healing Powers of Honey* by Cal Orey (New York: Kensington Books, 2011)

- *The Health Benefits of Cayenne* by John Heinerman (New York: McGraw-Hill, 1999)

- "Hiccups: Causes and Cures" by J. H. Lewis, *Journal of Clinical Gastroenterology*, December 1985, Volume 7, Number 6, pages 539–552

- "A High Molecular Mass Constituent of Cranberry Juice Inhibits *Helicobacter Pylori* Adhesion to Human Gastric Mucus" by Ora Burger, Itzhak Ofek, Mina Tabak, et al., *FEMS Immunology and Medical Microbiology*, December 2000, Volume 29, pages 295–301

- "Higher Serum Folate Levels Are Associated with a Lower Risk of Atopy and Wheeze" by Elizabeth C. Matsui and William Matsui, *Journal of Allergy and Clinical Immunology,* June 2009, Volume 123, Number 6, pages 1253–1259

- "Histatins Are the Major Wound-Closure Stimulating Factors in Human Saliva as Identified in a Cell Culture Assay" by Menno J. Oudhoff, Jan G. M. Bolscher, Kamran Nazmi, et al., *FASEB Journal*, November 1, 2008, Volume 22, Number 1, pages 3805–3812

- *Home Remedies* by Dr. Rekha Deshpandey (London, England: ibs Books, 2008)

- *Home Remedies from A to Z* by Tanja Hirschsteiner (Hauppauge, New York: Barron's Educational Series, 2000)

- *Home Remedies from the Country Doctor* by Jay Heinrichs, Dorothy Heinrichs, and the editors of *Yankee* magazine (Emmaus, Pennsylvania: Rodale, 1999)

- *Home Remedies: What Works: Thousands of Americans Reveal Their Favorite Home-Tested Cures for Everyday Health Problems* by Gale Maleskey, Brian Kaufman, and the editors of *Prevention* health books (Emmaus, Pennsylvania: Rodale, 1995)

- "Honey in the Treatment of Infantile Gastroenteritis" by I. E. Haffejee and A. Moosa, *British Medical Journal,* June 22, 1985, Volume 290, pages 1866–1867

- "How Many Days of Bed Rest for Acute Low Back Pain? A Randomized Clinical Trial" by R. A. Deyo, A. K. Diehl, and M. Rosenthal, *New England Journal of Medicine*, October 23, 1986, Volume 315, Number 17, pages 1064–1070

- *Human Sexuality* by William Masters, Virginia Johnson, and Robert C. Kolodny (New York: HarperCollins, 1995)

- "Inhibiting Interspecies Coaggregation of Plaque Bacteria with a Cranberry Juice Constituent" by El Weise, R. Lev-Dor, Y. Kashamn, et al., *Journal of the American Dental Association*, December 1998, Volume 129, Number 12, pages 1719–1723

- "Inhibition of the Adherence of P-Fimbriated *Escherichia coli* to Uroepithelial-Cell Surfaces by Proanthocyanidin Extracts from Cranberries" by Amy B. Howell, Ara Der Marderosian, and Lai Yeap Foo, *New England Journal of Medicine*, October 8, 1998, Volume 339, pages 1085–1086

- "Investigating the Antimicrobial Activity of Natural Honey and Its Effects on the Pathogenic Bacterial Infections of Surgical Wounds and Conjunctiva" by N. S. Al-Waili, *Journal of Medicinal Food*, Summer 2004, Volume 7, Number 2, pages 210–222

- "Isolation and Characterization of Two Antimicrobial Agents from Mace (*Myristica fragrans*)" by K. Y. Orabi, J. S. Mossa, and F. S. el-Feraly, *Journal of Natural Products,* May–June 1991, Volume 54, Number 3, pages 856–859

- *Kitchen Cures: Homemade Remedies for Your Health* by the editors of *Reader's Digest* (New York, NY: Reader's Digest Association, 2001)

- "Legume Consumption and Risk of Coronary Heart Disease in U.S. Men and Women" by Lydia A. Bazzano, Jiang He, Lorraine G. Ogden, et al., *Archives of Internal Medicine*, November 26, 2001, Volume 161, Number 21, pages 2573–2578

- *Lemon Magic: 200 Beauty and Household Uses for Lemons and Lemon Juice* by Patty Moosbrugger (New York: Three Rivers Press, 1999)

- "Local Hyperthermia Benefits Natural and Experimental Common Colds" by D. Tyrrell, I. Barrow, and J. Arthur, *BMJ,* May 13, 1989, Volume 298, Number 6683, pages 1280–1283

- "Lycopene-Rich Treatments Modify Noneosinophilic Airway Inflammation in Asthma: Proof of Concept" by Lisa G. Wood, Manohar L. Garg, Heather Powell, and Peter G. Gibson, *Free Radical Research,* January 2008, Volume 42, Number 1, pages 94–102

- "Magnesium Intake and Risk of Type 2 Diabetes in Men and Women" by R. Lopez-Ridaura, W. C. Willett, E. B. Rimm, et al., *Diabetes Care,* January 2004, Volume 27, Number 1, pages 134–140

- "Mechanisms Involved in the Antinociception Caused by Ethanolic Extract Obtained from the Leaves of *Melissa Officinalis* (Lemon Balm) in Mice" by Giselle Guginski, Ana Paula Luiz, Morgana Duarte Silva, et al., *Pharmacology, Biochemistry and Behavior,* July 2009, Volume 93, Number 1, pages 10–16

- *Menopause without Medicine: The Trusted Women's Resource with the Latest Information on HRT, Breast Cancer, Heart Disease, and Natural Estrogens* by Linda Ojeda (Alameda, California: Hunter House, 2003)

- "Micronutrients and the Premenstrual Syndrome: The Case for Calcium" by Susan Thys-Jacob, *Journal of the American College of Nutrition,* April 2000, Volume 19, Number 2, pages 220–227

- "Motion Sickness, Ginger, and Psychophysics" by D. Mowray and D. Clayson, *Lancet,* March 20, 1982, Volume 319, Number 8273, pages 655–657

- *Natural Prescriptions for Women: What to Do—And When to Do It—To Solve More Than 100 Female Health Problems—Without Drugs* by Susan Berg and the editors of *Prevention* health books (Emmaus, Pennsylvania: Rodale, 2000)

- "Neural Dynamics of Event Segmentation in Music: Converging Evidence for Dissociable Ventral and Dorsal Networks" by Devarajan Sridharan, Daniel J. Levitin, Chris H. Chafe, et al., *Neuron,* August 2, 2007, Volume 55, Number 3, pages 521–532

- *New Medicine: Complete Family Health Guide* edited by David Peters with Kenneth R. Pelletier (London: Dorling Kindersley, 2005)

- "Nut and Peanut Butter Consumption and Risk of Type 2 Diabetes in Women" by Rui Jiang, JoAnn E. Manson, Meir J. Stampfer, et al., *Journal of the American Medical Association,* November 27, 2002, Volume 288, Number 20, pages 2554–2560

- "Omega-3 Supplementation Lowers Inflammation and Anxiety in Medical Students: A Randomized Controlled Trial" by J. K. Kiecold-Glaser, M. A. Belury, R. Andridge, et al., *Brain, Behavior, and Immunity,* November 2011, Volume 25, Number 8, pages 1725–1734

- *1,801 Home Remedies: Trustworthy Treatments for Everyday Health Problems* by the editors of *Reader's Digest* (Pleasantville, NY: Reader's Digest, 2004)

- "Osteoporosis and Smoking" by M. Iki, *Clinical Calcium,* July 2005, Volume 15, Number 7, pages 156–158

- "Out of Control: A True Story of Binge Eating" by Jane Brody, *New York Times,* February 20, 2007

- *The People's Pharmacy: Quick and Handy Home Remedies: Q&As for Your Common Ailments* by Joe and Terry Graedon (Washington, DC: National Geographic, 2011)

- *Physiology of Sport and Exercise, Fifth Edition* by W. Larry Kenney, Jack Wilmore, and David Costi (Champaign, Illinois: Human Kinetics, 2012)

- "Plasma Lycopene, Other Carotenoids, and Retinol and the Risk of Cardiovascular Disease in Women" by Howard D. Sesso, Julie E. Buring, Edward P. Norkus, and J. Michael Gaziano, *American Journal of Clinical Nutrition,* January 2004, Volume 79, Number 1, pages 47–53

- *Power Sleep: The Revolutionary Program That Prepares Your Mind for Peak Performance* by James B. Maas with Megan L. Wherry, David J. Axelord, Barbara R. Hogan, and Jennifer A. Blumin (New York: HarperCollins, 1998)

- *Prescription for Herbal Healing* by Phyllis A. Balch (New York: Avery, 2002)

- "Prevention of Collagen-Induced Arthritis in Mice by a Polyphenolic Fraction from Green Tea" by T. M. Haqqi, D. D. Anthony, S. Gupta, et al., *Proceedings of the National Academy of Sciences,* April 13, 1999, Volume 96, Number 8, pages 4524–4529

- "Prevention of Ethanol-Induced Gastric Lesions in Rats by Natural Honey and Glucose-Fructose-Sucrose-Maltose Mixture" by K. Gharzouli, A. Gharzouli, S. Amira, and S. Khennouf, *Pharmacological Research*, February 1999, Volume 39, Number 2, pages 151–156

- *Prevention's Healing with Vitamins: The Most Effective Vitamin and Mineral Treatments for Everyday Health Problems and Serious Disease* by the editors of *Prevention* health books (Emmaus, Pennsylvania: Rodale, 1996)

- "Prospective Study of Beverage Use and the Risk of Kidney Stones" by Gary C. Curhan, Walter C. Willett, Eric B. Rimm, et al., *American Journal of Epidemiology*, 1996, Volume 143, Number 3, pages 240–247

- "Protection Against *Helicobacter Pylori* and Other Bacterial Infections by Garlic" by Gowsala P. Sivam, *Journal of Nutrition*, March 1, 2001, Volume 131, Number 3, pages 11065–11085

- "Protective Effect of Ginger Oil on Aspirin and Pylorus Ligation-Induced Gastric Ulcer Model in Rats" by M. Khushtar, V. Kumar, K. Javed, and Uma Bhandari, *Indian Journal of Pharmaceutical Sciences*, 2009, Volume 71, Number 5, pages 554–558

- "A Randomized Double Blind-Cross Over Trial of Soya Protein for the Treatment of Cyclical Breast Pain" by I. J. McFadyen, U. Chetty, K.D. Setchell, et al., *Breast*, October 2000, Volume 9, Number 5, pages 271–276

- "A Randomized, Double-Blind, Placebo-Controlled Trial of Oral *Matricaria Recutita* (Chamomile) Extract Therapy for Generalized Anxiety Disorder" by J. D. Amsterdam, L. Yimei, I. Soeller, et al., *Journal of Clinical Psychopharmacology*, August 2009, Volume 29, Number 4, pages 378–382

- "Red Blood Cell Magnesium and Chronic Fatigue Syndrome" by I. M. Cox, M. J. Campbell, and D. Downson, *Lancet*, March 30, 1991, Volume 337, Number 8744, pages 757–760

- "Relation Between Dietary N-3 and N-6 Fatty Acids and Clinically Diagnosed Dry Eye Syndrome in Women" by Biljana Miljanovic, Komal A. Trivedi, M. Reza Dana, et al., *American Journal of Clinical Nutrition*, October 2005, Volume 82, Number 4, pages 887–893

- "Relationship Between Intake of Green Tea and Periodontal Disease" by Mitoshi Kushiyama, Yoshihiro Shimazaki, Masatoshi Murakami, and Yoshihisa Yamashita, *Journal of Periodontology*, March 2009, Volume 80, Number 3, pages 372–377

- "Relief of Dental Pain by Ice Massage of the Hand" by R. Melzack, S. Guite, and A. Gonshor, *Canadian Medical Association Journal*, January 26, 1980, Volume 122, Number 2, pages 189–191

- "A Review of Human Carcinogens—Part D: Radiation" by Fatiha El Ghissassi, Robert Baan, Kurt Straif, et al., *Lancet Oncology*, August 2009, Volume 10, Number 8, pages 751–752

- "The Role of Breakfast in the Treatment of Obesity: A Randomized Clinical Trial" by D. G. Schlundt, J. O. Hill, T. Sbrocco, et al., *American Journal of Clinical Nutrition*, March 1992, Volume 55, Number 3, pages 645–651

- "Role of Magnesium in the Pathogenesis and Treatment of Migraines" by A. Mauskop and B. M. Altura, *Clinical Neuroscience*, 1998, Volume 5, Number 1, pages 24–27

- "Safety and Whole-Body Antioxidant Potential of a Novel Anthocyanin-Rich Formulation of Edible Berries" by D. Bagchi, S. Roy, V. Patel, et al., *Molecular Cell Biochemistry*, January 2006, Volume 281, Numbers 1–2, pages 197–209

- *Shoes in the Freezer, Beer in the Flower Bed* by Joan Wilen and Lydia Wilen (New York: Fireside, 1997)

- "Short-Term Germ-Killing Effect of Sugar-Sweetened Cinnamon Chewing Gum on Salivary Anaerobes Associated with Halitosis" by Min Zhu, Regina Carvalho, Aubrey Scher, and Christine D. Wu, *Journal of Clinical Dentistry*, January 2011, Volume 22, Number 1, pages 23–26

- "Soft Drinks, Fructose Consumption, and the Risk of Gout in Men: Prospective Cohort Study" by H. K. Choi and G. Curhan, *BMJ*, February 9, 2008, pages 309–312

- *Solve It with Salt* by Patty Moosbrugger (New York: Three Rivers Press, 1998)

- *Staying Healthy with Nutrition: The Complete Guide to Diet and Nutritional Medicine* by Elson M. Haas, MD, with Buck Levin (Berkeley, California: Ten Speed Press, 1992)

- "A Study of Caffeine Consumption and Symptoms: Indigestion, Palpitations, Tremor, Headache and Insomnia" by M. J. Shirlow and C. D. Mathers, *International Journal of Epidemiology*, June 1985, Volume 14, Number 2, pages 239–248

- *Supermarket Super Remedies* edited by Matthew Hoffman (New Hudson, Michigan: American Master Products/Jerry Baker, 2006)

- "Tart Cherry Juice: A Lip-Puckering Pain Remedy?" by Elena Conis, *Los Angeles Times*, July 6, 2009

- "Tea Consumption and Cognitive Impairment and Decline in Older Chinese Adults" by Tze-Pin Ng, Lei Feng, Mathew Niti, et al., *American Journal of Clinical Nutrition*, July 2008, Volume 88, Number 1, pages 224–231

- "Termination of Idiopathic Persistent Singultus (Hiccup) with Supra-Supramaximal Inspiration" by Luc G. Morris, Jennifer L. Marti, and David J. Ziff, *Anesthesia & Analgesia,* July 2004, Volume 99, Number 1, pages 305–306

- "Topical Capsaicin for Chronic Neck Pain: A Pilot Study" by B. J. Mathias, T. R. Dillingham, D. N. Zeigler, et al., *American Journal of Physical Medicine & Rehabilitation*, January–February 1995, Volume 74, Number 1, pages 39–44

- "Turmeric Extract May Improve Irritable Bowel Syndrome Symptomology in Otherwise Healthy Adults: A Pilot Study" by Rafe Bundy, Ann F. Walker, Richard W. Middleton, and Jonathan Booth, *Journal of Alternative and Complementary Medicine*, December 2004, Volume 10, Number 6, pages 1015–1018

- "Turmeric May Help Prevent Osteoporosis, UA Study Finds" by Janet Stark, *UANews*, September 27, 2010

- "Vinegar and Peanut Products as Complementary Foods to Reduce Postprandial Glycemia" by Carol S. Johnston and Amanda J. Buller, *Journal of the American Dietetic Association,* December 2005, Volume 105, Number 12, pages 1939–1942

- *Vinegar, Duct Tape, Milk Jugs & More: 1,001 Ingenious Ways to Use Common Household Items to Repair, Restore, Revive, or Replace Just About Everything in Your Life* by Earl Proulx and the editors of *Yankee* magazine (Emmaus, Pennsylvania: Rodale, 1999)

- "Vinegar Improves Insulin Sensitivity to a High-Carbohydrate Meal in Subjects with Insulin Resistance or Type 2 Diabetes" by Carol S. Johnston, Cindy M. Kim, and Amanda J. Buller, *Diabetes Care*, January 2004, Volume 27, Number 1, pages 281–282

- "Why Coffee Protects Against Diabetes" by Mark Wheeler, *UCLA Newsroom*, January 12, 2011

- "Why Fish Is Good for Your Brain: Study Suggests It Can Make Alzheimer's Far Less Likely" by Sadie Whitelocks, *Daily Mail*, December 1, 2001

- "Xylitol Chewing Gum in Prevention of Acute Otitis Media: Double Blind Randomised Trial" by M. Uhari, T. Kontiokari, M. Koskela, and Marjo Niemela, *BMJ*, November 9, 1996, Volume 313, Number 7066, pages 1180–1184

- "You Needn't Fear Poison Ivy—It's Easy to Cure," *Popular Mechanics,* August 1930, page 294

- *Your Best Medicine* by Marc A. Goldstein, Myrna Chandler Goldstein, and Larry P. Credit (Emmaus, Pennsylvania: Rodale, 2008)

Trademark Information

"Advil" is a registered trademark of Pfizer Consumer Healthcare.

"Afrin" is a registered trademark of MSD Consumer Care, Inc.

"Alberto VO5" is a registered trademark of Alberto-Culver USA, Inc.

"Aleve" is a registered trademark of Bayer HealthCare LLC.

"Alka-Seltzer" is a registered trademark of Bayer Corporation.

"Angostura" is a registered trademark of Angostura Bitters Limited.

"Arm & Hammer" is a registered trademark of Church & Dwight Co, Inc.

"Aunt Jemima" is a registered trademark of the Quaker Oats Company.

"Bacardi" is a registered trademark of Bacardi & Company, Limited.

"Bag Balm" is a registered trademark of Dairy Association, Co., Inc.

"Baker's" and "Angel Flake" are registered trademarks of Kraft Foods.

"Band-Aid" is a registered trademark of Johnson & Johnson Consumer Companies, Inc.

"Bayer" is a registered trademark of Bayer HealthCare LLC.

"Benadryl" is a registered trademark of McNeil-PPC, Inc.

"Betty Crocker" is a registered trademark of General Mills.

"Birds Eye" is a registered trademark of Pinnacle Foods Group LLC.

"Bounty" is a registered trademark of Procter & Gamble.

"Bubble Wrap" is a registered trademark of Sealed Air Corporation.

"Budweiser" is a registered trademark of Anheuser-Busch, Inc.

"Campbell" is a registered trademark of Campbell Soup Company.

"Canada Dry" and the Shield Design are registered trademarks of Dr Pepper/Seven Up Inc.

"Carnation" and "Nestlé" are registered trademarks of Société des Produits Nestlé S.A., Vevey, Switzerland.

"Certo" is a registered trademark of Kraft Foods.

"ChapStick" is a registered trademark of A. H. Robbins Company.

"CharcoCaps" is a registered trademark of W. F. Young, Inc.

"Cheerios" is a registered trademark of General Mills.

"Chicken of the Sea" is a registered trademark of Chicken of the Sea International.

"Clabber Girl" is a registered trademark of Clabber Girl Corporation.

"Clearasil" is a registered trademark of Reckitt Benckiser LLC.

"Clorox" is a registered trademark of the Clorox Company.

"Coca-Cola" and "Coke" are registered trademarks of the Coca-Cola Company.

"Colgate" is a registered trademark of Colgate-Palmolive Company.

"Colman's" is a registered trademark of World Finer Foods, Inc.

"Conair" is a registered trademark of Conair Corporation.

"Cool Whip" is a registered trademark of Kraft Foods.

"Coppertone" is a registered trademark of MSD Consumer Care, Inc.

"Corn Huskers" is a registered trademark of Johnson & Johnson Consumer Companies, Inc.

"Cortaid" is a registered trademark of Johnson & Johnson Consumer Companies, Inc.

"Country Time" and "Country Time Lemonade" are registered trademarks of Kraft Foods.

"Crayola" is a registered trademark of Binney & Smith Inc.

"Cream of Wheat" is a registered trademark of B&G Foods, Inc.

"Crisco" is a registered trademark of the J. M. Smucker Co.

"Dannon" is a registered trademark of the Dannon Company.

"Dawn" is a registered trademark of Procter & Gamble.

"Desitin" is a registered trademark of Johnson & Johnson Consumer Companies, Inc.

"Dial" is a registered trademark of Dial Corp.

"Dickinson's" is a registered trademark of Dickinson Brands Inc.

"Dixie" is a registered trademark of James River Corporation.

"Dole" is a registered trademark of Dole Food Company, Inc.

"Domino" is a registered trademark of Domino Foods, Inc.

"Dove" is a registered trademark of Unilever.

"Downy" is a registered trademark of Procter & Gamble.

"Dr. Bronner's" is a registered trademark of Dr. Bronner's Magic All-One!

"Dr. Teal's" is a registered trademark of Advanced Beauty Systems, Inc.

"Duck" is a registered trademark of ShurTech Brands, LLC.

"Dynasty" is a registered trademark of JFC International, Inc.

"Efferdent" is a registered trademark of Warner-Lambert.

"Elmer's Glue-All" and Elmer the Bull are registered trademarks of Elmer's Products, Inc.

"Fels-Naptha" is a registered trademark of the Dial Corporation.

"Fleischmann's" is a registered trademark of ACH Foods.

"Forster" is a registered trademark of Diamond Brands, Inc.

"French's" is a registered trademark of Reckitt Benckiser Inc.

"Fruit of the Earth" is a registered trademark of Fruit of the Earth, Inc.

"Gatorade" is a registered trademark of the Gatorade Company.

"General Mills," "Total," and "Fiber One" are registered trademarks of General Mills.

"Gerber" is a registered trademark of Société des Produits Nestlé S.A., Vevey, Switzerland.

"Gold Medal" is a registered trademark of General Mills, Inc.

"Gold's" is a registered trademark of Gold Pure Food Products Co., Inc.

"Grandma's" is a registered trademark of B&G Foods, Inc.

"Grapeola" is a registered trademark of Kusha, Inc.

"Hain" is a registered trademark of the Hain Celestial Group, Inc.

"Head & Shoulders" is a registered trademark of Procter & Gamble.

"Heinz" is a registered trademark of H.J. Heinz Company.

"Hennessy" is a registered trademark of Jas Hennessey & Co.

"Hershey's" is a registered trademark of Hershey Foods Corporation.

"Huggies" is a registered trademark of Kimberly-Clark Corporation.

"Hunt's" is a registered trademarks of Hunt-Wesson, Inc.

"Ivory" is a registered trademark of Procter & Gamble.

"Jell-O" is a registered trademark of Kraft Foods.

"Jif" is a registered trademark of the J. M. Smucker Co.

"Johnson's" and "Johnson & Johnson" are registered trademarks of Johnson & Johnson Consumer
      Companies, Inc.

"Karo" is a registered trademark of CPC International Inc.

"Kellogg's," "All-Bran," "Special K," and "Rice Krispies" are registered trademarks of the Kellogg Company.

"Kikkoman" is a registered trademark of Kikkoman Corporation.

"Kingsford's" is a registered trademark of ACH Food Companies.

"Kiwi" is a registered trademark of Sara Lee Corporation.

"Kleenex" is a registered trademark of Kimberly-Clark Corporation.

"Knorr" is a registered trademark of Unilever.

"Knox" is a registered trademark of Kraft Foods.

"Kraft" is a registered trademark of Kraft Foods.

"Krazy" is a registered trademark of Krazy Glue.

"Kretschmer" is a registered trademark of Sun Country Foods, Inc.

"K-Y" is a registered trademark of McNeil-PPC, Inc.

"Lakewood" is a registered trademark of a Florida Family Trust.

"Lewis Labs" is a registered trademark of Lewis Laboratories International, Ltd.

"Libby's" is a registered trademark of Société des Produits Nestlé S.A., Vevey, Switzerland.

"Life Savers" and "Pep-O-Mint" are registered trademarks of Wm. Wrigley Jr. Company.

"Lipton," "The 'Brisk' Tea," and "Flo-Thru" are registered trademarks of Unilever.

"Listerine" is a registered trademark of Warner-Lambert.

"Loriva" is a registered trademark of Loriva Supreme Foods, Inc.

"Lubriderm" is a registered trademark of Warner-Lambert.

"Lysol" is a registered trademark of Reckitt Benckiser.

"L'eggs" and "Sheer Energy" are registered trademarks of Sara Lee Corporation.

"Maxwell House" is a registered trademark of Maxwell House Coffee Company.

"McCormick" is a registered trademark of McCormick & Company, Incorporated.

"Metamucil" is a registered trademark of Procter & Gamble.

"Minute Maid" is a registered trademark of the Coca-Cola Company.

"Miracle Whip" is a registered trademark of Kraft Foods.

"Morton" is a registered trademark of Morton International, Inc.

"Motrin" is a registered trademark of McNeil-PPC, Inc.

"Mott's" is a registered trademark of Mott's Inc.

"Mr. Coffee" is a registered trademark of Mr. Coffee, Inc.

"Mylanta" is a registered trademark of McNeil Consumer Pharmaceuticals Co.

"Nabisco" and "Premium" are registered trademarks of Kraft Foods.

"Neosporin" is a registered trademark of Johnson & Johnson Consumer Companies, Inc.

"Nestea" and "Nestlé" are registered trademarks of Société des Produits Nestlé S.A., Vevey, Switzerland.

"Noxzema" is a registered trademark of Unilever.

"Now" is a registered trademark of Now Foods.

"Ocean Spray" and "Craisins" are registered trademarks of Ocean Spray Cranberries, Inc.

"Orajel" is a registered trademark of Church & Dwight Co., Inc.

"Oral-B" is a registered trademark of Oral-B Laboratories.

"Palmolive" is a registered trademark of Colgate-Palmolive Company.

"Pam" is a registered trademark of American Home Foods.

"Pampers" is a registered trademark of Procter & Gamble.

"Pepto-Bismol" is a registered trademark of Procter & Gamble.

"Pernod" is a registered trademark of Pernod Ricard USA.

"Phillips'" is a registered trademark of Bayer HealthCare LLC.

"Planters" is a registered trademark of Kraft Foods.

"Playtex" and "Living" are registered trademarks of Playtex Products, Inc.

"Popsicle" is a registered trademark of Unilever.

"Preparation H" is a registered trademark of Pfizer Consumer Healthcare.

"Progresso" is a registered trademark of General Mills.

"Purell" is a registered trademark of Johnson & Johnson Consumer Companies, Inc.

"Q-Tips" is a registered trademark of Chesebrough-Pond's USA Co.

"Quaker" is a registered trademark of the Quaker Oats Company.

"ReaLemon" is a registered trademark of Dr Pepper Snapple Group.

"ReaLime" is a registered trademark of Dr Pepper Snapple Group.

"Reddi-wip" is a registered trademark of Con Agra Foods, Inc.

"Requa" is a registered trademark of Requa Manufacturing Co., Inc.

"Revlon" is a registered trademark of Revlon.

"Rubbermaid" is a registered trademark of Newell Rubbermaid Inc.

"Saco" is a registered trademark of Saco Foods, Inc.

"Saran" and "Saran Wrap" are registered trademarks of S.C. Johnson & Sons, Inc.

"Scotch" is a registered trademark of 3M.

"Sea Breeze" is a registered trademark of Sea Breeze.

Index

About the Author

Joey Green—author of *Joey Green's Cleaning Magic, Joey Green's Fix-It Magic, Joey Green's Gardening Magic, Joey Green's Amazing Pet Cures*, and *Joey Green's Kitchen Magic*—got Meredith Vieira to rub French's Mustard on her chest to decongest a cold on *The View*, convinced Barbara Walters to put a wet Pampers diaper on her head to prevent dehydration, persuaded Jay Leno to shave with Jif Peanut Butter on *The Tonight Show*, got Rosie O'Donnell to moisturize her face with Miracle Whip, and showed Diane Sawyer how to polish furniture with Spam.

A walking encyclopedia of quirky yet ingenious household hints, he has appeared on dozens of national television shows to demonstrate offbeat uses for brand-name products, including *Good Morning America, Today, Fox and Friends, The 700 Club*, and many more. He has been profiled in the *New York Times*, the *Los Angeles Times*, the *Washington Post*, the *New York Daily News, People, USA Today*, the *Boston Globe*, and the *Miami Herald*, and he has been interviewed by literally hundreds of radio stations.

Green, a former contributing editor to *National Lampoon* and a former advertising copywriter at J. Walter Thompson, is the author of fifty books, including *Marx & Lennon: The Parallel Sayings, Contrary to Popular Belief, Dumb History*, and *Selling Out: If Famous Authors Wrote Advertising*. A native of Miami, Florida, and a graduate of Cornell University, he wrote television commercials for Burger King and Walt Disney World and won a Clio Award for a print ad he created for Eastman Kodak. He backpacked around the world for two years on his honeymoon and lives in Los Angeles with his wife, Debbie, and their two daughters, Ashley and Julia.

Visit Joey Green on the internet at

www.wackyuses.com